ENDOCRINE BOARD REVIEW 2022

Frances J. Hayes, MB BCh, BAO, Program Chair
Associate Clinical Chief of Endocrinology
Massachusetts General Hospital
Associate Professor of Medicine
Harvard Medical School

Natalie E. Cusano, MD, MS
Associate Professor of Medicine
Zucker School of Medicine
at Hofstra/Northwell
Director of the Bone
Metabolism Program
Division of Endocrinology
at Lenox Hill Hospital

Tobias Else, MD
Associate Professor
Division of Metabolism,
Endocrinology, and Diabetes
University of Michigan

Vivian A. Fonseca, MD
Professor of Medicine
Assistant Dean for Clinical Research
Tullis Tulane Alumni Chair in Diabetes
Chief, Section of Endocrinology
Tulane University Health
Sciences Center

Jacqueline Jonklaas, MD, PhD, MPH
Professor
Division of Endocrinology
Georgetown University Medical Center

Sangeeta R. Kashyap, MD
Professor of Medicine
Cleveland Clinic Lerner
College of Medicine
Physician Scientist
Endocrinology Institute
at Cleveland Clinic

Laurence Katznelson, MD
Professor of Neurosurgery
and Medicine
Division of Endocrinology
Stanford University School of Medicine

Kathryn A. Martin, MD
Assistant Professor of Medicine
Harvard Medical School
Faculty Clinician, Reproductive
Endocrine Unit
Massachusetts General Hospital
Senior Physician Editor,
Endocrinology and Diabetes
UpToDate

Marie E. McDonnell, MD
Section Chief, Diabetes Section
Division of Endocrinology
Diabetes and Hypertension
Brigham and Women's Hospital
Harvard Medical School

Stephanie Page, MD, PhD
Professor/Head, Division of
Metabolism, Endocrinology,
and Nutrition
Co-Director, UW Medicine
Diabetes Institute
Robert B. McMillen Professor
of Lipid Research
University of Washington
School of Medicine

Abbie L. Young, MS, CGC, ELS(D)
Medical Editor

Endocrine Society
2055 L Street NW, Suite 600, Washington, DC 20036
1-888-ENDOCRINE • www.endocrine.org

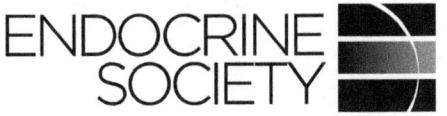

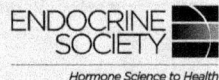

The Endocrine Society is the world's largest, oldest, and most active organization working to advance the clinical practice of endocrinology and hormone research. Founded in 1916, the Society now has more than 18,000 global members across a range of disciplines. The Society has earned an international reputation for excellence in the quality of its peer-reviewed journals, educational resources, meetings, and programs that improve public health through the practice and science of endocrinology.

For between-edition updates, visit us at:
https://www.endocrine.org/education-and-training/book-updates

Other publications:
endocrine.org/publications

ISBN: 978-1-943550-07-4
Library of Congress Control Number: 2022938699

On the Cover: © Shutterstock. Using a laptop to search information from a network. (panitanphoto)

OVERVIEW

Endocrine Board Review (EBR) 14th Edition (2022) is a board examination preparation book designed for endocrine fellows who have completed or are nearing completion of their fellowship and are preparing to sit for the board certification exam, and for practicing endocrinologists in search of a comprehensive self-assessment of endocrinology, either to prepare for recertification or to update their practice. EBR consists of approximately 220 case-based, American Board of Internal Medicine (ABIM) style, multiple-choice questions. Each section follows the ABIM Endocrinology, Diabetes, and Metabolism Certification Examination blueprint, covering the breadth and depth of the certification and recertification examinations. Each case is discussed in detail with detailed answer explanations and references provided.

The EBR 14th Edition (2022) reference book is intended primarily for consultation and self-assessment of knowledge relating to endocrinology. As a reference book, educational credits are not available upon completion of the multiple-choice questions included. For information on educational products that include educational credit, please visit endocrine.org/store.

LEARNING OBJECTIVES

Upon completion of this educational activity, learners will be able to demonstrate enhanced medical knowledge and clinical skills across all major areas of endocrinology; apply knowledge and skills in diagnosing, managing, and treating a wide spectrum of endocrine disorders; and successfully complete the board examination for certification or recertification in the subspecialty of endocrinology, diabetes, and metabolism.

TARGET AUDIENCE

This activity should be of substantial interest to endocrinologists, internists, and endocrine fellows preparing for the board examination or recertification; or endocrinologists and other health care practitioners seeking a review in endocrinology.

STATEMENT OF INDEPENDENCE

The Endocrine Society has a policy of ensuring that the content and quality of this educational activity are balanced, independent, objective, and scientifically rigorous. The scientific content of this activity was developed under the supervision of the Endocrine Society's EBR faculty. There are no commercial supporters of this activity and no commercial entities have had an influence over the planning of this activity.

DISCLOSURE POLICY

The faculty, committee members, and staff who are in position to control the content of this activity are required to disclose to the Endocrine Society and to learners any relevant financial relationship(s) of the individual or spouse/partner that have occurred within the last 12 months with any commercial interest(s) whose products or services are related to the content. Financial relationships are defined by remuneration in any amount from the commercial interest(s) in the form of grants; research support; consulting fees; salary; ownership interest (eg, stocks, stock options, or ownership interest excluding diversified mutual funds); honoraria or other payments for participation in speakers' bureaus, advisory boards, or boards of directors; or other financial benefits. The intent of this disclosure is not to prevent planners with relevant financial relationships from planning or delivery of content, but rather to provide learners with information that allows them to make their own judgments of whether these financial relationships may have influenced the educational activity with regard to exposition or conclusion.

The Endocrine Society has reviewed all disclosures and resolved or managed all identified conflicts of interest, as applicable.

The faculty reported the following relevant financial relationship(s) during the content development process for this activity:

Natalie E. Cusano, MD, MS, has served as a research investigator for Shire/Takeda, a speaker for Alexion Pharmaceuticals, and a consultant for Ascendis Pharma.

Tobias Else, MD, has served as an advisory board member to Corcept Therapeutics, HRA Pharma, Lantheus, and Merck, and his institution has received research support from Corcept Therapeutics, Merck, and Strongbridge Biopharma.

Sangeeta R. Kashyap, MD, has served as a consultant and coinvestigator to GI Dynamics and as a consultant to Fractyl, Inc; her institution has received research support from Fractyl, Inc, and Janssen Pharmaceuticals; and she is Chief Medical Officer of Gila Therapeutics.

Stephanie Page, MD, PhD, is an editor at UpToDate.

Laurence Katznelson, MD, has served as a consultant and principal investigator to Chiasma and Camarus, and he has served as an advisory board member to Novo Nordisk, Chiasma, Pfizer, Strongbridge Biopharma, and Recordati.

Marie E. McDonnell, MD, has served as a trial event adjudicator for a trial conducted by Eisai and received research funding from Lilly, Inc, that is paid to her institution.

Vivian A. Fonseca, MD, has received honoraria from consulting and lecturing from Asahi, Novo Nordisk, Sanofi, Bayer, and Abbott; his institution has received grants from Gilead, Boehringer Ingelheim, Fractyl, Jaguar Gene Therapy, and Sanofi; and he has stock in Amgen and stock options in Mellitus Health and BRAVO4Health.

Kathryn A. Martin, MD, is a senior physician editor at UpToDate.

The following faculty reported no relevant financial relationships: Frances J. Hayes, MB BCh, BAO, and Jacqueline Jonklaas, MD, PhD, MPH

The medical editor for this activity reported no relevant financial relationships: Abbie L. Young, MS, CGC, ELS(D)

Endocrine Society staff associated with the development of content for this activity reported no relevant financial relationships.

DISCLAIMERS

The information presented in this activity represents the opinion of the faculty and is not necessarily the official position of the Endocrine Society.

Use of professional judgment:

The educational content in this activity relates to basic principles of diagnosis and therapy and does not substitute for individual patient assessment based on the health care provider's examination of the patient and consideration of laboratory data and other factors unique to the patient. Standards in medicine change as new data become available.

Drugs and dosages:

When prescribing medications, the physician is advised to check the product information sheet accompanying each drug to verify conditions of use and to identify any changes in drug dosage schedule or contraindications.

POLICY ON UNLABELED/OFF-LABEL USE

The Endocrine Society has determined that disclosure of unlabeled/off-label or investigational use of commercial product(s) is informative for audiences and therefore requires this information to be disclosed to the learners at the beginning of the presentation. Uses of specific therapeutic agents, devices, and other products discussed in this educational activity may not be the same as those indicated in product labeling approved by the Food and Drug Administration (FDA). The Endocrine Society requires that any discussions of such "off-label" use be based on scientific research that conforms to generally accepted standards of experimental design, data collection, and data analysis. Before recommending or prescribing any therapeutic agent or device, learners should review the complete prescribing information, including indications, contraindications, warnings, precautions, and adverse events.

ACKNOWLEDGMENT OF COMMERCIAL SUPPORT

The activity is not supported by educational grant(s) or other funds from any commercial supporters.

Publication Date: August 2022

Contents

For between-edition updates, visit us at: https://www.endocrine.org/education-and-training/book-updates.

LABORATORY REFERENCE RANGES

Reference ranges vary among laboratories. Conventional units are listed first with SI units in parentheses.

Lipid Values

High-density lipoprotein (HDL) cholesterol

    Optimal ------------------------- >60 mg/dL (SI: >1.55 mmol/L)

    Normal------------------- 40-60 mg/dL (SI: 1.04-1.55 mmol/L)

    Low ---------------------------- <40 mg/dL (SI: <1.04 mmol/L)

Low-density lipoprotein (LDL) cholesterol

    Optimal --

        <100 mg/dL (SI: <2.59 mmol/L) (for primary prevention);

        <70 mg/dL (SI: <1.81 mmol/L) (for secondary prevention)

    Low --------------------100-129 mg/dL (SI: 2.59-3.34 mmol/L)

    Borderline-high --------130-159 mg/dL (SI: 3.37-4.12 mmol/L)

    High -------------------160-189 mg/dL (SI: 4.14-4.90 mmol/L)

    Very high ----------------------≥190 mg/dL (SI: ≥4.92 mmol/L)

Non-HDL cholesterol

    Optimal -----------------------<130 mg/dL (SI: <3.37 mmol/L)

    Borderline-high --------130-159 mg/dL (SI: 3.37-4.12 mmol/L)

    High --------------------------≥240 mg/dL (SI: ≥6.22 mmol/L)

Total cholesterol

    Optimal -----------------------<200 mg/dL (SI: <5.18 mmol/L)

    Borderline-high --------200-239 mg/dL (SI: 5.18-6.19 mmol/L)

    High --------------------------≥240 mg/dL (SI: ≥6.22 mmol/L)

Triglycerides

    Optimal -----------------------<150 mg/dL (SI: <1.70 mmol/L)

    Borderline-high --------150-199 mg/dL (SI: 1.70-2.25 mmol/L)

    High -------------------200-499 mg/dL (SI: 2.26-5.64 mmol/L)

    Very high ----------------------≥500 mg/dL (SI: ≥5.65 mmol/L)

Lipoprotein (a) ----------------------≤30 mg/dL (SI: ≤1.07 μmol/L)

Apolipoprotein B ------------------- 50-110 mg/dL (SI: 0.5-1.1 g/L)

Hematologic Values

Erythrocyte sedimentation rate -------------------------0-20 mm/h

Haptoglobin ------------------ 30-200 mg/dL (SI: 300-2000 mg/L)

Hematocrit---------------------- 41%-51% (SI: 0.41-0.51) (male);

    35%-45% (SI: 0.35-0.45) (female)

Hemoglobin A_{1c}--------------------- 4.0%-5.6% (20-38 mmol/mol)

Hemoglobin ------------- 13.8-17.2 g/dL (SI: 138-172 g/L) (male);

    12.1-15.1 g/dL (SI: 121-151 g/L) (female)

International normalized ratio -----------------------------0.8-1.2

Mean corpuscular volume (MCV ------80-100 μm^3 (SI: 80-100 fL)

Platelet count------------- 150-450 x 10^3/μL (SI: 150-450 x 10^9/L)

Protein (total) -------------------------6.3-7.9 g/dL (SI: 63-79 g/L)

Reticulocyte count -0.5%-1.5% of red blood cells (SI: 0.005-0.015)

White blood cell count------ 4500-11,000/μL (SI: 4.5-11.0 x 10^9/L)

Thyroid Values

Thyroglobulin ------ 3-42 ng/mL (SI: 3-42 μg/L) (after surgery and

    radioactive iodine treatment: <1.0 ng/mL [SI: <1.0 μg/L])

Thyroglobulin antibodies --------------- ≤4.0 IU/mL (SI: ≤4.0 kIU/L)

Thyrotropin (TSH) ------------------------------------0.5-5.0 mIU/L

Thyrotropin-receptor antibodies (TRAb) -----------------≤1.75 IU/L

Thyroid-stimulating immunoglobulin----- ≤120% of basal activity

Thyroperoxidase (TPO) antibodies ----- <2.0 IU/mL (SI: <2.0 kIU/L)

Thyroxine (T_4) (free) ------- 0.8-1.8 ng/dL (SI: 10.30-23.17 pmol/L)

Thyroxine (T_4) (total)---- 5.5-12.5 μg/dL (SI: 94.02-213.68 nmol/L)

Free thyroxine (T_4) index ------------------------------- 4-12

Triiodothyronine (T_3) (free)--- 2.3-4.2 pg/mL (SI: 3.53-6.45 pmol/L)

Triiodothyronine (T_3) (total) -- 70-200 ng/dL (SI: 1.08-3.08 nmol/L)

Triiodothyronine (T_3), reverse -- 10-24 ng/dL (SI: 0.15-0.37 nmol/L)

Triiodothyronine uptake, resin -------------------------- 25%-38%

Radioactive iodine uptake----------------------3%-16% (6 hours);

    15%-30% (24 hours)

Endocrine Values

Serum

Aldosterone------------------ 4-21 ng/dL (SI: 111.0-582.5 pmol/L)

Alkaline phosphatase ---------- 50-120 U/L (SI: 0.84-2.00 μkat/L)

Alkaline phosphatase (bone-specific) ----------------------------

    ≤20 μg/L (adult male); ≤14 μg/L (premenopausal female);

    ≤22 μg/L (postmenopausal female)

Androstenedione --

    65-210 ng/dL (SI: 2.27-7.33 nmol/L) (adult male);

    30-200 ng/dL (SI:1.05-6.98 nmol/L) (adult female)

Antimullerian hormone --

    0.7-19.0 ng/mL (SI: 5.0-135.7 pmol/L) (male, >12 years);

    0.9-9.5 ng/mL (SI: 6.4-67.9 pmol/L) (female, 13-45 years);

    <1.0 ng/mL (SI: <7.1 pmol/L) (female, >45 years)

Calcitonin -------------<16 pg/mL (SI: <4.67 pmol/L) (basal, male);

    <8 pg/mL (SI: <2.34 pmol/L) (basal, female);

    ≤130 pg/mL (SI: ≤37.96 pmol/L) (peak calcium infusion, male);

    ≤90 pg/mL (SI: ≤26.28 pmol/L) (peak calcium infusion, female)

Carcinoembryonic antigen ------------- <2.5 ng/mL (SI: <2.5 μg/L)

Chromogranin A ------------------------ <93 ng/mL (SI: <93 μg/L)

Corticosterone 53-1560 ng/dL (SI: 1.53-45.08 nmol/L) (>18 years)

Corticotropin (ACTH) ---------- 10-60 pg/mL (SI: 2.2-13.2 pmol/L)

Cortisol (8 AM) -------------- 5-25 µg/dL (SI: 137.9-689.7 nmol/L)

Cortisol (4 PM) ----------------2-14 µg/dL (SI: 55.2-386.2 nmol/L)

C-peptide -------------------- 0.5-2.0 ng/mL (SI: 0.17-0.66 nmol/L)

C-reactive protein ---------- 0.8-3.1 mg/L (SI: 7.62-29.52 nmol/L)

Cross-linked N-telopeptide of type 1 collagen --------------------

    5.4-24.2 nmol BCE/mmol creat (male);

    6.2-19.0 nmol BCE/mmol creat (female)

Dehydroepiandrosterone sulfate (DHEA-S)

Patient Age	Female	Male
18-29 years	44-332 µg/dL (SI: 1.19-9.00 µmol/L)	89-457 µg/dL (SI: 2.41-12.38 µmol/L)
30-39 years	31-228 µg/dL (SI: 0.84-6.78 µmol/L)	65-334 µg/dL (SI: 1.76-9.05 µmol/L)
40-49 years	18-244 µg/dL (SI: 0.49-6.61 µmol/L)	48-244 µg/dL (SI: 1.30-6.61 µmol/L)
50-59 years	15-200 µg/dL (SI: 0.41-5.42 µmol/L)	35-179 µg/dL (SI: 0.95-4.85 µmol/L)
≥60 years	15-157 µg/dL (SI: 0.41-4.25 µmol/L)	25-131 µg/dL (SI: 0.68-3.55 µmol/L)

Deoxycorticosterone ----<10 ng/dL (SI: <0.30 nmol/L) (>18 years)

1,25-Dihydroxyvitamin D$_3$---16-65 pg/mL (SI: 41.6-169.0 pmol/L)

Estradiol ------------- 10-40 pg/mL (SI: 36.7-146.8 pmol/L) (male);

    10-180 pg/mL (SI: 36.7-660.8 pmol/L) (follicular, female);

    100-300 pg/mL (SI: 367.1-1101.3 pmol/L) (midcycle, female);

    40-200 pg/mL (SI: 146.8-734.2 pmol/L) (luteal, female);

    <20 pg/mL (SI: <73.4 pmol/L) (postmenopausal, female)

Estrone ------------- 10-60 pg/mL (SI: 37.0-221.9 pmol/L) (male);

    17-200 pg/mL (SI: 62.9-739.6 pmol/L) (premenopausal female);

    7-40 pg/mL (SI: 25.9-147.9 pmol/L) (postmenopausal female)

α-Fetoprotein ------------------------------- <6 ng/mL (SI: <6 µg/L)

Follicle-stimulating hormone (FSH) ------------------------------

    1.0-13.0 mIU/mL (SI: 1.0-13.0 IU/L) (male);

    <3.0 mIU/mL (SI: <3.0 IU/L) (prepuberty, female);

    2.0-12.0 mIU/mL (SI: 2.0-12.0 IU/L) (follicular, female);

    4.0-36.0 mIU/mL (SI: 4.0-36.0 IU/L) (midcycle, female);

    1.0-9.0 mIU/mL (SI: 1.0-9.0 IU/L) (luteal, female);

    >30.0 mIU/mL (SI: >30.0 IU/L) (postmenopausal, female)

Free fatty acids -------------- 10.6-18.0 mg/dL (SI: 0.4-0.7 nmol/L)

Gastrin------------------------------- <100 pg/mL (SI: <100 ng/L)

Growth hormone (GH)-- 0.01-0.97 ng/mL (SI: 0.01-0.97 µg/L) (male);

    0.01-3.61 ng/mL (SI: 0.01-3.61 µg/L) (female)

Homocysteine ----------------------- ≤1.76 mg/L (SI: ≤13 µmol/L)

β-Human chorionic gonadotropin (β-hCG) -----------------------

    <3.0 mIU/mL (SI: <3.0 IU/L) (nonpregnant female);

    >25 mIU/mL (SI: >25 IU/L) indicates a positive pregnancy test

β-Hydroxybutyrate ----------------<3.0 mg/dL (SI: <288.2 µmol/L)

17-Hydroxypregnenolone --- 29-189 ng/dL (SI: 0.87-5.69 nmol/L)

17α-Hydroxyprogesterone ---

    <220 ng/dL (SI: <6.67 nmol/L) (adult male);

    <80 ng/dL (SI: <2.42 nmol/L) (follicular, female);

    <285 ng/dL (SI: <8.64 nmol/L) (luteal, female);

    <51 ng/dL (SI: <1.55 nmol/L) (postmenopausal, female)

25-Hydroxyvitamin D ---

    <20 ng/mL (SI: <49.9 nmol/L) (deficiency);

    21-29 ng/mL (SI: 52.4-72.4 nmol/L) (insufficiency);

    30-80 ng/mL (SI: 74.9-199.7 nmol/L) (optimal levels);

    >80 ng/mL (SI: >199.7 nmol/L) (toxicity possible)

Inhibin B ------------------------15-300 pg/mL (SI: 15-300 ng/L)

Insulinlike growth factor 1 (IGF-1)

Patient Age	Female	Male
18 years	162-541 ng/mL (SI: 21.2-70.9 nmol/L)	170-640 ng/mL (SI: 22.3-83.8 nmol/L)
19 years	138-442 ng/mL (SI: 18.1-57.9 nmol/L)	147-527 ng/mL (SI: 19.3-69.0 nmol/L)
20 years	122-384 ng/mL (SI: 16.0-50.3 nmol/L)	132-457 ng/mL (SI: 17.3-59.9 nmol/L)
21-25 years	116-341 ng/mL (SI: 15.2-44.7 nmol/L)	116-341 ng/mL (SI: 15.2-44.7 nmol/L)
26-30 years	117-321 ng/mL (SI: 15.3-42.1 nmol/L)	117-321 ng/mL (SI: 15.3-42.1 nmol/L)
31-35 years	113-297 ng/mL (SI: 14.8-38.9 nmol/L)	113-297 ng/mL (SI: 14.8-38.9 nmol/L)
36-40 years	106-277 ng/mL (SI: 13.9-36.3 nmol/L)	106-277 ng/mL (SI: 13.9-36.3 nmol/L)
41-45 years	98-261 ng/mL (SI: 12.8-34.2 nmol/L)	98-261 ng/mL (SI: 12.8-34.2 nmol/L)
46-50 years	91-246 ng/mL (SI: 11.9-32.2 nmol/L)	91-246 ng/mL (SI: 11.9-32.2 nmol/L)
51-55 years	84-233 ng/mL (SI: 11.0-30.5 nmol/L)	84-233 ng/mL (SI: 11.0-30.5 nmol/L)
56-60 years	78-220 ng/mL (SI: 10.2-28.8 nmol/L)	78-220 ng/mL (SI: 10.2-28.8 nmol/L)
61-65 years	72-207 ng/mL (SI: 9.4-27.1 nmol/L)	72-207 ng/mL (SI: 9.4-27.1 nmol/L)
66-70 years	67-195 ng/mL (SI: 8.8-25.5 nmol/L)	67-195 ng/mL (SI: 8.8-25.5 nmol/L)
71-75 years	62-184 ng/mL (SI: 8.1-24.1 nmol/L)	62-184 ng/mL (SI: 8.1-24.1 nmol/L)

Patient Age	Female	Male
76-80 years	57-172 ng/mL (SI: 7.5-22.5 nmol/L)	57-172 ng/mL (SI: 7.5-22.5 nmol/L)
>80 years	53-162 ng/mL (SI: 6.9-21.2 nmol/L)	53-162 ng/mL (SI: 6.9-21.2 nmol/L)

Insulinlike growth factor binding protein 3 ----------- 2.5-4.8 mg/L

Insulin----------------------- 1.4-14.0 µIU/mL (SI: 9.7-97.2 pmol/L)

Islet-cell antibody assay---- 0 Juvenile Diabetes Foundation units

Luteinizing hormone (LH)-------------------------------------

    1.0-9.0 mIU/mL (SI: 1.0-9.0 IU/L) (male);

    <1.0 mIU/mL (SI: <1.0 IU/L) (prepuberty, female);

    1.0-18.0 mIU/mL (SI: 1.0-18.0 IU/L) (follicular, female);

    20.0-80.0 mIU/mL (SI: 20.0-80.0 IU/L) (midcycle, female);

    0.5-18.0 mIU/mL (SI: 0.5-18.0 IU/L) (luteal, female);

    >30.0 mIU/mL (SI: >30.0 IU/L) (postmenopausal, female)

Metanephrines (plasma fractionated)

    Metanephrine--------------------<99 pg/mL (SI: <0.50 nmol/L)

    Normetanephrine-------------- <165 pg/mL (SI: <0.90 nmol/L)

75-g oral glucose tolerance test blood glucose values -----------

    60-100 mg/dL (SI: 3.3-5.6 mmol/L) (fasting);

    <200 mg/dL (SI: <11.1 mmol/L) (1 hour);

    <140 mg/dL (SI: <7.8 mmol/L) (2 hour);

    between 140-200 mg/dL (SI: 7.8-11.1 mmol/L) is considered impaired glucose tolerance or prediabetes; greater than 200 mg/dL (SI: >11.1 mmol/L) is a sign of diabetes mellitus

50-g oral glucose tolerance test for gestational diabetes --------

    <140 mg/dL (SI: <7.8 mmol/L) (1 hour)

100-g oral glucose tolerance test for gestational diabetes -------

    <95 mg/dL (SI: <5.3 mmol/L) (fasting);

    <180 mg/dL (SI: <10.0 mmol/L) (1 hour);

    <155 mg/dL (SI: <8.6 mmol/L) (2 hour);

    <140 mg/dL (SI: <7.8 mmol/L) (3 hour)

Osteocalcin ---------------------9.0-42.0 ng/mL (SI: 9.0-42.0 µg/L)

Parathyroid hormone, intact (PTH) - 10-65 pg/mL (SI: 10-65 ng/L)

Parathyroid hormone–related protein (PTHrP) -------- <2.0 pmol/L

Progesterone -----------------≤1.2 ng/mL (SI: ≤3.8 nmol/L) (male);

    ≤1.0 ng/mL (SI: ≤3.2 nmol/L) (follicular, female);

    2.0-20.0 ng/mL (SI: 6.4-63.6 nmol/L) (luteal, female);

    ≤1.1 ng/mL (SI: ≤3.5 nmol/L) (postmenopausal, female);

    >10.0 ng/mL (SI: >31.8 nmol/L) (evidence of ovulatory adequacy)

Proinsulin ----------------- 26.5-176.4 pg/mL (SI: 3.0-20.0 pmol/L)

Prolactin ----------------4-23 ng/mL (SI: 0.17-1.00 nmol/L) (male);

    4-30 ng/mL (SI: 0.17-1.30 nmol/L) (nonlactating female);

    10-200 ng/mL (SI: 0.43-8.70 nmol/L) (lactating female)

Prostate-specific antigen (PSA) -------------------------------

    <2.0 ng/mL (SI: <2.0 µg/L) (≤40 years);

    <2.8 ng/mL (SI: <2.8 µg/L) (≤50 years);

    <3.8 ng/mL (SI: <3.8 µg/L) (≤60 years);

    <5.3 ng/mL (SI: <5.3 µg/L) (≤70 years);

    <7.0 ng/mL (SI: <7.0 µg/L) (≤79 years);

    <7.2 ng/mL (SI: <7.2 µg/L) (≥80 years)

Renin activity, plasma, sodium replete, ambulatory --------------

    0.6-4.3 ng/mL per h

Renin, direct concentration ------- 4-44 pg/mL (SI: 0.1-1.0 pmol/L)

Sex hormone–binding globulin (SHBG) ---------------------------

    1.1-6.7 µg/mL (SI: 10-60 nmol/L) (male);

    2.2-14.6 µg/mL (SI: 20-130 nmol/L) (female)

α-Subunit of pituitary glycoprotein hormones --------------------

    <1.2 ng/mL (SI: <1.2 µg/L)

Testosterone (bioavailable)-------------------------------------

    0.8-4.0 ng/dL (SI: 0.03-0.14 nmol/L)

    (20-50 years, female on oral estrogen);

    0.8-10.0 ng/dL (SI: 0.03-0.35 nmol/L)

    (20-50 years, female not on oral estrogen);

    83.0-257.0 ng/dL (SI: 2.88-8.92 nmol/L) (male 20-29 years);

    72.0-235.0 ng/dL (SI: 2.50-8.15 nmol/L) (male 30-39 years);

    61.0-213.0 ng/dL (SI: 2.12-7.39 nmol/L) (male 40-49 years);

    50.0-190.0 ng/dL (SI: 1.74-6.59 nmol/L) (male 50-59 years);

    40.0-168.0 ng/dL (SI: 1.39-5.83 nmol/L) (male 60-69 years)

Testosterone (free)-- 9.0-30.0 ng/dL (SI: 0.31-1.04 nmol/L) (male);

    0.3-1.9 ng/dL (SI: 0.01-0.07 nmol/L) (female)

Testosterone (total) - 300-900 ng/dL (SI: 10.4-31.2 nmol/L) (male);

    8-60 ng/dL (SI: 0.3-2.1 nmol/L) (female)

Vitamin B$_{12}$ ------------------ 180-914 pg/mL (SI: 133-674 pmol/L)

Chemistry Values

Alanine aminotransferase ------- 10-40 U/L (SI: 0.17-0.67 µkat/L)

Albumin--------------------------------3.5-5.0 g/dL (SI: 35-50 g/L)

Amylase ----------------------- 26-102 U/L (SI: 0.43-1.70 µkat/L)

Anion gap -------------------------- 3-11 mEq/L (SI: 3-11 mmol/L)

Aspartate aminotransferase ---- 20-48 U/L (SI: 0.33-0.80 µkat/L)

Bicarbonate ---------------------- 21-28 mEq/L (SI: 21-28 mmol/L)

Bilirubin (total)---------------- 0.3-1.2 mg/dL (SI: 5.1-20.5 µmol/L)

Blood gases

    Po_2, arterial blood ---------80-100 mm Hg (SI: 10.6-13.3 kPa)

    Pco_2, arterial blood ------------35-45 mm Hg (SI: 4.7-6.0 kPa)

Blood pH--- 7.35-7.45

Calcium -----------------------8.2-10.2 mg/dL (SI: 2.1-2.6 mmol/L)

Calcium (ionized) ----------- 4.60-5.08 mg/dL (SI: 1.2-1.3 mmol/L)

Carbon dioxide ------------------- 22-28 mEq/L (SI: 22-28 mmol/L)

CD$_4$ cell count--------------------500-1400/µL (SI: 0.5-1.4 x 10^9/L)

Chloride---------------------- 96-106 mEq/L (SI: 96-106 mmol/L)

Creatine kinase ----------------- 50-200 U/L (SI: 0.84-3.34 µkat/L)

Creatinine-----------0.7-1.3 mg/dL (SI: 61.9-114.9 µmol/L) (male);
   0.6-1.1 mg/dL (SI: 53.0-97.2 µmol/L) (female)

Ferritin ---------------------- 15-200 ng/mL (SI: 33.7-449.4 pmol/L)

Folate ------------------------------------ ≥4.0 ng/mL (SI: ≥4.0 µg/L)

Glucose ------------------------- 70-99 mg/dL (SI: 3.9-5.5 mmol/L)

γ-Glutamyltransferase ------------ 2-30 U/L (SI: 0.03-0.50 µkat/L)

Iron --
   50-150 µg/dL (SI: 9.0-26.8 µmol/L) (male);
   35-145 µg/dL (SI: 6.3-26.0 µmol/L) (female)

Lactate dehydrogenase --------- 100-200 U/L (SI: 1.7-3.3 µkat/L)

Lactic acid --------------------5.4-20.7 mg/dL (SI: 0.6-2.3 mmol/L)

Lipase ------------------------- 10-73 U/L (SI: 0.17-1.22 µkat/L)

Magnesium --------------------- 1.5-2.3 mg/dL (SI: 0.6-0.9 mmol/L)

Osmolality ------------275-295 mOsm/kg (SI: 275-295 mmol/kg)

Phosphate --------------------- 2.3-4.7 mg/dL (SI: 0.7-1.5 mmol/L)

Potassium --------------------- 3.5-5.0 mEq/L (SI: 3.5-5.0 mmol/L)

Prothrombin time --8.3-10.8 s

Serum urea nitrogen--------------8-23 mg/dL (SI: 2.9-8.2 mmol/L)

Sodium --------------------- 136-142 mEq/L (SI: 136-142 mmol/L)

Transferrin saturation ----------------------------------- 14%-50%

Troponin I ------------------------------ <0.6 ng/mL (SI: <0.6 µg/L)

Tryptase --------------------------- <11.5 ng/mL (SI: <11.5 µg/L)

Uric acid ------------------ 3.5-7.0 mg/dL (SI: 208.2-416.4 µmol/L)

Urine

Albumin-----------30-300 µg/mg creat (SI: 3.4-33.9 µg/mol creat)

Albumin-to-creatinine ratio ----------------------- <30 mg/g creat

Aldosterone-------------------- 3-20 µg/24 h (SI: 8.3-55.4 nmol/d)
   (should be <12 µg/24 h [SI: <33.2 nmol/d] with oral sodium
   loading—confirmed with 24-hour urinary sodium >200 mEq)

Calcium -------------------- 100-300 mg/24 h (SI: 2.5-7.5 mmol/d)

Catecholamine fractionation
   Normotensive normal ranges:
      Dopamine -------------------- <400 µg/24 h (SI: <2610 nmol/d)
      Epinephrine ----------------------<21 µg/24 h (SI: <115 nmol/d)
      Norepinephrine -----------------<80 µg/24 h (SI: <473 nmol/d)

Citrate ----------------- 320-1240 mg/24 h (SI: 16.7-64.5 mmol/d)

Cortisol ------------------------ 4-50 µg/24 h (SI: 11-138 nmol/d)

Cortisol following dexamethasone suppression test
   (low-dose: 2 day, 2 mg daily)-- <10 µg/24 h (SI: <27.6 nmol/d)

Creatinine-------------------- 1.0-2.0 g/24 h (SI: 8.8-17.7 mmol/d)

Glomerular filtration rate (estimated) ----->60 mL/min per 1.73 m^2

5-Hydroxyindole acetic acid---2-9 mg/24 h (SI: 10.5-47.1 µmol/d)

Iodine (random)--->100 µg/L

17-Ketosteroids - 6.0-21.0 mg/24 h (SI: 20.8-72.9 µmol/d) (male);
   4.0-17.0 mg/24 h (SI: 13.9-59.0 µmol/d) (female)

Metanephrine fractionation
   Normotensive normal ranges:
      Metanephrine -------- <261 µg/24 h (SI: <1323 nmol/d) (male);
      <180 µg/24 h (SI: <913 nmol/d) (female)
      Normetanephrine --------------------- age and sex dependent
      Total metanephrine ------------------ age and sex dependent

Osmolality ---------- 150-1150 mOsm/kg (SI: 150-1150 mmol/kg)

Oxalate -------------------------- <40 mg/24 h (SI: <456 mmol/d)

Phosphate ------------------ 0.9-1.3 g/24 h (SI: 29.1-42.0 mmol/d)

Potassium ---------------------17-77 mEq/24 h (SI: 17-77 mmol/d)

Sodium -------------------- 40-217 mEq/24 h (SI: 40-217 mmol/d)

Uric acid ------------------------- <800 mg/24 h (SI: <4.7 mmol/d)

Saliva

Cortisol (salivary), midnight --------- <0.13 µg/dL (SI: <3.6 nmol/L)

Semen

Semen analysis --------------->20 million sperm/mL; >50% motility

COMMON ABBREVIATIONS USED IN ENDOCRINE BOARD REVIEW

ACTH = corticotropin

ACE inhibitor = angiotensin-converting enzyme inhibitor

ALT = alanine aminotransferase

AST = aspartate aminotransferase

BMI = body mass index

CNS = central nervous system

CT = computed tomography

DHEA = dehydroepiandrosterone

DHEA-S = dehydroepiandrosterone sulfate

DNA = deoxyribonucleic acid

DPP-4 inhibitor = dipeptidyl-peptidase 4 inhibitor

DXA = dual-energy x-ray absorptiometry

FDA = Food and Drug Administration

FGF-23 = fibroblast growth factor 23

FNA = fine-needle aspiration

FSH = follicle-stimulating hormone

GH = growth hormone

GHRH = growth hormone–releasing hormone

GLP-1 receptor agonist = glucagonlike peptide 1 receptor agonist

GnRH = gonadotropin-releasing hormone

hCG = human chorionic gonadotropin

HDL = high-density lipoprotein

HIV = human immunodeficiency virus

HMG-CoA reductase inhibitor = 3-hydroxy-3-methylglutaryl coenzyme A reductase inhibitor

IGF-1 = insulinlike growth factor 1

LDL = low-density lipoprotein

LH = luteinizing hormone

MCV = mean corpuscular volume

MIBG = *meta*-iodobenzylguanidine

MRI = magnetic resonance imaging

NPH insulin = neutral protamine Hagedorn insulin

PCSK9 inhibitor = proprotein convertase subtilisin/kexin 9 inhibitor

PET = positron emission tomography

PSA = prostate-specific antigen

PTH = parathyroid hormone

PTHrP = parathyroid hormone–related protein

SGLT-2 inhibitor = sodium-glucose cotransporter 2 inhibitor

SHBG = sex hormone–binding globulin

T_3 = triiodothyronine

T_4 = thyroxine

TPO antibodies = thyroperoxidase antibodies

TRH = thyrotropin-releasing hormone

TRAb = TSH-receptor antibodies

TSH = thyrotropin

VLDL = very low-density lipoprotein

ENDOCRINE
BOARD
REVIEW

Adrenal Board Review

Tobias Else, MD

1 A 24-year-old man is referred for evaluation of hypertension and low-normal potassium levels. He reports that he has a family history of hypertension and states that his blood pressure has been "high" since he was 16 years old. His current antihypertensive treatment regimen is amlodipine, 5 mg daily, and metoprolol, 25 mg daily. Both of his parents have hypertension; his father had a stroke at age 54 years. Adrenal imaging shows a 1.2-cm nodule in the right adrenal gland and 0.6-cm and 0.8-cm nodules in the left adrenal gland.

On physical examination, his blood pressure is 172/98 mm Hg and pulse rate is 72 beats/min.

Laboratory test results (sample collected at 9:00 AM):

Sodium = 138 mEq/L (136-142 mEq/L)
  (SI: 138 mmol/L [136-142 mmol/L])
Potassium = 3.5 mEq/L (3.5-5.0 mEq/L)
  (SI: 3.5 mmol/L [3.5-5.0 mmol/L])
Aldosterone = 24.2 ng/dL (4-21 ng/dL)
  (SI: 671.3 pmol/L [111.0-582.5 pmol/L])
Plasma renin activity = 0.1 ng/mL per h
  (0.6-4.3 ng/mL per h)
Plasma ACTH = 38 pg/mL (10-60 pg/mL)
  (SI: 8.4 pmol/L [2.2-13.2 pmol/L])
Cortisol = 12 µg/dL (5-25 µg/dL) (SI: 331.1 nmol/L
  [137.9-689.7 nmol/L])

Results of adrenal venous sampling are shown (done under cosyntropin stimulation in the early afternoon; peripheral vein baseline aldosterone concentration = 11 ng/dL [305.1 pmol/L] and cortisol = 8 µg/dL [220.7 nmol/L]).

Measurement	Right adrenal vein	Left adrenal vein	Inferior vena cava
Aldosterone	9220 ng/dL (SI: 255,762 pmol/L)	22,520 ng/dL (SI: 624,704 pmol/L)	118 ng/dL (SI: 3273 pmol/L)
Cortisol	539 µg/dL (SI: 14,869 nmol/L)	1247 µg/dL (SI: 34,402 nmol/L)	37 µg/dL (SI: 1020 nmol/L)
Aldosterone-to-cortisol ratio	17	18	3

Which of the following is the best next step in this patient's care?

A. Measure metanephrines
B. Perform 1-mg dexamethasone-suppression test with next-morning aldosterone measurement
C. Perform left adrenalectomy
D. Start spironolactone, 12.5 mg daily
E. Stop metoprolol and repeat screening

2 A 68-year-old man is referred for an incidentally discovered adrenal mass. He underwent CT-urography 2 years ago for an episode of nephrolithiasis, at which time a 10.4-cm adrenal tumor was identified. The result was not communicated to the patient. However, he recently switched primary care physicians and MRI was ordered, which identified an 11.2-cm adrenal mass. He has no symptoms of bloating, early satiety, abdominal fullness, or pain. He has had no recent changes in weight or overall well-being.

He also has a diagnosis of hypertension and coronary artery disease and had a stent placed 3 years ago. He has moderate left ventricular hypertrophy and is treated with losartan, 25 mg daily; carvedilol, 6.25 mg twice daily; furosemide, 20 mg daily; and acetylsalicylic acid, 81 mg daily.

On physical examination, his blood pressure is 122/78 mm Hg and pulse rate is 70 beats/min. His height is 69 in (175 cm), and weight is 230.6 lb (104.6 kg) (BMI = 34 kg/m^2).

Laboratory test results:
Sodium = 138 mEq/L (136-142 mEq/L)
 (SI: 138 mmol/L [136-142 mmol/L])
Potassium = 4.5 mEq/L (3.5-5.0 mEq/L)
 (SI: 4.5 mmol/L [3.5-5.0 mmol/L])
Aldosterone = 3.2 ng/dL (4-21 ng/dL)
 (SI: 88.8 pmol/L [111.0-582.5 pmol/L])
Plasma renin activity = 1.1 ng/mL per h
Plasma ACTH = 38 pg/mL (10-60 pg/mL)
 (SI: 8.4 pmol/L [2.2-13.2 pmol/L])
Cortisol = 12 μg/dL (5-25 μg/dL) (SI: 331.1 nmol/L
 [137.9-689.7 nmol/L])
Plasma normetanephrine = 85 pg/mL
 (<165 pg/mL) (SI: 0.46 nmol/L [<0.90 nmol/L])
Plasma metanephrine = 20 pg/mL (<99 pg/mL)
 (SI: 0.10 nmol/L [<0.50 nmol/L])

A 1-mg dexamethasone-suppression test results in a cortisol value of 1.1 μg/dL (30.3 nmol/L).

Noncontrast CT   **MRI (in phase)**   **MRI (out-of-phase)**

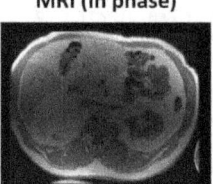 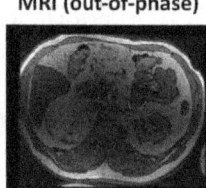

Which of the following is the best next step in this patient's care?

  A. Measure 24-hour urinary aldosterone, sodium, and creatinine after 3-day salt loading
  B. Measure 24-hour urinary cortisol
  C. Perform biopsy of the right adrenal gland
  D. Perform 18FDG-PET
  E. Recommend further clinical observation and imaging as indicated

3 A 35-year-old man presents with fatigue, malaise, loss of appetite, nausea, and night sweats. He was born in Myanmar and immigrated last year to the United States. He has a positive interferon-gamma release assay result for tuberculosis and is started on isoniazid, rifampicin, ethambutol, and pyrazinamide. Six weeks later, the patient is referred for evaluation of adrenal imaging findings. CT from initial diagnosis (*see image*) shows an enlarged right adrenal gland (2.8 cm) and bilateral adrenal calcifications.

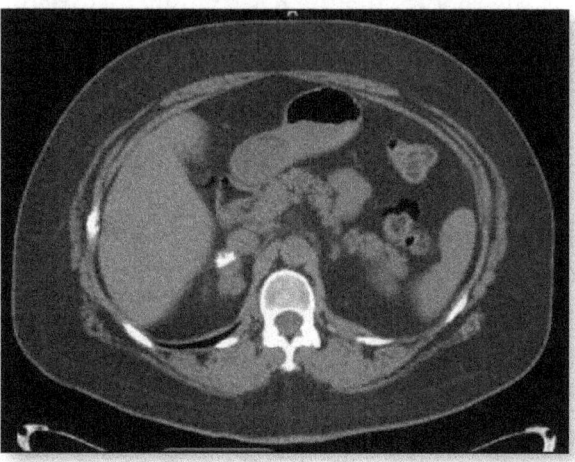

The patient reports that despite starting therapy, he has had increasing loss of appetite and nausea but no vomiting or diarrhea. He feels tired and weak.

On physical examination, he is thin and appears chronically ill. His blood pressure is 90/58 mm Hg, pulse rate is 87 beats/min, and temperature is 101.3°F (38.5°C). His height is 70 in (178 cm), and weight is 128 lb (58 kg) (BMI = 18.4 kg/m^2).

Laboratory test results from the time of initial presentation 6 weeks earlier:
Sodium = 131 mEq/L (136-142 mEq/L)
 (SI: 131 mmol/L [136-142 mmol/L])
Potassium = 5.2 mEq/L (3.5-5.0 mEq/L)
 (SI: 5.2 mmol/L [3.5-5.0 mmol/L])
Plasma ACTH = 72 pg/mL (10-60 pg/mL)
 (SI: 15.8 pmol/L [2.2-13.2 pmol/L])
Cortisol = 12 μg/dL (5-25 μg/dL) (SI: 331.1 nmol/L
 [137.9-689.7 nmol/L])

Which of the following is the best next step in this patient's care?

A. Hold rifampicin
B. Measure 21-hydroxylase antibodies
C. Perform biopsy of the right adrenal gland
D. Start hydrocortisone, 10 mg in the morning and 5 mg in the early afternoon
E. Start hydrocortisone, 50 mg oral 3 times a day, and fludrocortisone, 0.1 mg daily

4 A 22-year-old man has transferred his care for management of adrenal insufficiency following bilateral adrenalectomy at age 12 years for adrenal Cushing syndrome. He does not have any symptoms or signs of adrenal insufficiency and has adequate replacement therapy with hydrocortisone, 15 mg in the morning and 10 mg in the early afternoon. He had recent scrotal ultrasonography by a urologist for a left testicular varicocele and was incidentally found to have small testicular calcifications but normal testicular size.

He feels well and has no immediate plans for family planning.

On physical examination, he appears healthy. His blood pressure is 125/69 mm Hg, pulse rate is 64 beats/min, and temperature is 98.1°F (36.7°C). His height is 70.1 in (178 cm), and weight is 171.5 lb (78 kg) (BMI = 24.5 kg/m^2). He has perioral freckling, freckling of the lips, and white striae on his lower abdomen. Muscle bulk and strength are normal.

Laboratory test results:
Sodium = 139 mEq/L (136-142 mEq/L)
(SI: 139 mmol/L [136-142 mmol/L])
Potassium = 4.2 mEq/L (3.5-5.0 mEq/L)
(SI: 4.2 mmol/L [3.5-5.0 mmol/L])
Plasma ACTH = 98 pg/mL (10-60 pg/mL)
(SI: 21.6 pmol/L [2.2-13.2 pmol/L])
Cortisol (omitted dose in the morning of blood draw) = 0.1 μg/dL (5-25 μg/dL)
(SI: 2.8 nmol/L [137.9-689.7 nmol/L])
Plasma renin activity = 9.1 ng/mL per h (0.6-4.3 ng/mL per h)
Total testosterone = 560 ng/dL (300-900 ng/dL)
(SI: 19.4 nmol/L [10.4-31.2 nmol/L])
Prolactin = 20 ng/mL (4-23 ng/mL)
(SI: 0.87 nmol/L [0.17-1.00 nmol/L])

FSH = 22.3 mIU/mL (1.0-13.0 mIU/mL)
(SI: 22.3 IU/L [1.0-13.0 IU/L])
LH = 4.1 mIU/mL (1.0-9.0 mIU/mL)
(SI: 4.1 IU/L [1.0-9.0 IU/L])

Which of the following is the most important immediate next step in this patient's care?

A. Measurement of IGF-1
B. Measurement of morning 17-hydroxyprogesterone, androstenedione, and DHEA-S
C. Testicular biopsy
D. Thyroid ultrasonography
E. Transthoracic echocardiography

5 A 59-year-old man is referred for evaluation of an adrenal nodule and possible adrenal insufficiency. He had a recent abdominal CT for pain as part of an emergency department evaluation. The homogeneous nodule measures 1.2 cm and has a density of –2 Hounsfield units. No prior imaging is available.

The patient has chronic back pain and has received multiple facet joint injections over the last 3 years. He has been on long-term opioid therapy with oxycodone extended release, 20 mg daily, for the last 5 years. He also takes carbamazepine and gabapentin as adjunct pain medications. He had a steady weight gain of 62 lb (28.2 kg) over the last 3 years and is treated for hypertension with amlodipine, 5 mg daily, and hydrochlorothiazide, 25 mg daily. Type 2 diabetes mellitus was diagnosed 2 years ago. He was initially treated with lifestyle changes but was subsequently prescribed glipizide and metformin. His last hemoglobin A$_{1c}$ measurement 6 months ago was 7.1% (54 mmol/mol).

He has no nausea, vomiting, or diarrhea. Aside from chronic back pain, he has no other symptoms.

On physical examination, he appears healthy. His blood pressure is 138/77 mm Hg, pulse rate is 68 beats/min, and temperature is 98.1°F (36.7°C). His height is 71.5 in (182 cm), and weight is 262 lb (119 kg) (BMI = 36 kg/m^2). He has central fat distribution and normal muscle strength. There is no bruising and no increased pigmentation.

Laboratory test results (sample drawn while fasting at 8 AM):

Sodium = 140 mEq/L (136-142 mEq/L)
(SI: 140 mmol/L [136-142 mmol/L])

Potassium = 4.2 mEq/L (3.5-5.0 mEq/L)
(SI: 4.2 mmol/L [3.5-5.0 mmol/L])

Plasma ACTH = 22 pg/mL (10-60 pg/mL)
(SI: 4.8 pmol/L [2.2-13.2 pmol/L])

Cortisol = 1.4 μg/dL (5-25 μg/dL)
(SI: 38.6 nmol/L [137.9-689.7 nmol/L])

Plasma renin activity = 3.1 ng/mL per h
(0.6-4.3 ng/mL per h)

Aldosterone = 14.8 ng/dL (4-21 ng/dL)
(SI: 410.6 pmol/L [111.0-582.5 pmol/L])

Hemoglobin A_{1c} = 8.1% (4.0%-5.6%)
(SI: 65 mmol/mol [20-38 mmol/mol])

Which of the following is the best next step in this patient's care?

A. Counsel to seek alternatives to facet injections
B. Discuss alternatives to opioid medication
C. Measure 24-hour urinary aldosterone after 3 days of salt loading
D. Perform a cosyntropin-stimulation test
E. Start hydrocortisone replacement with 10 mg in the morning and 5 mg in the early afternoon

6 A 25-year-old Asian woman is referred by her primary care physician for an elevated DHEA-S concentration of 630 μg/dL (17.1 μmol/L) documented 6 months ago. DHEA-S was measured as part of a workup for 3 years of oligomenorrhea. She does not have a diagnosis of diabetes mellitus. She reports undergoing normal puberty and having regular periods as an undergraduate student. She takes no medications. She lost 33 lb (15 kg) in the last year while following a low-carbohydrate diet, restricting caloric intake, and increasing her exercise. Her periods are now regular with normal flow. She continues to have very mild acne but is not bothered by it. She has no plans for pregnancy in the near future.

Findings on CT of the adrenal glands are normal.

On physical examination, she appears healthy. Her blood pressure is 110/62 mm Hg, pulse rate is 62 beats/min, and temperature is 97.9ºF (36.6ºC). Her height is 64.5 in (164 cm), and weight is 132 lb (60 kg) (BMI = 22.3 kg/m²). She has normal muscle strength, no bruising, and no increased pigmentation. There is no increased hair growth, but she has very mild acne on her chin.

Laboratory test results:

Sodium = 141 mEq/L (136-142 mEq/L)
(SI: 141 mmol/L [136-142 mmol/L])

Potassium = 4.2 mEq/L (3.5-5.0 mEq/L)
(SI: 4.2 mmol/L [3.5-5.0 mmol/L])

Plasma ACTH = 10 pg/mL (10-60 pg/mL)
(SI: 2.2 pmol/L [2.2-13.2 pmol/L])

Cortisol (random at 12 PM) = 10.8 μg/dL
(2-14 μg/dL) (SI: 298.0 nmol/L
[55.2-386.2 nmol/L])

Cortisol (following 1-mg dexamethasone-suppression test) = 1.4 μg/dL (SI: 38.6 nmol/L)

DHEA-S (repeated measurement) = 477 μg/dL
(44-332 μg/dL) (SI: 12.9 μmol/L
[1.19-9.00 μmol/L])

Testosterone = 30 ng/dL (8-60 ng/dL)
(SI: 1.0 nmol/L [0.3-2.1 nmol/L])

Prolactin = 11 ng/mL (4-23 ng/mL)
(SI: 0.48 nmol/L [0.17-1.00 nmol/L])

SHBG = 9.0 μg/mL (2.2-14.6 μg/mL)
(SI: 80 nmol/L [20-130 nmol/L])

Measurement	Without cosyntropin stimulation	With cosyntropin stimulation
17-Hydroxyprogesterone	45 ng/dL (SI: 1.36 nmol/L)	80 ng/dL (SI: 2.42 nmol/L)
17-Hydroxypregnenolone	108 ng/dL (SI: 3.25 nmol/L)	1170 ng/dL (SI: 35.33 nmol/L)
Cortisol	10.8 μg/dL (SI: 298.0 nmol/L) (random, at 12 PM)	24.7 μg/dL (SI: 681.4 nmol/L)

Which of the following is the best next step in this patient's care?

A. Measure gonadotropins
B. Recommend no intervention now
C. Start hydrocortisone replacement
D. Start low-dosage dexamethasone, 0.5 mg at night
E. Start spironolactone

7 A 23-year-old woman with congenital adrenal hyperplasia due to 21-hydroxylase deficiency diagnosed at birth is transitioning to adult care from her pediatric endocrinologist. Her current treatment consists of hydrocortisone, 10 mg 3 times daily with meals, and fludrocortisone acetate, 0.2 mg every evening. She has regular menses, is not sexually active, and is not attempting to become pregnant.

On physical examination, she has no acne, unwanted facial hair, purple striae, or skin thinning. Her BMI is 25 kg/m², and blood pressure is 117/74 mm Hg. She feels well and has no concerns.

She took hydrocortisone today at 6 AM and 12 PM, and her blood is drawn at 5:30 PM.

Laboratory test results (5:30 PM blood draw):
Sodium = 138 mEq/L (136-142 mEq/L)
(SI: 138 mmol/L [136-142 mmol/L])
Potassium = 4.2 mEq/L (3.5-5.0 mEq/L)
(SI: 4.2 mmol/L [3.5-5.0 mmol/L])
Serum DHEA-S = <15 μg/dL (44-332 μg/dL)
(SI: <0.4 μmol/L [1.19-9.00 μmol/L])
Serum total testosterone = 40 ng/dL (8-60 ng/dL)
(SI: 1.4 nmol/L [0.3-2.1 nmol/L])
Plasma renin activity = 2.4 ng/mL per h
(0.6-4.3 ng/mL per h)
Serum androstenedione = 90 ng/dL (80-240 ng/dL)
(SI: 3.14 nmol/L [2.79-8.38 nmol/L])
Serum 17-hydroxyprogesterone = 4500 ng/dL
(<80 ng/dL) (SI: 136.4 nmol/L [<2.42 nmol/L])

Which of the following changes to her management should be recommended?
  A. Divide hydrocortisone as 7.5 mg 4 times daily
  B. Increase the second dose of hydrocortisone to 15 mg
  C. Recommend no changes
  D. Stop fludrocortisone acetate
  E. Switch hydrocortisone to dexamethasone, 1 mg at bedtime

8 A 38-year-old woman is referred for evaluation of adrenal nodularity. She reports weight gain of 11 lb (5 kg), poor sleep, and easy bruising over the last 2 years.

On physical examination, her blood pressure is 144/92 mm Hg. She has moderate facial plethora with rounding, dermal atrophy, and disproportionate supraclavicular fat pads. She cannot rise from a squat, and she has several 2- to 3-cm bruises on her legs.

Laboratory test results:
Serum cortisol after 1 mg dexamethasone = 8.0 μg/dL (SI: 220.7 nmol/L)
Serum DHEA-S = 110 μg/dL (31-228 μg/dL)
(SI: 2.98 μmol/L [0.84-6.78 μmol/L])
Hemoglobin A₁c = 7.3% (4.0%-5.6%) (56 mmol/mol [20-38 mmol/mol])
Plasma ACTH = 5 pg/mL (10-60 pg/mL)
(SI: 1.1 pmol/L [2.2-13.2 pmol/L])
Urinary free cortisol = 62 μg/24 h (4-50 μg/24 h)
(SI: 171 nmol/d [11-138 nmol/d])
Abdominal CT shows bilateral adrenal nodularity, 4 × 3 cm on the right side and 2 × 2 cm on the left side (*see image*).

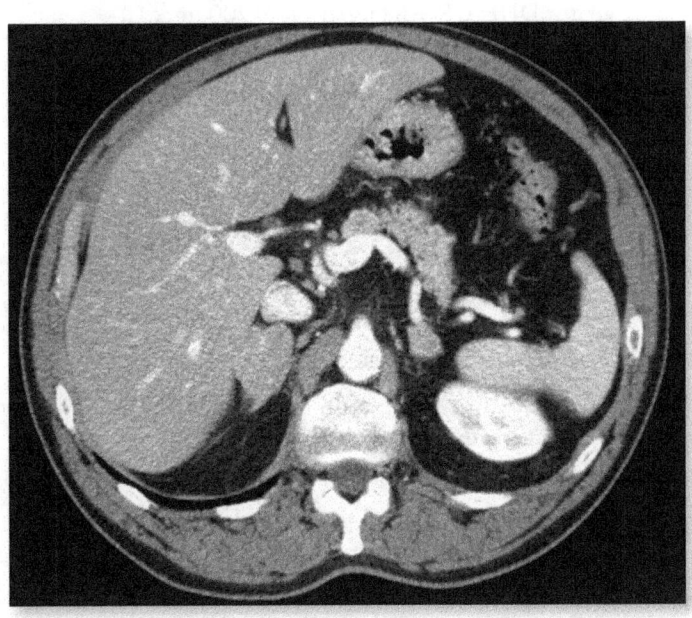

Courtesy of Rich Auchus.

Which of the following should be recommended as the best next step in this patient's management?
  A. Laparoscopic right adrenalectomy
  B. MRI of the adrenal glands
  C. Observation
  D. Pasireotide
  E. Spironolactone and metformin

9 A 55-year-old woman is referred for evaluation of an incidentally discovered right adrenal mass. The mass measures 3.4 cm in diameter, the precontrast attenuation value is –5 Hounsfield units, and there is more than 60% contrast medium washout 15 minutes after contrast administration. The left adrenal gland has no nodularity. Her only medication is alendronate for osteoporosis.

On physical examination, she has borderline hypertension (144/92 mm Hg). Her weight is 169 lb (76.8 kg) (BMI = 29 kg/m²). She has no facial plethora, dermal atrophy, bruising, or supraclavicular fat pads.

Initial laboratory test results:
  Plasma ACTH (8 AM) = 7 pg/mL (10-60 pg/mL)
    (SI: 1.5 pmol/L [2.2-13.2 pmol/L])
  Repeated plasma ACTH = 8 pg/mL (SI: 1.8 pmol/L)
  Serum DHEA-S = 58 µg/dL (15-200 µg/dL)
    (SI: 1.57 µmol/L [0.41-5.42 µmol/L])
  Serum cortisol after 1 mg dexamethasone = 4.2 µg/dL (SI: 115.9 nmol/L)
  Repeated serum cortisol = 4.2 µg/dL
    (SI: 115.9 nmol/L)
  Urinary free cortisol = 22 µg/24 h (4-50 µg/24 h)
    (SI: 60.7 nmol/d [11-138 nmol/d])

Two years later, the patient has gained 32 lb (14.5 kg) (BMI = 34 kg/m²). She has no facial plethora, dermal atrophy, bruising, or supraclavicular fat pads. Hypertension is controlled on amlodipine and losartan (132/80 mm Hg). She is still taking alendronate and has started metformin to treat diabetes (hemoglobin A_{1c} = 6.9% [52 mmol/mol]).

Repeated laboratory test results:
  Plasma ACTH (8 AM) = 8 pg/mL (SI: 1.8 pmol/L)
  Repeated plasma ACTH = 6 pg/mL (SI: 1.3 pmol/L)
  Serum DHEA-S = <15 µg/dL (SI: <0.41 µmol/L)
  Serum cortisol after 1 mg dexamethasone = 4.1 µg/dL (SI: 113.1 nmol/L)
  Urinary free cortisol = 28 µg/24 h (SI: 77.3 nmol/d)
  Dexamethasone = 230 ng/dL

Which of the following is the best recommendation for this patient's care?
  A. Delay medical or surgical therapy until urinary free cortisol is clearly elevated
  B. Perform fluorodeoxyglucose-PET scan to evaluate for malignant transformation
  C. Refer for laparoscopic right adrenalectomy
  D. Refer for petrosal sinus sampling
  E. Start medical treatment with mifepristone, 300 mg daily

10 A 34-year-old woman presents with rapidly progressive hirsutism, secondary amenorrhea, balding, voice deepening, and hypertension over the last 6 months. Her primary care physician has obtained some initial laboratory test results:
  Sodium = 143 mEq/L (136-142 mEq/L)
    (SI: 143 mmol/L [136-142 mmol/L])
  Potassium = 3.1 mEq/L (3.5-5.0 mEq/L)
    (SI: 3.1 mmol/L [3.5-5.0 mmol/L])
  Serum aldosterone = <4 ng/dL (4-21 ng/dL)
    (SI: <111.0 pmol/L [111.0-582.5 pmol/L])
  Plasma renin activity = <0.6 ng/mL per h
    (0.6-4.3 ng/mL per h)
  Plasma ACTH = 11 pg/mL (10-60 pg/mL)
    (SI: 2.4 pmol/L [2.2-13.2 pmol/L])
  Serum cortisol (8 AM) = 14 µg/dL (5-25 µg/dL)
    (SI: 386.2 nmol/L [137.9-689.7 nmol/L])
  Serum DHEA-S = 2833 µg/dL (44-352 µg/dL)
    (SI: 76.8 µmol/L [1.2-9.5 µmol/L])
  Serum 11-deoxycortisol = 282 ng/dL (10-79 ng/dL)
    (SI: 8.5 nmol/L [0.30-2.39 nmol/L])
  Serum total testosterone = 310 ng/dL (8-60 ng/dL)
    (SI: 10.8 nmol/L [0.3-2.1 nmol/L])
  SHBG = 1.0 µg/mL (2.2-14.6 µg/mL)
    (SI: 8.9 nmol/L [20-130 nmol/L])

Which of the following is this patient's most likely diagnosis?
  A. Anabolic steroid abuse
  B. Adrenocortical carcinoma
  C. Macronodular adrenocortical hyperplasia
  D. Nonclassic 11β-hydroxylase deficiency
  E. Ovarian hyperthecosis

11 A 22-year-old woman is referred for evaluation of severe hypertension and adrenal masses. She has new-onset hypertension and mild hyperglycemia. Her mother and a maternal uncle also developed severe hypertension before age 40 years. The uncle died of a myocardial infarction, and the patient's mother underwent adrenalectomy for bilateral pheochromocytoma and ultimately died of metastatic renal cell cancer.

Laboratory test results:
Sodium = 138 mEq/L (136-142 mEq/L)
(SI: 138 mmol/L [136-142 mmol/L])
Potassium = 3.8 mEq/L (3.5-5.0 mEq/L)
(SI: 3.8 mmol/L [3.5-5.0 mmol/L])
Plasma normetanephrine = 1502 pg/mL
(<165 pg/mL) (SI: 8.2 nmol/L [<0.90 nmol/L])
Plasma metanephrine = 60 pg/mL (<99 pg/mL)
(SI: 0.30 nmol/L [<0.50 nmol/L])
Serum aldosterone = 5 ng/dL (4-21 ng/dL)
(SI: 138.7 pmol/L [111.0-582.5 pmol/L])
Plasma renin activity = 2.4 ng/mL per h
(0.6-4.3 ng/mL per h)

CT scan after intravenous contrast is shown (*see image*).

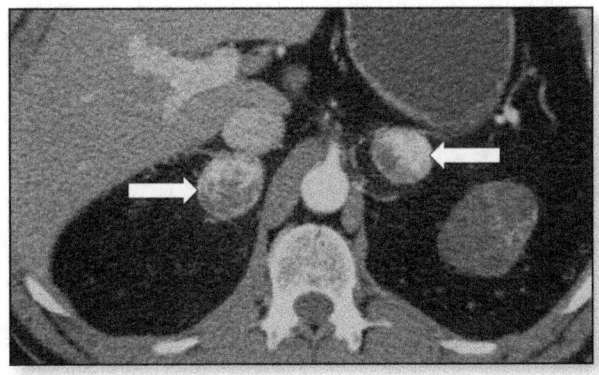

A pathogenic variant in which of the following genes is most likely responsible for pheochromocytoma in this kindred?

A. *KCNJ5*
B. *PRKAR1A*
C. *RET*
D. *SDHD*
E. *VHL*

12 A 57-year-old woman was diagnosed with a pancreatic gastrinoma 6 years ago when she presented with duodenal ulcers and abdominal pain. At the time of resection, CT demonstrated a 1.3-cm pancreatic primary tumor and a single 4-cm hepatic metastasis. She underwent resection of the primary tumor and liver metastasis and was treated with lanreotide injections, 120 mg every 4 weeks. Pathology showed a well-differentiated neuroendocrine tumor with a Ki-67 index (reflecting mitotic rate) of 1%. She remained well, but serial imaging demonstrated gradual appearance of multiple liver metastases (all <1 cm) with slight interval growth each year. In the 3 months since her last CT, she abruptly developed hypertension and hypokalemia, diabetes mellitus, poor sleep, muscle weakness, and depression.

On physical examination, her blood pressure is 167/96 mm Hg. She has a flat affect with slow response to commands, 2+ bilateral pedal edema, and muscle weakness.

Laboratory test results:
Serum potassium = 2.8 mEq/L (3.5-5.0 mEq/L)
(SI: 2.8 mmol/L [3.5-5.0 mmol/L])
Serum cortisol (random) = 120 μg/dL (5-25 μg/dL)
(SI: 3311 nmol/L [138-390 nmol/L])
Plasma ACTH = 750 pg/mL (10-60 pg/mL)
(SI: 165.0 pmol/L [2.2-13.2 pmol/L])
Fasting serum gastrin = 95 pg/mL (<100 pg/mL)
(SI: 95 ng/L [<100 ng/L])
Serum albumin = 4.1 g/dL (3.5-5.0 g/dL)
(SI: 41 g/L [35-50 g/L])
Hemoglobin A$_{1c}$ = 8.2% (4.0%-5.6%) (66 mmol/mol [20-38 mmol/mol])

On repeated CT, the liver metastases are not measurably changed from 3 months ago. The adrenal glands are somewhat thickened but have no tumors.

Which of the following is the most appropriate immediate next step in this patient's management?

    A. Change therapy to depot octreotide, 30 mg every 3 weeks

    B. Initiate ketoconazole therapy

    C. Initiate lutetium-DOTATATE therapy

    D. Perform bilateral adrenalectomy

    E. Refer to oncology for cytotoxic chemotherapy

13 A 49-year-old woman has been referred with a history of estrogen receptor–positive breast cancer diagnosed 3 years earlier. Her only medication is tamoxifen. She has not had any evidence of breast cancer recurrence, but recent abdominal CT showed a 2.8-cm right adrenal nodule with an attenuation value of 46 Hounsfield units. Fluorodeoxyglucose PET demonstrated accumulation of fluorodeoxyglucose in the right adrenal nodule, but no significant accumulation in other sites. The patient is asymptomatic and has never had hypertension.

On physical examination, her height is 64 in (162.6 cm) and weight is 110 lb (50 kg) (BMI = 18.9 kg/m²). Her blood pressure is 122/76 mm Hg, and pulse rate is 68 beats/min.

Laboratory test results:
    Potassium = 4.4 mEq/L (3.5-5.0 mEq/L)
      (SI: 4.4 mmol/L [3.5-5.0 mmol/L])
    Sodium = 138 mEq/L (136-142 mEq/L)
      (SI: 138 mmol/L [136-142 mmol/L])
    Aldosterone = 16 ng/dL (4-21 ng/dL)
      (SI: 443.8 pmol/L [111.0-582.5 pmol/L])
    Plasma renin activity = 3.5 ng/mL per h
      (0.6-4.3 ng/mL per h)
    Cortisol after overnight 1-mg dexamethasone-suppression test = 2.2 μg/dL (SI: 60.7 nmol/L)

Which of the following is the best next step in this patient's management?

    A. Bilateral adrenal venous sampling for aldosterone, cortisol, and epinephrine

    B. High-dose dexamethasone-suppression test

    C. Measurement of plasma free fractionated metanephrines

    D. Percutaneous CT-guided aspiration biopsy of the right adrenal nodule

    E. Surgical removal of the right adrenal nodule

14 A 37-year-old woman would like a second opinion regarding her endocrine status. In the last 4 years, she has gained 56 lb (25.5 kg) and developed secondary amenorrhea, hypertension, depression, and diabetes. She has a very cushingoid appearance, with facial fullness and plethora, as well as a marked increase in supraclavicular and dorsocervical fat accumulation. She has truncal obesity (BMI = 37 kg/m²) and wide, violaceous striae on her abdomen and in her axillae. Her medications include insulin glargine, insulin lispro, metformin, sitagliptin, lisinopril, furosemide, and fluoxetine.

Laboratory test results:
    Sodium = 138 mEq/L (136-142 mEq/L)
      (SI: 138 mmol/L [136-142 mmol/L])
    Potassium = 3.6 mEq/L (3.5-5.0 mEq/L)
      (SI: 3.6 mmol/L [3.5-5.0 mmol/L])
    Chloride = 100 mEq/L (96-106 mEq/L)
      (SI: 100 mmol/L [96-106 mmol/L])
    Bicarbonate = 26 mEq/L (21-28 mEq/L)
      (SI: 26 mmol/L [21-28 mmol/L])
    Serum urea nitrogen = 16 mg/dL (8-23 mg/dL)
      (SI: 5.7 mmol/L [2.9-8.2 mmol/L])
    Calcium = 9.6 mg/dL (8.2-10.2 mg/dL)
      (SI: 2.4 mmol/L [2.1-2.6 mmol/L])
    Hemoglobin A$_{1c}$ = 6.9% (4.0%-5.6%) (52 mmol/mol [20-38 mmol/mol])
    Urinary free cortisol = 68 μg/24 h and 74 μg/24 h (4-50 μg/24 h) (SI: 187.7 nmol/d and 204.2 nmol/d [11.0-138 nmol/d])
    Late-night salivary cortisol = 0.43 μg/dL and 0.62 μg/dL (<0.13 μg/dL) (SI: 11.9 nmol/L and 17.1 nmol/L [<3.6 nmol/L])

Cortisol after overnight 1-mg dexamethasone-suppression test = 8.2 μg/dL (SI: 226.2 nmol/L)

Which of the following studies should be ordered next?
- A. Adrenal-directed CT
- B. Dexamethasone corticotropin-releasing hormone test
- C. High-dose dexamethasone-suppression test
- D. Plasma ACTH measurement
- E. Pituitary-directed MRI

15 A 56-year-old man is referred for evaluation of an incidentally discovered adrenal mass. He had not seen a physician in 10 years, and he sought medical attention for postprandial abdominal pain. Abdominal CT without contrast was obtained (*see image*). The official interpretation was "1.2-cm left adrenal mass (8 Hounsfield units); MRI can further characterize." His abdominal pain has since resolved with a 6-week course of omeprazole. His medical history is unremarkable.

On physical examination, he has no cushingoid stigmata. Blood pressure measurements obtained in the clinic since he first presented have ranged as follows: systolic 144 to 162 mm Hg and diastolic 92 to 98 mm Hg (even after resolution of abdominal pain).

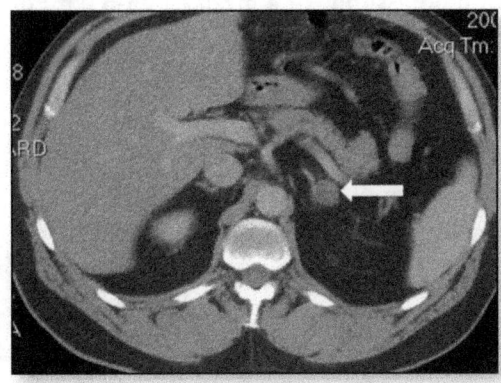

Laboratory test results:
Potassium = 3.8 mEq/L (3.5-5.0 mEq/L) (SI: 3.8 mmol/L [3.5-5.0 mmol/L])
Plasma normetanephrine = 150 pg/mL (<165 pg/mL) (SI: 0.82 nmol/L [<0.90 nmol/L])
Plasma metanephrine = 40 pg/mL (<99 pg/mL) (SI: 0.20 nmol/L [<0.50 nmol/L])

Serum cortisol (8 AM) after overnight 1-mg dexamethasone-suppression test = 0.4 μg/dL (SI: 11.0 nmol/L)
Fasting glucose = 80 mg/dL (70-99 mg/dL) (SI: 4.4 mmol/L [3.9-5.5 mmol/L])

Which of the following is the best next step in this patient's management?
- A. Measure serum aldosterone and plasma renin activity
- B. Measure serum DHEA-S and plasma ACTH
- C. Obtain 24-hour urine collection to measure metanephrines
- D. Perform adrenal MRI
- E. Repeat adrenal CT in 1 year

16 An 18-year-old man is referred for follow-up of adrenal insufficiency, which he developed at age 13 years. He takes hydrocortisone, 15 mg upon waking and 5 mg in the early afternoon, plus fludrocortisone acetate, 0.2 mg daily. He also takes fluconazole, 150 mg once weekly, for recurrent episodes of oral thrush since age 10 years. An older sibling died suddenly at age 5 years of unknown causes.

On physical examination, his height is 64 in (162.6 cm) and weight is 110 lb (50 kg) (BMI = 18.9 kg/m²). He has thin nails and brown horizontal bands on his teeth without oral thrush (*see image*). His blood pressure is 115/75 mm Hg, and pulse rate is 70 beats/min. He has no hyperpigmentation or vitiligo.

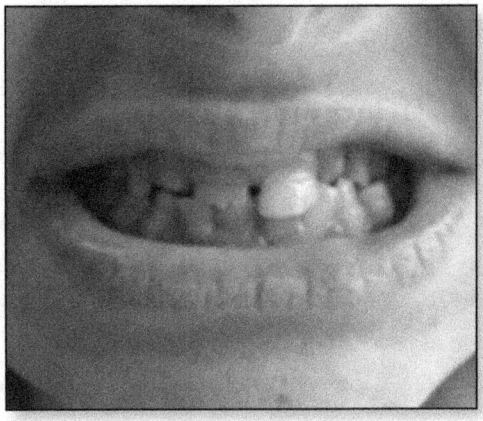

Orlova EM, et al. *J Clin Endocrinol Metab*, 2017;102(9) © Endocrine Society.

Laboratory test results (sample drawn at 9 AM):
  Serum sodium = 142 mEq/L (136-142 mEq/L)
    (SI: 142 mmol/L [136-142 mmol/L])
  Serum potassium = 3.9 mEq/L (3.5-5.0 mEq/L)
    (SI: 3.9 mmol/L [3.5-5.0 mmol/L])
  Plasma ACTH = 250 pg/mL (10-60 pg/mL)
    (SI: 55.0 pmol/L [2.2-13.2 pmol/L])
  Plasma direct renin = 33 pg/mL (30-40 pg/mL)
    (SI: 0.8 pmol/L [0.7-1.0 pmol/L])
  Serum 21-hydroxylase antibodies = 70 U/mL
    (<1 U/mL)

Which of the following other endocrinopathies is he most at risk to develop?
  A. Gonadal failure
  B. Graves disease
  C. Hypoparathyroidism
  D. Hypothyroidism
  E. Type 1 diabetes mellitus

17 A 48-year-old man with a history of stage IV small cell lung cancer is referred for rapid onset of cushingoid features, hypertension, and hypokalemia.

Laboratory test results:
  Serum cortisol = 80 μg/dL (5-25 μg/dL)
    (SI: 2207.0 nmol/L [137.9-689.7 nmol/L])
  Plasma ACTH = 580 pg/mL (10-60 pg/mL)
    (SI: 127.6 pmol/L [2.2-13.2 pmol/L])
  Serum glucose = 402 mg/dL (70-99 mg/dL)
    (SI: 22.3 mmol/L [3.9-5.5 mmol/L])

Eplerenone, 100 mg twice daily, is started to control the hypokalemia and hypertension, with good response. Ketoconazole is initiated and advanced to the dosage of 200 mg 3 times daily. He is tolerating this regimen well, and improvements in glucose and cortisol levels are noted.

Which of the following changes should this patient anticipate as a result of ketoconazole therapy?
  A. Decrease in corticosteroid-binding globulin
  B. Decrease in testosterone
  C. Increase in ACTH
  D. Increase in 11-deoxycortisol
  E. Increase in estradiol

18 A 68-year-old man is diagnosed with primary aldosteronism after having difficult-to-control hypertension with intermittent hypokalemia for at least 10 years and microalbuminuria for the last 2 years. Adrenal venous sampling demonstrates bilateral hyperaldosteronism, and medical therapy is started with eplerenone, 50 mg daily, added to amlodipine, 10 mg daily. Over 6 weeks, his blood pressure falls from 158/96 mm Hg to 135/88 mm Hg, and the eplerenone dosage is increased to 50 mg twice daily. After another 8 weeks, his blood pressure is 125/82 mm Hg.

Laboratory test results (baseline before eplerenone):
  Serum potassium = 3.1 mEq/L (3.5-5.0 mEq/L)
    (SI: 3.1 mmol/L [3.5-5.0 mmol/L])
  Serum creatinine = 1.4 mg/dL (0.7-1.3 mg/dL)
    (SI: 123.8 μmol/L [61.9-114.9 μmol/L])
  Serum aldosterone = 28 ng/dL (4-21 ng/dL)
    (SI: 777 pmol/L [111-583 pmol/L])
  Plasma renin activity = <0.6 ng/mL per h
    (0.6-4.3 ng/mL per h)

Laboratory test results (after 8 weeks taking eplerenone, 50 mg twice daily):
  Serum potassium = 4.4 mEq/L (3.5-5.0 mEq/L)
    (SI: 4.4 mmol/L [3.5-5.0 mmol/L])
  Serum creatinine = 1.8 mg/dL (0.7-1.3 mg/dL)
    (SI: 159.1 μmol/L [61.9-114.9 μmol/L])
  Serum aldosterone = 33 ng/dL (4-21 ng/dL)
    (SI: 915 pmol/L [111-583 pmol/L])
  Plasma renin activity = 1.3 ng/mL per h
    (0.6-4.3 ng/mL per h)

Repeated testing 2 weeks later shows equivalent results.

On the basis of these results, which of the following changes should be made to his blood pressure therapy?
  A. Change eplerenone to spironolactone, 100 mg daily
  B. Discontinue amlodipine
  C. Discontinue eplerenone and add atenolol, 50 mg daily
  D. Reduce the eplerenone dosage to 50 mg daily
  E. No changes

19 A nephrology colleague asks for an opinion regarding a 32-year-old woman who underwent successful left laparoscopic adrenalectomy for a 2.1-cm aldosterone-secreting adenoma 4 months earlier. The patient had presented with hypokalemia (potassium = 2.9 mEq/L [2.9 mmol/L]) and severe hypertension (initial blood pressure was 162/102 mm Hg). She was not seen by an endocrinologist before surgery. After surgery, her hypokalemia resolved and her blood pressure normalized without any medications. Since her operation, she has been easily fatigued and has had a decreased appetite; she has lost 6.5 lb (3 kg). Her only medication is an oral contraceptive.

On physical examination, she is a healthy appearing woman with obesity (BMI = 31.3 kg/m²). Her blood pressure is 124/82 mm Hg, and pulse rate is 82 beats/min. She has upper-body obesity, with some increase in supraclavicular and dorsocervical fat. The rest of her examination findings are normal.

Laboratory test results (sample drawn in the morning):
    Sodium = 134 mEq/L (136-142 mEq/L)
        (SI: 134 mmol/L [136-142 mmol/L])
    Potassium = 4.7 mEq/L (3.5-5.0 mEq/L)
        (SI: 4.7 mmol/L [3.5-5.0 mmol/L])
    Glucose = 91 mg/dL (70-99 mg/dL)
        (SI: 5.1 mmol/L [3.9-5.5 mmol/L])
    Creatinine = 0.8 mg/dL (0.6-1.1 mg/dL)
        (SI: 70.7 μmol/L [53.0-97.2 μmol/L])
    Cortisol = 3.8 μg/dL (5-25 μg/dL)
        (SI: 104.8 nmol/L [137.9-689.7 nmol/L])
    Plasma ACTH = 98 pg/mL (10-60 pg/mL)
        (SI: 21.6 pmol/L [2.2-13.2 pmol/L])
    Aldosterone = 5 ng/dL (4-21 ng/dL)
        (SI: 138.7 pmol/L [111.0-582.5 pmol/L])
    Plasma renin activity = 0.4 ng/mL per h
        (0.6-4.3 ng/mL per h)

In addition to initiating hydrocortisone replacement therapy, which of the following is the best recommendation?
    A. DHEA-S measurement
    B. Measurement of 21-hydroxylase antibodies
    C. MRI of the pituitary gland
    D. No further diagnostic studies

20 A 42-year-old woman with a history of Cushing disease asks for an opinion regarding the possibility of recurrence. Six years earlier, she underwent transsphenoidal pituitary microsurgery for removal of a 5-mm corticotroph adenoma (confirmed with immunocytochemistry). Postoperatively, she had well-documented secondary adrenal insufficiency requiring glucocorticoid support for 11 months. She had complete recovery of her pituitary-adrenal axis. Her signs and symptoms of hypercortisolism resolved, with a 30-lb (13.6-kg) weight loss, resolution of hypertension, decreased facial fullness and plethora, and resumption of normal menses.

During the past 6 months, she has gained 25 lb (11.4 kg) and had a slight increase in her blood pressure. Her menses have been normal. She feels more depressed and is having difficulty dealing with the stress of her job. She is not taking any medication. She is convinced that she has Cushing syndrome again. However, her primary care physician measured a urinary cortisol excretion of 28 μg/24 h (77.3 nmol/d).

On physical examination, she has some facial rounding, but no plethora. Her blood pressure is 148/96 mm Hg, and her pulse rate is 78 beats/min. Her height is 64.5 in (163.8 cm), and weight is 164 lb (74.5 kg) (BMI = 27.7 kg/m²). She has some nonviolaceous striae. She has good muscle strength and no edema.

Which of the following is the best next step to exclude recurrent Cushing disease?
    A. 2-Day low-dose dexamethasone-suppression test (0.5 mg every 6 hours for 48 hours)
    B. Late-night salivary cortisol measurement
    C. Pituitary-directed MRI
    D. Plasma ACTH measurement
    E. No further tests are needed; patient should be reassured

21 A 38-year-old woman with a history of Cushing disease presents to the emergency department with nausea, weakness, and malaise. The diagnosis of an ACTH-secreting pituitary tumor with endogenous hypercortisolism was established 5 years ago. She had 2 unsuccessful pituitary operations and stereotactic radiosurgery. Despite these treatments, hypercortisolism persisted. Mifepristone therapy was started 10 weeks ago with dosage escalation from 300 to 900 mg daily.

She has type 2 diabetes mellitus treated with metformin and glimepiride (hemoglobin A_{1c}, 7.3% [56 mmol/mol]) and hypertension treated with lisinopril and hydrochlorothiazide, 10 to 12.5 mg daily. Since starting mifepristone, she has lost 12 lb (5.4 kg), and her glucose levels have dramatically decreased. One week ago, her oral hypoglycemic therapy and antihypertensive medication were discontinued. Her last menstrual period was 3 months ago. She saw her primary care physician yesterday, and the following laboratory test results were documented:

Sodium = 134 mEq/L (136-142 mEq/L)
 (SI: 134 mmol/L [136-142 mmol/L])
Potassium = 2.8 mEq/L (3.5-5.0 mEq/L)
 (SI: 2.8 mmol/L [3.5-5.0 mmol/L])
Chloride = 93 mEq/L (96-106 mEq/L)
 (SI: 93 mmol/L [96-106 mmol/L])
Bicarbonate = 30 mEq/L (21-28 mEq/L)
 (SI: 30 mmol/L [21-28 mmol/L])
Glucose = 68 mg/dL (70-99 mg/dL)
 (SI: 3.8 mmol/L [3.9-5.5 mmol/L])
Serum urea nitrogen = 22 mg/dL (8-23 mg/dL)
 (SI: 7.8 mmol/L [2.9-8.2 mmol/L])
Creatinine = 1.0 mg/dL (0.6-1.1 mg/dL)
 (SI: 88.4 μmol/L [53.0-97.2 μmol/L])
Calcium = 9.8 mg/dL (8.2-10.2 mg/dL)
 (SI: 2.5 mmol/L [2.1-2.6 mmol/L])
Cortisol = 57 μg/dL (5-25 μg/dL) (SI: 1573 nmol/L [137.9-689.7 nmol/L])
ACTH = 124 pg/mL (10-60 pg/mL)
 (SI: 27.3 pmol/L [2.2-13.2 pmol/L])
TSH = 8.3 mIU/L (0.5-5.0 mIU/L)
Free T_4 = 1.1 ng/dL (0.8-1.8 ng/dL)
 (SI: 14.16 pmol/L [10.30-23.17 pmol/L])

On physical examination, she is a lethargic woman with upper body obesity (BMI = 36.3 kg/m²). Her blood pressure is 88/68 mm Hg, pulse rate is 102 beats/min, and temperature is 99.3°F (37.4°C). She has some facial fullness, but no plethora. There is increased supraclavicular and dorsocervical fat accumulation. Her skin pigmentation is normal. Her visual fields are full to confrontation. She has generalized weakness and slight pretibial edema.

The emergency department physician has initiated intravenous isotonic fluids with potassium, and he calls to ask for directions regarding her continued care.

Which of the following is the best recommendation?
 A. Discontinue mifepristone and administer dexamethasone, 4 mg every 8 hours
 B. Initiate ketoconazole, 200 mg every 8 hours
 C. Initiate levothyroxine, 50 mcg, in combination with liothyronine, 5 mcg daily
 D. Perform a pregnancy test
 E. Perform pituitary MRI immediately

22 A 66-year-old woman presents to her local physician with hypertension of 20 years' duration, which has been poorly controlled for the past 6 years. She does not use tobacco or drink alcohol. She takes amlodipine, 10 mg daily; losartan, 100 mg daily; and hydrochlorothiazide, 12.5 mg daily. Her blood pressure is 155/93 mm Hg. She is referred to endocrinology after the following laboratory values are obtained:

Sodium = 140 mEq/L (136-142 mEq/L)
 (SI: 140 mmol/L [136-142 mmol/L])
Potassium = 4.1 mEq/L (3.5-5.0 mEq/L)
 (SI: 4.1 mmol/L [3.5-5.0 mmol/L])
Serum creatinine = 1.1 mg/dL (0.6-1.1 mg/dL)
 (SI: 97.2 μmol/L [53.0-97.2 μmol/L])
Serum aldosterone = 14 ng/dL (4-21 ng/dL)
 (SI: 388.4 pmol/L [111.0-582.5 pmol/L])
Plasma renin activity = <0.6 ng/mL per h
 (0.6-4.3 ng/mL per h)

Which of the following should be ordered first?
 A. Adrenal-directed CT
 B. Adrenal venous sampling
 C. 24-Hour urinary aldosterone and sodium measurement on the third day of a high-salt diet
 D. MR-angiography of the renal arteries
 E. Overnight (1 mg) dexamethasone-suppression test measuring cortisol and aldosterone

Calcium and Bone Board Review

Natalie Cusano, MD, MS

1 A 55-year-old woman sustains a rib fracture during a severe coughing episode. She has no personal history of fracture and no parental history of hip fracture. She is healthy other than asthma treated with albuterol as needed. Menopause occurred at age 51 years, and she currently has no hot flashes or other menopausal symptoms. She consumes 3 servings of dairy per day supplemented with vitamin Assessment of bone mineral density is notable for T-scores of −2.0 at the lumbar spine, −1.8 at the femoral neck, and −1.6 at the total hip. Metabolic evaluation for secondary causes of bone loss is unremarkable.

Her 25-hydroxyvitamin D concentration is 31 ng/mL (30-80 ng/mL [optimal]) (SI: 77.4 nmol/L [74.9-199.7 nmol/L]).

Which of the following is the best next step?
   A. Calculate her FRAX score
   B. Repeat a bone density test in 2 years
   C. Start alendronate
   D. Start calcium supplementation with vitamin D
   E. Start hormone therapy

2 A 65-year-old woman presents to establish care for osteoporosis. Osteoporosis was diagnosed at age 58 years in the setting of a low-trauma vertebral fracture at T12. She has been treated with denosumab since that time, with her last dose 8 months ago before her move from another state. Her most recent bone density assessment 2 years ago demonstrated significant improvements at the lumbar spine and total hip from baseline. She also has a history of stage 1 breast cancer diagnosed at age 61 years status post lumpectomy, radiation therapy, and tamoxifen therapy (she was not able to tolerate aromatase inhibitor treatment). She was feeling in her usual state of health until recently when she was lifting a heavy pot of soup and developed acute back pain. Vertebral fractures at T10, T11, and L1 were subsequently diagnosed.

Laboratory test results:
   Serum calcium = 9.8 mg/dL (8.2-10.2 mg/dL)
      (SI: 2.5 mmol/L [2.1-2.6 mmol/L])
   PTH = 45 pg/mL (10-65 pg/
      mL) (SI: 45 ng/L [10-65 ng/L])
   25-Hydroxyvitamin D = 31 ng/mL (30-80 ng/mL
      [optimal]) (SI: 77.4 nmol/L [74.9-199.7 nmol/L])
   Creatinine = 0.8 mg/dL (0.6-1.1 mg/dL)
      (SI: 70.2 μmol/L [53.0-97.2 μmol/L])
   Albumin = 3.8 g/dL (3.5-5.0 g/dL)
      (SI: 38 g/L [35-50 g/L])
   Alkaline phosphatase = 200 U/L (50-120 U/L)
      (SI: 3.3 μkat/L [0.84-2.00 μkat/L])
   Bone-specific alkaline phosphatase = 42 mg/L
      (≤22 mg/L)
   Phosphate = 3.0 mg/dL (2.3-4.7 mg/dL)
      (SI: 1.0 mmol/L [0.7-1.5 mmol/L])

Which of the following is the most likely contributor to her vertebral fractures?
   A. Adverse effect of prolonged antiresorptive therapy
   B. Adverse effect of tamoxifen
   C. Breast cancer
   D. Missed denosumab dose
   E. Paget disease

3 A 60-year-old American woman with osteopenia asks what nutritional or supplemental approaches may be beneficial for her bone health.

Which of the following nonpharmacologic therapies has/have been shown to reduce fracture risk in similar patients?

A. Calcium and vitamin D supplementation
B. Calcium alone
C. Strontium citrate
D. Vitamin D alone
E. Vitamin K_2

4 A 28-year-old G1P0 woman at 11 weeks' gestation presents with nausea and vomiting. She recalls being told she had mild hypercalcemia a few years ago, but she did not follow-up at that time. She is tired but arousable.

Laboratory test results:
  Serum calcium = 13.9 mg/dL (8.2-10.2 mg/dL) (SI: 3.5 mmol/L [2.1-2.6 mmol/L])
  PTH = 75 pg/mL (10-65 pg/mL) (SI: 75 ng/L [10-65 ng/L])
  25-Hydroxyvitamin D = 26 ng/mL (30-80 ng/mL [optimal]) (SI: 64.9 nmol/L [74.9-199.7 nmol/L])
  1,25-Dihydroxyvitamin D = 82 pg/mL (16-65 pg/mL) (SI: 213.2 pmol/L [41.6-169.0 pmol/L])
  Creatinine = 0.8 mg/dL (0.6-1.1 mg/dL) (SI: 70.7 µmol/L [53.0-97.2 µmol/L])
  Albumin = 3.4 g/dL (3.5-5.0 g/dL) (SI: 34 g/L [35-50 g/L])
  Phosphate = 3.0 mg/dL (2.3-4.7 mg/dL) (SI: 1.0 mmol/L [0.7-1.5 mmol/L])
  Urinary calcium = 321 mg/24 h (100-250 mg/24 h) (SI: 8.0 mmol/d [2.5-7.5 mmol/d])

Her serum-corrected calcium level remains elevated at 12.9 mg/dL (3.2 mmol/L) after intravenous fluids. Her nausea has improved.

Which of the following is the best next step for management of this patient's disorder?

A. Cinacalcet
B. Denosumab
C. Parathyroidectomy in the second trimester
D. Parathyroidectomy now
E. Prednisone

5 A 28-year-old woman is referred by her primary care physician for endocrine evaluation after abnormal findings on an x-ray performed because of right shoulder pain (*see image*). She has a history of precocious puberty and recurrent ovarian cysts. Previous evaluation by a pediatric endocrinologist when she was a child did not result in a clear diagnosis.

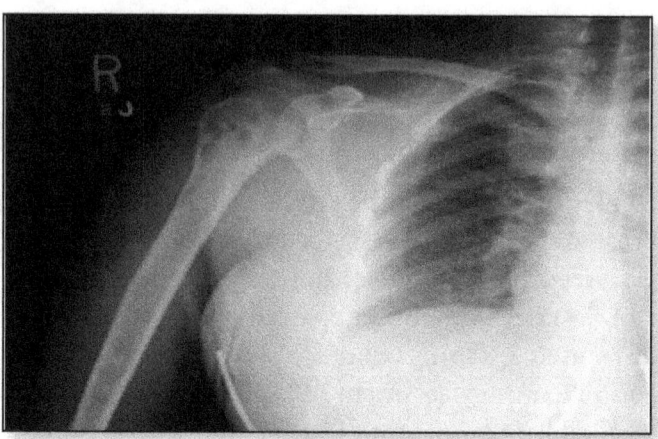

On physical examination, her height is 61 in (154.9 cm) and weight is 130 lb (59 kg) (BMI = 24.6 kg/m²). She has normal facies, an enlarged and nodular thyroid gland, and a flat hyperpigmented brown macule with rough borders on her mid-back.

Laboratory test results:
  TSH = 0.2 mIU/L (0.5-5.0 mIU/L)
  Calcium, normal
  PTH, normal,
  Alkaline phosphatase, normal
  Phosphate, normal
  25-Hydroxyvitamin D, normal
  1,25-Dihydroxyvitamin D, normal

Kidney function is normal.

Which of the following best explains this patient's clinical presentation?

A. Albright hereditary osteodystrophy
B. Fibrodysplasia ossificans progressiva
C. McCune-Albright syndrome
D. Monostotic fibrous dysplasia
E. Oncogenic osteomalacia (tumor-induced osteomalacia)

6 A 65-year-old woman with a history of multiple low-trauma vertebral fractures is initiating treatment with romosozumab. She inquires about monitoring for treatment effect.

What are the expected changes in bone turnover markers with romosozumab therapy?

Answer	Bone formation	Bone resorption
A.	↑	☐
B.	↑	↑
C.	↑	↓
D.	☐	↓
E.	↓	↓

7 A 51-year-old man with newly diagnosed HIV infection is admitted to the hospital with nausea, vomiting, and altered mental status. According to friends, he has been ill for 3 months with fever, weight loss, night sweats, malaise, and cough. He is an undocumented immigrant from Central America who has avoided seeking traditional medical care because of concerns about deportation. He is found to have active pulmonary *Mycobacterium bovis* with multiple opacities on chest x-ray. He has been taking an over-the-counter "vitamin" supplement found in the Dominican Republic and upper Manhattan that contains massive doses of vitamin D (864,000 IU) and vitamin A (123,000 IU) in a 5-mL bottle (much higher than the listed dosage).

On physical examination, he is a lethargic, cachectic man with tachycardia and diffuse lymphadenopathy.

Laboratory test results:
Calcium = 17.1 mg/dL (8.2-10.2 mg/dL) (SI: 4.3 mmol/L [2.1-2.6 mmol/L])
Albumin = 3.3 g/dL (3.5-5.0 g/dL) (SI: 33 g/L [35-50 g/dL])
Intact PTH = <10 pg/mL (10-65 pg/mL) (SI: <10 ng/L [10-65 ng/L])
PTHrP, undetectable

25-Hydroxyvitamin D = 525 ng/mL (30-80 ng/mL [optimal]) (SI: 1310.4 nmol/L [74.9-199.7 nmol/L])
1,25-Dihydroxyvitamin D = >180 pg/mL (16-65 pg/mL) (SI: >468 pmol/L [41.6-169.0 pmol/L])

Over what timeframe is this patient's 25-hydroxyvitamin D concentration expected to decrease to around 30 ng/mL (74.9 nmol/L)?
A. 2 to 3 days
B. 2 to 3 weeks
C. 2 to 3 months
D. 8 to 12 months
E. 24 to 36 months

8 A 62-year-old woman with a history of stage 4 chronic kidney disease due to uncontrolled hypertension presents to establish care after a recent right distal radius fracture. Results of bone density testing are significant for T-scores of −2.3 at the lumbar spine, −2.4 at the femoral neck, −2.4 at the total hip, and −3.2 at the distal radius.

Laboratory test results:
Serum calcium = 8.2 mg/dL (8.2-10.2 mg/dL) (SI: 2.1 mmol/L [2.1-2.6 mmol/L])
Creatinine = 3.2 mg/dL (0.6-1.1 mg/dL) (SI: 282.9 μmol/L [53.0-97.2 μmol/L])
Estimated glomerular filtration rate = 20 mL/min per 1.73 m² (>60 mL/min per 1.73 m²)
Intact PTH = 175 pg/mL (10-65 pg/mL) (SI: 175 ng/L [10-65 ng/L])
25-Hydroxyvitamin D = 14 ng/mL (30-80 ng/mL [optimal]) (SI: 34.9 nmol/L [74.9-199.7 nmol/L])
Phosphate = 5.4 mg/dL (2.3-4.7 mg/dL) (SI: 1.7 mmol/L [0.7-1.5 mmol/L])
Alkaline phosphatase = 320 U/L (50-120 U/L) (SI: 5.3 μkat/L [0.84-2.00 μkat/L])
Bone-specific alkaline phosphatase = 75 mg/L (≤22 mg/L)

In consultation with her nephrologist, the decision is made to treat with denosumab to decrease her fracture risk.

In this patient, which of the following is the most likely adverse effect of denosumab therapy?

    A. Impaired fracture healing

    B. Osteonecrosis of the jaw

    C. Severe flulike syndrome

    D. Severe hypocalcemia

    E. Worsening kidney function

9 An 82-year-old woman has a history of multiple medical problems, including primary hyperparathyroidism. Despite a history of nephrolithiasis and meeting criteria for parathyroidectomy, she has declined surgery. Her bone mineral density is notable for T-scores of –1.8 at the lumbar spine, –2.1 at the femoral neck, –1.8 at the total hip, and –2.4 at the distal radius. Her serum calcium concentration has been in the range of 11.3 to 11.6 mg/dL (2.8 to 2.9 mmol/L) with symptoms of nausea and constipation. Therapy with cinacalcet is considered.

What are the expected effects on this patient's biochemical and bone density parameters with cinacalcet therapy?

Answer	Serum calcium	PTH	Bone density
A.	↓↓	☐	↑
B	↓	☐	☐
C.	↓↓	↓	☐
D.	↓↓	↓	↑
E.	↓	↓	↑

10 A 55-year-old woman with postoperative hypoparathyroidism presents for follow-up. She has a history of Graves disease and is status post total thyroidectomy at age 39 years complicated by hypoparathyroidism. She currently takes levothyroxine, 125 mcg daily; calcium, 500 mg 3 times daily; and calcitriol, 0.25 mcg twice daily. She has no symptoms of hypocalcemia and otherwise feels well.

Laboratory test results:

    Serum calcium = 8.0 mg/dL (8.2-10.2 mg/dL)
      (SI: 2.0 mmol/L [2.1-2.6 mmol/L])
    25-Hydroxyvitamin D = 31 ng/mL (30-80 ng/mL
      [optimal]) (SI: 77.4 nmol/L [74.9-199.7 nmol/L])
    Creatinine = 1.2 mg/dL (0.6-1.1 mg/dL)
      (SI: 106.1 μmol/L [53.0-97.2 μmol/L])
    Albumin = 3.8 g/dL (3.5-5.0 g/dL)
      (SI: 38 g/L [35-50 g/L])
    Phosphate = 4.7 mg/dL (2.3-4.7 mg/dL)
      (SI: 1.5 mmol/L [0.7-1.5 mmol/L])

Which of the following is the best next step for monitoring this patient?

    A. Bone density assessment

    B. Dental examination

    C. Imaging of the basal ganglia

    D. Kidney ultrasonography

    E. Measurement of intraocular pressure

11 A 38-year-old woman is referred after passing a kidney stone. Imaging studies show bilateral kidney stones. Metabolic evaluation is consistent with primary hyperparathyroidism as illustrated by the following laboratory test results:

    Serum calcium = 11.9 mg/dL (8.2-10.2 mg/dL)
      (SI: 3.0 mmol/L [2.1-2.6 mmol/L])
    Serum PTH = 112 pg/mL (10-65 pg/mL)
      (SI: 112 ng/L [10-65 ng/L])
    Urinary calcium excretion = 400 mg/24 h
      (100-300 mg/24 h) (SI: 10 mmol/d
      [2.5-7.5 mmol/d])

Following a sestamibi scan demonstrating a "probable" adenoma in the right lower pole, the patient undergoes minimally invasive parathyroidectomy with resection of a single enlarged parathyroid gland. Pathologic examination confirms a parathyroid adenoma. Two weeks later, she returns for blood work while taking elemental calcium, 600 mg twice daily.

Laboratory test results 2 weeks after surgery:

    Calcium = 11.8 mg/dL (8.2-10.2 mg/dL)
      (SI: 3.0 mmol/L [2.1-2.6 mmol/L])
    Phosphate = 2.2 mg/dL (2.3-4.7 mg/dL)
      (SI: 0.7 mmol/L [0.7-1.5 mmol/L])

Albumin = 4.2 g/dL (3.5-5.0 g/dL)
   (SI: 42 g/L [35-50 g/L])
PTH = 120 pg/mL (10-65 pg/mL)
   (SI: 120 ng/L [10-65 ng/L])
Serum creatinine = 1.0 mg/dL (0.6-1.1 mg/dL)
   (SI: 88.4 μmol/L [53.0-97.2 μmol/L])

Which of the following is the best next step?
   A. 4D CT of the neck
   B. Cessation of calcium supplementation and recheck of laboratory tests in 1 month
   C. Genetic testing for pathogenic variants in the calcium-sensing receptor gene (*CASR*)
   D. Genetic testing for pathogenic variants in the multiple endocrine neoplasia type 1 gene (*MEN1*)
   E. Repeated sestamibi scan

12 A 22-year-old woman presents for follow-up of hypoparathyroidism. She was initially diagnosed at age 9 years when severe hypocalcemia caused a seizure. She has been maintained on calcium and calcitriol since that time. Over the past several months, she has noted anorexia, 10-lb (4.5-kg) weight loss, weakness, diarrhea, and dizziness.

   Physical examination reveals a supine blood pressure of 80/60 mm Hg, pulse rate of 120 beats/min, and dystrophic fingernails and toenails.

Which of the following laboratory measurements is key to this patient's diagnosis?
   A. 24-Hour urine 5-hydroxyindoleacetic acid (5-HIAA)
   B. Islet-cell and glutamic acid decarboxylase antibodies
   C. Serum cortisol and ACTH
   D. Serum TSH and TRAb-receptor antibody
   E. Transglutaminase antibodies

13 A 75-year-old man presents for evaluation after diagnosis of an L1 fracture that occurred when lifting his grandchild. He underwent pelvic irradiation for bladder cancer 5 years ago. He is otherwise in good health. He has regular follow-up with his oncologist.

On physical examination, he has tenderness over his lower spine. Four years ago, DXA revealed T-scores of −2.0 at the lumbar spine and −1.5 at the femoral neck with FRAX scores that did not meet treatment thresholds.

   Current laboratory test results, including complete blood cell count, routine chemistries, alkaline phosphatase, PSA, 25-hydroxyvitamin D, serum/urine protein electrophoresis, and PTH, are all normal. Serum testosterone on a morning specimen is 270 ng/dL (300-900 ng/dL) (SI: 9.4 nmol/L [10.4-31.2 nmol/L]). SHBG is within the reference range.

Which of the following is the best next step in this patient's care?
   A. Begin alendronate
   B. Begin teriparatide
   C. Begin testosterone
   D. Refer for kyphoplasty
   E. Refer for nuclear medicine bone scan

14 Paget disease of bone was recently diagnosed in a 72-year-old woman with chronic left hip pain. Her alkaline phosphatase concentration is 250 U/L (40-120 U/L) (SI: 4.2 μkat/L [0.7-2.0 μkat/L]), and her γ-glutamyltranspeptidase level is normal. Bone scan shows intense increased uptake in the left ilium, acetabulum, and femoral head. Radiographs show Paget disease in her left hemipelvis and femoral head, as well as moderate degenerative arthritis in the left hip. Treatment with zoledronic acid is recommended. She wonders what to expect in the next few years.

Which of the following is most likely to occur?
   A. Hearing loss due to Paget disease
   B. Osteonecrosis of the femoral neck
   C. Spread of Paget disease to the right hip
   D. Total resolution of all hip pain
   E. Worsening arthritis in the hip

15 A 42-year-old woman presents with bilateral hip pain and the radiographic findings shown (*see image*).

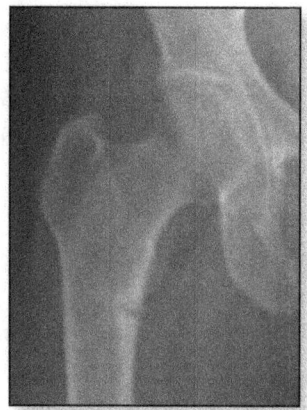

Laboratory test results:

Serum calcium = 8.2 mg/dL (8.2-10.2 mg/dL)
(SI: 2.1 mmol/L [2.1-2.6 mmol/L])

Phosphate = 2.2 mg/dL (2.3-4.7 mg/dL)
(SI: 0.7 mmol/L [0.7-1.5 mmol/L])

Creatinine = 0.9 mg/dL (0.7-1.3 mg/dL)
(SI: 79.6 µmol/L [61.9-114.9 µmol/L])

Serum alkaline phosphatase = 346 U/L
(50-120 U/L) (SI: 5.78 µkat/L [0.84-2.00 µkat/L])

Measurement of which of the following is most likely to provide this patient's diagnosis?

A. 1,25-Dihydroxyvitamin D
B. 25-Hydroxyvitamin D
C. FGF-23
D. Intact PTH
E. Serum protein electrophoresis

16 A 55-year-old man with rheumatoid arthritis has been on a stable dosage of methotrexate and prednisone, 5 mg daily, for the past 3 years. DXA performed last month shows his lowest T-score to be −2.0 at the femoral neck. According to the FRAX calculator, his risk for major osteoporosis-related fracture is 12% and his risk for hip fracture is 1.1%. His only other health issue is Barrett esophagus for which he takes long-term proton-pump inhibitor therapy.

In addition to optimizing calcium and vitamin D, which of the following is the best therapeutic intervention?

A. Denosumab
B. Ibandronate
C. Teriparatide
D. Zoledronic acid
E. No intervention needed now

17 A 23-year-old man is referred for a second opinion regarding hypercalcemia. He was noted to have a serum calcium concentration of 12.5 mg/dL (3.1 mmol/L) in the emergency department after presenting with nausea and vomiting due to gastrointestinal illness. Hypercalcemia has persisted in the subsequent months after recovery with calcium concentrations ranging from 11.9 to 12.3 mg/dL (3.0 to 3.1 mmol/L). He is otherwise healthy and has no history of kidney stones or fractures. He brings the following laboratory test results to his appointment:

Serum calcium = 12.3 mg/dL (8.2-10.2 mg/dL)
(SI: 3.1 mmol/L [2.1-2.6 mmol/L])

PTH = 60 pg/mL (10-65 pg/mL) (SI: 60 ng/L
[10-65 ng/L])

25-Hydroxyvitamin D = 31 ng/mL (30-80 ng/mL
[optimal]) (SI: 77.4 nmol/L [74.9-199.7 nmol/L])

Magnesium = 2.3 mg/dL (1.5-2.3 mg/dL)
(SI: 0.95 mmol/L [0.6-0.9 mmol/L])

Phosphate = 2.3 mg/dL (2.3-4.7 mg/dL)
(SI: 0.7 mmol/L [0.7-1.5 mmol/L])

24-hour urinary calcium clearance-to-creatinine
clearance ratio = 0.006

Calcium-sensing receptor *(CASR)* gene testing,
negative for pathogenic variants

His mother is normocalcemic. His father is deceased, and the patient has no siblings or children. Neck ultrasonography and parathyroid sestamibi scan are negative for parathyroid abnormalities.

Which of the following is the best next step in this patient's management?
- A. 4D CT of the neck and mediastinum
- B. MRI of the neck and mediastinum
- C. Genetic testing for *GNA11* and *AP2S1* pathogenic variants
- D. Genetic testing for *PHEX* pathogenic variants
- E. Referral to a surgeon for 4-gland parathyroid exploration

18 A 45-year-old man has had a single episode of a calcium-containing kidney stone. His evaluation reveals normal serum calcium and PTH levels, with a 24-hour urinary calcium excretion of 335 mg/24 h (100-300 mg/24 h) (SI: 8.4 mmol/d [2.5-7.5 mmol/d]), but normal 24-hour urinary oxalate, uric acid, sodium, and citrate levels. His urine volume is 1450 mL/24 h. The kidney stone analysis reveals calcium oxalate.

Which of the following recommendations would provide the greatest reduction in his risk of future calcium oxalate stone disease?
- A. Hydrochlorothiazide
- B. Increased fluid intake
- C. Potassium citrate
- D. Reduced dietary oxalate
- E. Reduced dietary sodium

19 A 71-year-old man is referred after DXA documented a femoral neck T-score of −2.9. His only other medical issue is mild benign prostatic hypertrophy. He thinks he has a healthy sex drive and has no problems achieving or maintaining erections for intercourse. His overall strength and energy are good, and he is still working full time. His current height is 1.5 in (3.8 cm) less than his peak height.

On physical examination, his BMI is 24 kg/m². He has no kyphosis, and there is room for 2 fingers in the space between the ribs and iliac crests in the midaxillary line.

Laboratory test results:
Complete blood cell count, normal
Chemistry panel, normal

25-Hydroxyvitamin D = 35 ng/mL (30-80 ng/mL [optimal]) (SI: 87.4 nmol/L [62.4-199.7 nmol/L])
Urinary calcium excretion = 285 mg/24 h (100-300 mg/24 h) (SI: 7.1 mmol/d [2.5-7.5 mmol/d])
Serum testosterone (8 AM) = 285 ng/dL (300-900 ng/dL) (SI: 9.9 nmol/L [10.4-31.2 nmol/L])
SHBG, normal
LH = 6.0 mIU/mL (1.0-9.0 mIU/mL) (SI: 6.0 IU/L [1.0-9.0 IU/L])
Prolactin = 6 ng/mL (4-23 ng/mL) (SI: 0.26 nmol/L [0.17-1.00 nmol/L])
PSA = 6.5 ng/mL (<7.0 ng/mL) (SI: 6.5 μg/L [<7 μg/L])

Which of the following treatments should be recommended?
- A. Hydrochlorothiazide
- B. Risedronate
- C. Teriparatide
- D. Testosterone gel
- E. Testosterone gel plus finasteride

20 A 32-year-old woman with a 5-year history of postsurgical hypoparathyroidism is evaluated in the emergency department. She presented with perioral numbness and tingling and muscle spasms. She has been nonadherent to her regimen of oral calcium and calcitriol. Her weight is 154 lb (70 kg).

Laboratory test results:
Calcium = 6.5 mg/dL (8.2-10.2 mg/dL) (SI: 1.6 mmol/L [2.1-2.6 mmol/L])
Albumin = 3.8 mg/dL (3.5-5.0 g/dL) (SI: 38 g/L [35-50 g/L])
Phosphate = 5.3 mg/dL (2.3-4.7 mg/dL) (SI: 1.7 mmol/L [0.7-1.5 mmol/L])
Magnesium = 1.9 mg/dL (1.5-2.3 mg/dL) (SI: 0.78 mmol/L [0.6-0.9 mmol/L])
Creatinine = 0.9 mg/dL (0.6-1.1 mg/dL) (SI: 79.6 μmol/L [53.0-97.2 μmol/L])

In addition to restarting treatment with oral calcium and calcitriol, which additional treatment regimen would be best? (see table on the following page)

Answer	Initial therapy	Subsequent therapy
A.	Intravenous bolus of 100 mg calcium chloride	Continuous calcium chloride infusion of 0.5 mg/kg per h
B.	Intravenous bolus of 1 g calcium chloride	Continuous calcium chloride infusion of 2 mg/kg per h
C.	Intravenous bolus of 150 mg calcium gluconate	Continuous calcium gluconate infusion of 1 mg/kg per h
D.	Intravenous bolus of 150 mg calcium gluconate	Continuous calcium gluconate infusion of 1 mg/kg per h + teriparatide 20 mcg subcutaneously daily
E.	Intravenous bolus of 500 mg calcium gluconate	Continuous calcium gluconate infusion to achieve a total dose of 2000 mg calcium over 24 hours

21 A 56-year-old man is referred for evaluation of muscle and bone pain, fatigue, weakness, spontaneous fractures, and difficulty walking. Symptoms began 2 years ago. Physical examination reveals diffuse bony tenderness, proximal muscle weakness, and ataxic gait. DXA documents T-scores of –3 to –4 at all sites.

Laboratory test results:
  Chemistry panel, normal
  Serum 25-hydroxyvitamin D = 28 ng/mL
    (30-80 ng/mL [optimal])
    (SI: 69.9 nmol/L [62.4-199.7 nmol/L])
  Serum 1,25-dihydroxyvitamin D = 12 pg/mL
    (16-65 pg/mL) (SI: 31.2 pmol/L
    [41.6-169.0 pmol/L])
  PTH = 98 pg/mL (10-65 pg/mL)
    (SI: 98 ng/L [10-65 ng/L])
  Serum phosphate = measurements ranging from 1.1
    to 1.3 mg/dL (2.3 to 4.7 mg/dL) (SI: 0.36 to
    0.42 mmol/L [0.74 to 1.52 mmol/L])
  Maximum tubular phosphate reabsorption
    (phosphorus tubule maximum/glomerular
    filtration rate), low

Which of the following is the key diagnostic test to order next?
  A. 24,25-Dihydroxyvitamin D measurement
  B. 24-Hour urine collection for calcium,
     electrolytes, amino acids, glucose, and creatinine
  C. FGF-23 measurement
  D. *PHEX* gene testing
  E. Sestamibi scan

22 A 36-year-old woman undergoes total thyroidectomy for papillary thyroid carcinoma and subsequently has permanent surgical hypoparathyroidism. She takes elemental calcium, 1200 mg 3 times daily with meals; calcitriol, 0.5 mcg twice daily; and levothyroxine, 150 mcg daily. She feels well.

On physical examination, she has a well-healed thyroidectomy scar and negative Chvostek and Trousseau signs.

Laboratory test results 6 months after surgery:
  Serum calcium = 10.0 mg/dL (8.2-10.2 mg/dL)
    (SI: 2.5 mmol/L [2.1-2.6 mmol/L])
  Albumin = 4.0 g/dL (3.5-5.0 g/dL)
    (SI: 40 g/L [35-50 g/L])
  Phosphate = 4.9 mg/dL (2.3-4.7 mg/dL)
    (SI: 1.6 mmol/L [0.7-1.5 mmol/L])
  Urinary calcium = 380 mg/24 h (100-300 mg/24 h)
    (SI: 9.5 mmol/d [2.5-7.5 mmol/d])

Which of the following should be recommended now?
  A. Add hydrochlorothiazide
  B. Add recombinant human PTH (1-84)
  C. Add sevelamer (oral phosphate binder)
  D. Continue current regimen
  E. Decrease calcium supplementation

23 A 59-year-old postmenopausal woman with stage 1 breast cancer and no evidence of metastatic disease has completed surgery and radiation therapy to the breast. She has no history of fractures. Her oncologist would now like to treat her with anastrozole (an aromatase inhibitor) for at least 5 years. The oncologist orders DXA, which demonstrates T-scores of –2.2 at the lumbar spine, –1.7 at the femoral neck, and −1.5 at the total hip. Vertebral fracture assessment is negative for fracture. The FRAX results do not meet treatment thresholds for either major osteoporotic fractures or hip fractures. The oncologist refers the patient for advice regarding bone health.

In addition to optimizing calcium and vitamin D, which of the following interventions should be recommended?

A. Calcitonin
B. Raloxifene
C. Teriparatide
D. Zoledronic acid
E. No pharmacologic intervention needed

24 A 69-year-old woman presents for follow-up of osteoporosis. Evaluation for secondary causes of bone loss at her initial visit last year was unremarkable, including a normal serum calcium and concurrent PTH concentration. She has had 2 injections of denosumab, 60 mg subcutaneously 6 months apart, with the last injection 1 month before her current visit. She is taking calcium, 500 mg twice daily, and vitamin D, 2000 IU daily. She has no other medical problems and takes no other medications.

Laboratory test results:

Calcium = 9.4 mg/dL (8.2-10.2 mg/dL) (SI: 2.4 mmol/L [2.1-2.6 mmol/L])
PTH = 121 pg/mL (10-65 pg/mL) (SI: 121 ng/L [10-65 ng/L])
25-Hydroxyvitamin D = 44 ng/mL (30-80 ng/mL [optimal]) (SI: 109.8 nmol/L [74.9-199.7 nmol/L])
Serum urea nitrogen = 13 mg/dL (8-23 mg/dL) (SI: 4.6 mmol/L [2.9-8.2 mmol/L])
Creatinine = 0.5 mg/dL (0.6-1.1 mg/dL) (SI: 44.2 µmol/L [53.0-97.2 µmol/L])
Estimated glomerular filtration rate = 94 mL/min per 1.73 m^2 (>60 mL/min per 1.73 m^2)

Which of the following is the best next step?

A. Increase vitamin D supplementation to 4000 IU daily
B. Measure PTH again in 5 months (before her next denosumab injection)
C. Order a parathyroid sestamibi scan
D. Refer to a parathyroid surgeon
E. Stop denosumab therapy

25 A 20-year-old woman is referred from orthopedics after a recent tibial stress fracture. Her fracture has successfully healed, and she has resumed regular activities. She runs 25 miles per week, with no increase in physical activity before her fracture. She follows a healthy diet rich in protein and fiber, although she avoids fats. She has amenorrhea.

Physical examination findings are notable for a BMI of 19.1 kg/m^2 and are otherwise normal, including findings on pelvic examination. Bone density is significant for Z-scores of −2.6 at the lumbar spine, −1.6 at the femoral neck, and −1.5 at the total hip. Laboratory evaluation is notable for low levels of estradiol and FSH but is otherwise negative for secondary causes of amenorrhea and bone loss.

Which of the following is the best treatment for this patient's bone health?

A. Alendronate, 70 mg weekly
B. Combined oral contraceptive pill
C. Denosumab, 60 mg subcutaneously every 6 months
D. Teriparatide, 20 mcg daily
E. Working with a dietician to resolve energy deficiency

26 A 55-year-old woman with end-stage kidney disease due to hypertension has been receiving hemodialysis for 10 years. She is referred for evaluation because of multiple vertebral fractures and a femoral neck T-score of −3.8 on DXLong-term medications include calcitriol, 0.5 mcg twice daily, and cinacalcet, 60 mg twice daily.

Laboratory test results:

Serum calcium = 8.1 mg/dL (8.2-10.2 mg/dL)
(SI: 2.0 mmol/L [2.1-2.6 mmol/L])

Phosphate = 5.2 mg/dL (2.3-4.7 mg/dL)
(SI: 1.7 mmol/L [0.7-1.5 mmol/L])

25-Hydroxyvitamin D = 24 ng/mL (25-80 ng/mL
[optimal]) (SI: 59.9 nmol/L [62.4-199.7 nmol/L])

PTH = 78 pg/mL (10-65 pg/mL)
(SI: 78 ng/L [10-65 ng/L])

Total alkaline phosphatase = 48 U/L (50-120 U/L)
(SI: 0.80 μkat/L [0.84-2.00 μkat/L])

An iliac crest biopsy is done after double-tetracycline labeling.

While awaiting bone biopsy results, which of the following changes in management should be made immediately?

A. Begin denosumab
B. Begin teriparatide
C. Decrease the calcitriol dosage
D. Decrease the cinacalcet dosage
E. Increase the calcitriol dosage

27 A 50-year-old man with a history of postoperative hypoparathyroidism following total thyroidectomy for benign goiter presents to the emergency department for perioral numbness and tingling. His treatment regimen for hypoparathyroidism has remained stable over many years and includes calcium carbonate, 600 mg 3 times daily; calcitriol, 0.5 mcg twice daily; and vitamin D, 1000 IU daily. He states that he has had good treatment adherence. His medical history is otherwise remarkable only for gastroesophageal reflux disease, and 3 days ago his treatment was changed from ranitidine to omeprazole, 20 mg twice daily.

Laboratory test results:

Serum calcium = 6.8 mg/dL (8.2-10.2 mg/dL)
(SI: 1.7 mmol/L [2.1-2.6 mmol/L])

Albumin = 3.8 mg/dL (3.5-5.0 g/dL)
(SI: 38 g/L [35-50 g/L])

Intact PTH = <3 pg/mL (10-65 pg/mL)
(SI: <3 ng/L [10-65 ng/L])

25-Hydroxyvitamin D = 32 ng/mL (30-80 ng/mL
[optimal]) (SI: 79.9 nmol/L [62.4-199.7 nmol/L])

Phosphate = 5.3 mg/dL (2.3-4.7 mg/dL)
(SI: 1.7 mmol/L [0.7-1.5 mmol/L])

Magnesium = 1.5 mEq/L (1.5-2.2 mEq/L)
(SI: 0.6 mmol/L [0.6-0.9 mmol/L])

In addition to intravenous calcium gluconate infusion and calcitriol, 0.5 mg twice daily, which of the following therapies should this patient receive?

A. Calcium carbonate, 600 mg 4 times daily
B. Calcium carbonate, 600 mg 4 times daily, and hydrochlorothiazide, 25 mg daily
C. Calcium citrate, 600 mg 4 times daily
D. Teriparatide, 20 mcg subcutaneously daily, and calcium carbonate, 600 mg 4 times daily
E. Teriparatide, 20 mcg subcutaneously daily, and calcium citrate, 600 mg 4 times daily

28 A 61-year-old man is referred for evaluation of possible Paget disease. He was found to have elevated alkaline phosphatase on recent laboratory studies done before cataract surgery. He had bariatric surgery 15 years ago and takes cholecalciferol, 2000 IU daily. He has no chronic medical problems and has not been to a physician in the past 5 years. He feels generally well.

Laboratory test results:

Alkaline phosphatase = 220 U/L (50-120 U/L)
(SI: 3.7 μkat/L [0.8-2.0 μkat/L])

Serum calcium = 8.6 mg/dL (8.2-10.2 mg/dL)
(SI: 2.2 mmol/L [2.1-2.6 mmol/L])

Serum creatinine = 1.3 mg/dL (0.7-1.3 mg/dL)
(SI: 114.9 μmol/L [61.9-114.9 μmol/L])

γ-Glutamyltranspeptidase, normal

Which of the following is the best next step in this patient's evaluation?

A. 1,25-Dihydroxyvitamin D measurement
B. 25-Hydroxyvitamin D measurement
C. Serum C-telopeptide measurement
D. Skeletal survey
E. Whole-body bone scan

29 A 57-year-old woman seeks advice regarding osteoporosis and fractures. She entered menopause 5 years ago and has not taken hormone therapy. During childhood, she sustained several long-bone fractures that were attributed to her active lifestyle and participation in sports. Her last childhood fracture was at age 15 years. Since menopause, however, she has sustained fractures at the wrist, humerus, and femur in low-trauma falls. Recent DXA reveals T-scores of −3.0 at the spine, −2.8 at the femoral neck, and −2.7 at the total hip. Her mother was diagnosed with osteoporosis at age 65 years.

On physical examination, she is a well-appearing woman with no dysmorphic features. Her height is 65 in (165.1 cm). Sclerae appear slightly greyish. She has no joint deformities or laxity. Her dentition appears normal. She wears bilateral hearing aids.

Laboratory test results are normal for complete blood cell count, electrolytes, calcium, creatinine, liver function, alkaline phosphatase, TSH, 25-hydroxyvitamin D, 1,25-dihydroxyvitamin D, and intact PTH.

Sequencing which of the following genes will most likely establish this patient's diagnosis?

A. LDL receptor-related protein 5 (*LRP5*)
B. Osteoprotegerin gene (*TNFRSF11B*)
C. Sclerostin gene (*SOST*)
D. Type 1 collagen α 1 and 2 genes (*COL1A1/COL1A2*)
E. Vitamin D receptor gene (*VDR*)

30 A 78-year-old woman is referred for evaluation of hypercalcemia incidentally noted on routine laboratory testing. She feels well and has no concerns. She was treated for tuberculosis 40 years ago, and a basal cell skin cancer was excised 20 years ago. There is no personal or family history of hypercalcemia. Physical examination findings are unremarkable.

Laboratory test results:

Serum calcium = 11.1 mg/dL (8.2-10.2 mg/dL) (SI: 2.8 mmol/L [2.1-2.6 mmol/L])

PTH = 40 pg/mL (10-65 pg/mL) (SI: 40 ng/L [10-65 ng/L])

25-Hydroxyvitamin D = 18 ng/mL (30-80 ng/mL [optimal]) (SI: 44.9 nmol/L [74.9-199.7 nmol/L])

1,25-Dihydroxyvitamin D = 75 pg/mL (16-65 pg/mL) (SI: 195 pmol/L [41.6-169.0 pmol/L])

Creatinine = 1.2 mg/dL (0.6-1.1 mg/dL) (SI: 106.1 μmol/L [53.0-97.2 μmol/L])

Urinary calcium = 90 mg/24 h (100-300 mg/24 h) (SI: 2.3 mmol/d [2.5-7.5 mmol/d])

24-Hour urine calcium clearance-to-creatinine clearance ratio = 0.011

Which of the following is the most likely diagnosis for this patient's hypercalcemia?

A. Calcitriol toxicity
B. Familial hypocalciuric hypercalcemia
C. Granulomatous disease
D. Hypercalcemia of malignancy
E. Primary hyperparathyroidism

Diabetes Mellitus, Section 1 Board Review

Vivian A. Fonseca, MD

1 A 54-year-old man who has acromegaly and impaired glucose tolerance has an elevated IGF-1 concentration despite having had pituitary surgery. He is unable to tolerate the gastrointestinal adverse effects of long-acting octreotide, and his fasting blood glucose concentration has increased from 105 mg/dL (5.83 mmol/L) to 116 mg/dL (6.44 mmol/L). Octreotide is changed to pegvisomant.

Which of the following is the expected outcome in this patient after he has taken pegvisomant for 3 months?

- A. Decrease in insulin secretion
- B. Improvement in glucose tolerance
- C. Onset of type 2 diabetes mellitus
- D. Reduction in GH concentration
- E. Worsening insulin resistance

2 A 43-year-old man with a strong family history of diabetes mellitus and heart disease is concerned that he is at risk of developing these conditions and would like to explore screening options. He has mild fatigue, does not exercise, and has a poor diet.

On physical examination, his BMI is 33.2 kg/m². There are no other relevant findings.

Laboratory testing documents a fasting glucose concentration of 109 mg/dL (6.0 mmol/L).

Apart from fasting glucose, which of the following laboratory measurements is the best predictor of this patient's risk for developing type 2 diabetes mellitus?

- A. Glutamic acid decarboxylase antibodies
- B. LDL cholesterol
- C. Liver enzymes
- D. Microalbuminuria
- E. Testosterone

3 A 54-year-old woman who is overweight is evaluated for diabetes after a recent routine laboratory evaluation revealed a fasting plasma glucose concentration of 114 mg/dL (6.3 mmol/L) and a hemoglobin A_{1c} value of 6.7% (50 mmol/mol). The patient feels well, and her only medication is lisinopril. Her mother has type 2 diabetes mellitus.

On physical examination, her height is 63.5 in (161.3 cm) and weight is 160 lb (73 kg) (BMI = 27 kg/m²). Her blood pressure is 135/82 mm Hg, and pulse rate is 80 beats/min.

Laboratory test results:
Hemoglobin = 11.3 g/dL (13.8-17.2 g/dL) (SI: 113 g/L [138-172 g/L])
Hematocrit = 35% (41%-51%) (SI: 0.35 [0.41-0.51])

Which of the following is the most appropriate recommendation for determining whether this patient has diabetes?

- A. No additional testing is needed; she has diabetes based on her hemoglobin A_{1c} value
- B. Perform hemoglobin electrophoresis
- C. Perform oral glucose tolerance testing
- D. Repeat hemoglobin A_{1c} measurement
- E. Repeat plasma glucose measurement

4 A 36-year-old woman who recently started using continuous glucose monitoring reports a discrepancy between her sensor readings and results from her blood glucose meter. Because of the discrepancy, her monitor alarm does not signal when her blood glucose falls into the hypoglycemic range. Type 1 diabetes mellitus was diagnosed at age 8 years, and she was treated with insulin injection therapy until age 30 years when she started using an insulin pump. She began continuous glucose monitoring in an effort to reduce her hemoglobin A_{1c} to target. Her most recent hemoglobin A_{1c} measurement is 7.5% (58 mmol/mol). She changes the sensor according to the recommended schedule. A review of her sensor tracings reveals that her sensor readings lag behind her fingerstick readings by 20 to 30 minutes when her blood glucose concentrations decrease.

Which of the following should improve the ability of the continuous glucose monitor to alert the patient to episodes of hypoglycemia?
   A. Change the sensor more frequently
   B. Change the site of the sensor application
   C. Increase the calibration frequency for the sensor
   D. Lower the low-alarm threshold level
   E. Raise the low-alarm threshold level

5 A 35-year-old woman who has had type 1 diabetes mellitus since childhood is evaluated because of severe weakness and recurrent falls. During the past 10 years, she has had diabetes-related complications including retinopathy, neuropathy, and nephropathy. She uses an insulin pump and takes lisinopril, 20 mg daily. She reports dizziness when standing, and on multiple occasions she has fallen while trying to stand, resulting in several fractures.

On physical examination, the patient appears thin and uses a wheelchair. Her blood pressure is 90/60 mm Hg sitting and 70/40 mm Hg standing. Laser scars are noted on the retinas. Sensation in the feet is diminished, and ankle reflexes are absent.

Laboratory test results:
   Serum creatinine = 1.6 mg/dL (0.6-1.1 mg/dL)
      (SI: 141.4 µmol/L [53.0-97.2 µmol/L])
   Proteinuria, 4+
   Cortisol (8 AM) = 12.5 µg/dL (5-25 µg/dL)
      (SI: 344.9 nmol/L [137.9-689.7 nmol/L])

Which of the following is the best recommendation?
   A. Add midodrine hydrochloride
   B. Add phentermine
   C. Decrease sodium intake to prevent worsening nephropathy
   D. Stop lisinopril

6 An 18-year-old woman is referred for management of type 1 diabetes mellitus. She lives in a rural community with limited health care access. Her family does not have much faith in the medical system and rarely seeks care at the community health center. Type 1 diabetes was diagnosed at age 3 months. Her treatment regimen is insulin 70/30, 20 units twice daily. She refuses to take more injections and rarely monitors blood glucose. She has had 5 episodes of severe hypoglycemia in the last year. She has no siblings. Neither of her parents has diabetes or thyroid disease. She has a first cousin with type 1 diabetes. In her medical record, 2 hospital admissions for hypoglycemia with seizures are documented, but there have been no admissions for ketoacidosis.

On physical examination, she has moderate lipohypertrophy at injection sites but no evidence of diabetes-related complications.

Laboratory test results:
   Hemoglobin A_{1c} = 8.5% (4.0%-5.6%) (69 mmol/mol [20-38 mmol/mol])
   Glucose = 256 mg/dL (70-99 mg/dL)
      (SI: 14.2 mmol/L [3.9-5.5 mmol/L])
   C-peptide, negative
   Glutamic acid decarboxylase antibodies, negative

Which of the following genes is most likely to harbor a pathogenic variant?
   A. *GCK*
   B. *HNF1A*
   C. *HNF4A*
   D. *KCNJ11*
   E. *SLC2A2* (formerly *GLUT2*)

7 A 34-year-old woman who has had type 1 diabetes mellitus for 15 years seeks an opinion after her primary care physician suggested that she begin taking an ACE inhibitor and an SGLT-2 inhibitor to prevent nephropathy. The patient has had reasonable glycemic control on a multiple-daily injection regimen; her hemoglobin A_{1c} values have ranged from 6.5% to 7.5% (48 to 58 mmol/mol).

On physical examination, her blood pressure is 128/74 mm Hg.

Laboratory test results:

Hemoglobin A$_{1c}$ = 6.8% (4.0%-5.6%) (mmol/mol [20-38 mmol/mol])

Serum creatinine = 0.8 mg/dL (0.6-1.1 mg/dL) (SI: 70.7 μmol/L [53.0-97.2 μmol/L])

Urine albumin-to-creatinine ratio = 5 mg/g creat (<30 mg/g creat)

Estimated glomerular filtration rate = 85 mL/min per 1.73 m^2 (>60 mL/min per 1.73 m^2)

In addition to maintaining good glycemic control, which of the following is the best next step for this patient?

A. Begin an ACE inhibitor
B. Begin an angiotensin-receptor blocker
C. Begin an SGLT-2 inhibitor
D. Recommend no additional therapy

8 A 57-year-old man who has had type 1 diabetes mellitus since age 10 years is evaluated for a swollen right foot. He is unable to wear shoes, but his foot is otherwise pain free. He has had tingling and numbness in his feet for the past 10 to 12 years.

On physical examination, significant swelling on the right side of the foot is noted. The foot is hot, and the swelling extends beyond the ankle joint. There is callus formation on both feet but no ulceration. Pedal pulses are strong. He has marked sensory loss on both feet, and all reflexes are absent.

Results of blood tests reveal a normal serum uric acid level and a hemoglobin A$_{1c}$ value of 7.2% (55 mmol/mol). Radiography of the foot shows disorganization of the ankle joint and tarsal bones.

Which of the following tests is the most appropriate next step to determine whether this patient has osteomyelitis?

A. Biopsy
B. Bone scan
C. CT
D. MRI

9 A 46-year-old man with a 10-year history of type 1 diabetes mellitus and a BMI of 33 kg/m^2 asks about possible adjunctive treatments that will improve his blood glucose control and not increase his weight. He has had reasonable glycemic control, and his most recent hemoglobin A$_{1c}$ measurement is 7.4% (57 mmol/mol). His estimated glomerular filtration rate is 76 mL/min per m^2, and urinary albumin is undetectable. He has no diabetes-related complications.

Which of the following therapies are approved by the US FDA to add to this patient's insulin regimen?

A. Empagliflozin
B. Metformin
C. Miglitol
D. Pramlintide
E. Semaglutide

10 A 67-year-old woman presents with questions about new treatments for type 2 diabetes mellitus. Since her diagnosis 6 years ago, she has been treated with a sulfonylurea because of intolerance to metformin. She is now taking glipizide, 10 mg twice daily, and she documents blood glucose values that are generally less than 150 mg/dL (<8.3 mmol/L) with home glucose monitoring. However, since starting therapy, she has gained 15 lb (6.8 kg) and is frustrated with her inability to lose weight. Findings on hepatic ultrasonography performed last year were consistent with steatosis. She recently saw an ad in a magazine touting empagliflozin and is very interested in a "diabetes pill that causes weight loss." She takes hydrochlorothiazide and lisinopril for hypertension and atorvastatin for elevated cholesterol. She has no history of diabetes-related complications.

On physical examination, her weight is 208 lb (94.5 kg) (BMI = 35 kg/m^2), and blood pressure is 136/84 mm Hg. She has no signs of neuropathy.

Laboratory test results (sample drawn while fasting):

Glucose = 166 mg/dL (70-99 mg/dL) (SI: 9.2 mmol/L [3.9-5.5 mmol/L])

Hemoglobin A$_{1c}$ = 8.4% (4.0%-5.6%) (68 mmol/mol [20-38 mmol/mol])

Triglycerides = 217 mg/dL (<150 mg/dL [optimal]) (SI: 2.45 mmol/L [<1.70 mmol/L])

LDL cholesterol = 92 mg/dL (<100 mg/dL [for primary prevention]) (SI: 2.38 mmol/L [<2.59 mmol/L])

Creatinine = 1.9 mg/dL (0.6-1.1 mg/dL) (SI: 168.0 μmol/L [53.0-97.2 μmol/L])

Estimated glomerular filtration rate = 38 mL/min per m² (>60 mL/min per 1.73 m²)

AST = 47 U/L (20-48 U/L) (SI: 0.78 μkat/L [0.33-0.80 μkat/L])

ALT = 41 U/L (10-40 U/L) (SI: 0.68 μkat/L [0.17-0.67 μkat/L])

Albumin = 3.9 (3.5-5.0 g/dL) (SI: 39 g/L [35-50 g/L])

Calcium = 8.9 mg/dL (8.2-10.2 mg/dL) (SI: 2.2 mmol/L [2.1-2.6 mmol/L])

Phosphate = 3.7 mg/dL (2.3-4.7 mg/dL) (SI: 1.2 mmol/L [0.7-1.5 mmol/L])

TSH = 2.3 mIU/L (0.5-5.0 mIU/L)

Urinary albumin-to-creatinine ratio = 110 mg/g creat (<30 mg/g creat)

The patient is eager to start an SGLT-2 inhibitor.

In this patient, empagliflozin's main limitation would be that it would:

A. Cause only transient weight loss with weight regain in 1 to 2 months

B. Exacerbate hepatic steatosis

C. Improve proteinuria but worsen estimated glomerular filtration in the long term

D. Interfere with the effectiveness of her antihypertensive regimen

E. Not sufficiently decrease blood glucose levels

11 A 26-year-old woman with a 13-year history of type 1 diabetes mellitus and β-thalassemia requests help with her diabetes management. Despite being on a basal-bolus regimen with insulins glargine and aspart for 5 years and checking her blood glucose 5 to 7 times daily with appropriate insulin adjustments, she has been unable to reduce her hemoglobin A_{1c} level below 8.0% (<64 mmol/mol). This is mainly because she has had frequent mild hypoglycemia with any increases in her insulin dosage, mostly during daylight hours. Her weight is 122 lb (55.5 kg), and her current hemoglobin A_{1c} value is 8.2% (66 mmol/mol). Her serum creatinine concentration and urinary albumin-to-creatinine ratio are normal. The accuracy of her meter readings is confirmed by comparing with a laboratory glucose measurement. Her insurance has denied coverage for continuous glucose monitoring without an unaffordable high copay. Review of her glucose meter for the last 30 days shows 181 values, which are averaged in the Table.

Which of the following is the best next management option?

A. Add a twice-daily GLP-1 receptor agonist before breakfast and her evening meal

B. Increase the insulin glargine dosage by 2 units every 3 days to maintain fasting blood glucose concentrations between 80 and 130 mg/dL (4.4 and 7.2 mmol/L)

C. Initiate insulin pump therapy

D. Refer her to a dietitian to adjust the insulin-to-carbohydrate ratio

E. Use professional diagnostic continuous glucose monitoring to guide treatment

12 A 53-year-old woman with a 13-year history of type 2 diabetes has known chronic kidney disease. Her kidney function has been deteriorating, and at the last clinic visit, metformin was discontinued. Her glucose concentrations have increased despite adding glimepiride and continuing canagliflozin. She has an estimated glomerular filtration rate of 25 mL/min per 1.73 m².

	Morning	Lunch	Dinner	Bedtime	Overnight	Overall
Mean glucose	136 mg/dL (±20) (7.6 mmol/L [±1.1])	142 mg/dL (±34) (7.9 mmol/L [±1.9])	133 mg/dL (±27) (7.4 mmol/L [±1.5])	132 mg/dL (±31) (7.3 mmol/L [±2.3])	96 mg/dL (±19) (5.3 mmol/L [±1.1])	128 mg/dL (±21) (7.1 mmol/L [±1.2])

Values are presented with standard deviation in parentheses.

Which of the following medications/class of medications used to treat type 2 diabetes mellitus would be contraindicated in this setting?

    A. Detemir insulin

    B. Exenatide

    C. Pioglitazone

    D. SGLT-2 inhibitors

    E. Sulfonylureas

13

A 49-year-old man with stage 3 chronic kidney disease related to polycystic kidney disease has a 2-year history of type 2 diabetes mellitus treated with glipizide and liraglutide. He recently underwent segmental left colonic resection for complications of diverticulitis. On postoperative days 1 and 2, his blood glucose concentration climbed into the range of 250 to 300 mg/dL (13.9-16.7 mmol/L) for which he was given regular insulin. He remains on nothing-by-mouth status in the surgical ward.

On physical examination, his temperature is 99.5°F (37.5°C), blood pressure is 142/86 mm Hg, and pulse rate is 104 beats/min. His abdomen is distended with decreased bowel sounds. His current blood glucose concentration is 135 mg/dL (7.5 mmol/L).

Which of the following options is the best glycemic management regimen for this patient now?

    A. Aspart premixed insulin twice daily beginning at a blood glucose value >180 mg/dL (>10.0 mmol/L)

    B. Basal insulin daily plus rapid-acting insulin analogue (eg, insulin aspart) every 6 hours when his blood glucose is >180 mg/dL (>10.0 mmol/L) to achieve most blood glucose values between 140 and 180 mg/dL (7.8-10.0 mmol/L)

    C. Intravenous insulin infusion titrated to achieve blood glucose values between 80 and 110 mg/dL (4.4-6.1 mmol/L)

    D. Regular insulin sliding scale beginning at a blood glucose value >150 mg/dL (>8.3 mmol/L)

    E. Reinitiation of liraglutide; hold glipizide until eating

14

A 68-year-old man with type 2 diabetes mellitus describes tingling in his hands and legs over the last 6 months. These sensations are different from his longstanding foot numbness. He also feels unsteady when he gets up at night to void. He eats a well-balanced diet. He has taken metformin since diabetes was diagnosed 11 years ago. He also takes glipizide twice daily and NPH insulin at night.

On physical examination, his blood pressure is 126/74 mm Hg and BMI is 28 kg/m². Cranial nerves II through XII are intact, muscle bulk and strength are normal, and coordination in the upper and lower extremities is normal. He has reduced sharp sensation to the knee, decreased vibratory sense in the great toes, and loss of patellar and Achilles reflexes.

Laboratory test results:

    Hemoglobin A$_{1c}$ = 7.3% (4.0%-5.6%) (56 mmol/mol [20-38 mmol/mol])

    Hematocrit = 40% (41%-51%) (SI: 0.40 [0.41-0.51])

    Hemoglobin = 12.3 g/dL (3.8-17.2 g/dL) (SI: 123 g/L [138-172 g/L])

    Creatinine = 1.5 mg/dL (0.7-1.3 mg/dL) (SI: 132.6 μmol/L [61.9-114.9 μmol/L])

    AST = 55 U/L (20-48 U/L) (SI: 1.20 μkat/L [0.33-0.80 μkat/L])

    ALT = 72 U/L (10-40 U/L) (SI: 1.20 μkat/L [0.17-0.67 μkat/L])

Which of the following is the best next step in this patient's management?

    A. Measure γ-glutamyltransferase

    B. Measure serum vitamin B$_6$

    C. Measure serum vitamin B$_{12}$

    D. Perform MRI of the spine

    E. Refer for electromyography and nerve conduction studies

15 A 65-year-old man presents for a follow-up visit after kidney transplant 2 months ago. He is currently feeling well and is adherent to his posttransplant immunosuppressant regimen, including glucocorticoids. He reports both polyuria and polydipsia. He has obesity (BMI = 31.8 kg/m^2) with mild edema over his ankles. He has a family history of type 2 diabetes mellitus, but he has not been previously diagnosed with type 2 diabetes.

Laboratory test results:
Fasting plasma glucose = 145 mg/dL (70-99 mg/dL) (SI: 8.0 mmol/L [3.9-5.5 mmol/L])
Hemoglobin A$_{1c}$ = 8.2% (4.0%-5.6%) (66 mmol/mol [20-38 mmol/mol])

In addition to lifestyle therapy, which of the following options is the most appropriate next step in the management of this patient's condition?
A. Add sulfonylurea therapy
B. Add thiazolidinedione therapy
C. Increase the dosage of glucocorticoids to prevent rejection of kidney transplant
D. Initiate insulin therapy and maintain hemoglobin A$_{1c}$ levels below 8.0% (<64 mmol/mol)

16 A 65-year-old man is referred by his primary care physician for a 12-year history of suboptimally controlled type 2 diabetes mellitus. Diet, exercise, and 3 agents (metformin, glimepiride, and canagliflozin) have been unsuccessful. One year ago, oral agents were discontinued and he was prescribed intensive insulin therapy with multiple daily injections. Currently, he is on a regimen of 80 units of insulin glargine twice daily and 120 units daily of insulin lispro with meals. However, his hemoglobin A$_{1c}$ levels have ranged from 9.4% to 10.7% (79-93 mmol/mol).

On physical examination, his BMI is 46 kg/m^2 and blood pressure is 130/79 mm Hg.

Laboratory test results:
Hemoglobin A$_{1c}$ = 9.8% (4.0%-5.6%) (84 mmol/mol [20-38 mmol/mol])

Estimated glomerular filtration rate = 68 mL/min per 1.73 m^2 (>60 mL/min per 1.73 m^2)

Which of the following is the best next step to improve this patient's glycemic control?
A. Add linagliptin to current insulin therapy
B. Continue insulin glargine and change insulin lispro to regular U500 insulin 3 times daily
C. Convert multiple daily injections to insulin pump therapy with insulin lispro
D. Discontinue insulins glargine and lispro and switch to regular U500 insulin 3 times daily
E. Switch insulin glargine to insulin degludec, 110 units in the morning and evening

17 A 52-year-old woman with type 2 diabetes mellitus treated at home with metformin and a GLP-1 receptor agonist is currently on postoperative day 1 after a surgical procedure. Before surgery, her blood glucose values ranged from 150 to 180 mg/dL (8.3-10.0 mmol/L) and now they range from 170 to 250 mg/dL (9.4-13.9 mmol/L).

On physical examination, her vital signs are unremarkable. She is nauseated and has been unable to eat meals. She remains on nothing-by-mouth status in the surgical ward.

Which of the following is the best diabetes management regimen for this patient?
A. Continuous intravenous insulin infusion
B. Once-daily basal insulin, plus correction insulin dose regimen every 4 to 6 hours
C. Once-daily basal insulin, plus correction insulin dose regimen every 8 to 10 hours
D. Restarting home medications without insulin
E. Sliding-scale insulin regimen administered every 4 to 6 hours

18 A 46-year-old Hispanic man presents for follow-up after he was admitted to an outside hospital 3 months ago with hyperglycemia. His hemoglobin A$_{1c}$ level was 12.0% (108 mmol/mol). He was also told he had marked metabolic acidosis and ketonemia on admission, which is confirmed when hospital records are reviewed. He was treated with intravenous insulin and discharged 3 days later on a regimen of insulin glargine, 10 units once daily at bedtime. He has not been monitoring his blood glucose values at home, but he reports feeling that his blood glucose is "low" in the morning. His medical history is otherwise unremarkable, and his family history is notable only for type 2 diabetes diagnosed in his father at age 65 years.

On physical examination, his blood pressure is 122/73 mm Hg and BMI is 29 kg/m². The rest of his examination findings are unremarkable.

Which of the following measurements would most accurately establish the diagnosis and guide this patient's long-term insulin management?

Answer	C-peptide	Hemoglobin A$_{1c}$	Glutamic acid decarboxylase antibodies	Insulinoma-associated protein 2 antibodies
A.	☐	☐		
B.	☐		☐	☐
C.			☐	☐
D.		☐	☐	☐

19 A 58-year-old woman with type 2 diabetes mellitus presents for follow-up. She recently began walking to work and is eager to safely take on a more vigorous exercise regimen. Her type 2 diabetes is managed with insulin glargine. In the past year, her hemoglobin A$_{1c}$ values have ranged from 7.0% to 8.0% (53-64 mmol/mol) and she rarely has hypoglycemia. Her family history is positive for type 2 diabetes and hypertension and is negative for premature coronary heart disease.

On physical examination, her BMI is 27 kg/m² and blood pressure is 130/88 mm Hg.

Laboratory test results:
Hemoglobin A$_{1c}$ = 7.4% (4.0%-5.6%) (57 mmol/mol [20-38 mmol/mol])
LDL cholesterol = 122 mg/dL (<100 mg/dL [optimal]) (SI: 3.16 mmol/L [<2.59 mmol/L])
HDL cholesterol = 39 mg/dL (>60 mg/dL [optimal]) (SI: 1.01 mmol/L [>1.55 mmol/L])

Kidney function and findings on electrocardiography are normal.

Which of the following should be recommended regarding her exercise plans?
A. Enroll in a cardiac rehabilitation program to initiate more vigorous exercise
B. Perform an exercise tolerance test before starting more vigorous exercise
C. Perform stress echocardiography before starting more vigorous exercise
D. Progressively initiate more vigorous regular exercise

20 A 62-year-old man with a 10-year history of type 2 diabetes mellitus presents for a follow-up visit. He has a personal history of cardiovascular disease, with a myocardial infarction that occurred at age 58 years. He also has a family history of heart disease. His current medications are rosuvastatin, 20 mg daily; lisinopril, 20 mg daily; metformin, 1000 mg daily; insulin lispro, 4 units before each meal; and insulin glargine, 20 units in the morning. He quit smoking cigarettes 5 years ago after a 20 pack-year history. He has been unable to tolerate GLP-1 receptor agonists or SGLT-2 inhibitors. He had muscle cramps on atorvastatin, 80 mg daily, but is able to take his current dosage of rosuvastatin.

On physical examination, his seated blood pressure is 140/90 mm Hg and BMI is 30 kg/m².

Recent laboratory test results:
Hemoglobin A$_{1c}$ = 6.8% (4.0%-5.6%) (51 mmol/mol [20-38 mmol/mol])
Fasting plasma glucose = 94 mg/dL (70-99 mg/dL) (SI: 5.2 mmol/L [3.9-5.5 mmol/L])
Total cholesterol = 189 mg/dL (<200 mg/dL [optimal]) (SI: 4.90 mmol/L [<5.18 mmol/L])
Triglycerides = 120 mg/dL (<150 mg/dL [optimal]) (SI: 1.36 mmol/L [<1.70 mmol/L])
LDL cholesterol = 103 mg/dL (<100 mg/dL [optimal]) (SI: 2.67 mmol/L [<2.59 mmol/L])
HDL cholesterol = 40 mg/dL (>60 mg/dL [optimal]) (SI: 1.04 mmol/L [>1.55 mmol/L])

Which of the following is the best treatment to address his lipid profile?

A. Alirocumab, 75 mg every 2 weeks
B. Atorvastatin, 60 mg daily
C. Ezetimibe, 10 mg daily
D. Icosapent ethyl, 2 g twice daily
E. Pravastatin, 40 mg daily

21 A 20-year-old woman with cystic fibrosis affecting her lungs and liver would like to discuss her risk of having cystic fibrosis–related diabetes (CFRD) and how to screen for it. She has a family history of cystic fibrosis with CFRD. Her cystic fibrosis has been moderately controlled, although she has recurrent infections. Her BMI is 23 kg/m².

Which of the following is the best next step to screen her for CFRD?

A. Fasting plasma glucose measurement
B. Fructosamine measurement
C. Hemoglobin A_{1c} measurement
D. Oral glucose tolerance test
E. Random plasma glucose measurement when symptoms start

22 A 58-year-old man with no notable medical history presents to his primary care physician after unintentionally losing 10 lb (4.5 kg) over the last few months, as well as having a 2-week history of polyuria and nocturia. His family history includes diabetes mellitus in a maternal aunt and hypothyroidism and rheumatoid arthritis in his mother.

On physical examination, his blood pressure is 110/72 mm Hg, weight is 163 lb (74.1 kg), and BMI is 24 kg/m². His examination findings are unremarkable, with no localizing signs of infection.

Laboratory test results:
Random serum glucose = 254 mg/dL (70-99 mg/dL)
  (SI: 14.1 mmol/L [3.9-5.5 mmol/L])
Hemoglobin A_{1c} = 8.3% (4.0%-5.6%) (67 mmol/mol
  [20-38 mmol/mol])
Creatinine = 0.7 mg/dL (0.7-1.3 mg/dL)
  (SI: 61.9 µmol/L [61.9-114.9 µmol/L])
Complete blood cell count, normal
Electrolytes, normal

He is referred 3 months later, while he is taking metformin, 1000 mg twice daily. He has lost an additional 5 lb (2.3 kg).

Laboratory test results:
Random serum glucose = 233 mg/dL
  (SI: 12.9 mmol/L)
Hemoglobin A_{1c} = 9.1% (76 mmol/mol)
C-peptide = 1.2 ng/mL (0.9-4.3 ng/mL)
  (SI: 0.40 nmol/L [0.30-1.42 nmol/L])

Review of his twice-daily self-monitoring blood glucose log reveals most values in the range of the high 100s to low 200s (mg/dL) (5.6-11.1 mmol/L), with an average of 189 mg/dL (10.5 mmol/L).

Which of the following is the best next step to manage this patient's glycemia?

A. Add an SGLT-2 inhibitor
B. Add a once-weekly GLP-1 receptor agonist
C. Add a sulfonylurea
D. Start insulin

23 A 43-year-old woman with a 32-year history of type 1 diabetes mellitus is feeling stressed and frustrated because she is having unpredictable hypoglycemia occurring at various times of the day, often within an hour or two after eating. She reports adherence to her insulin regimen (multiple daily injections) and has had nutrition education (carbohydrate counting) in the past and again a few months ago. She has a history of diabetic peripheral neuropathy and diabetic retinopathy.

Review of systems reveals blurred vision and fluctuating weight. Her blood pressure is 121/79 mm Hg.

Results from a basic metabolic panel are unremarkable. Her glucose meter reveals glucose checks 6 to 7 times daily and highly variable glucose levels ranging from 40 mg/dL (2.2 mmol/L) to more than 300 mg/dL (>16.7 mmol/L) at various times during the day, with no appreciable pattern. Her current hemoglobin A_{1c} measurement is 8.0% (64 mmol/mol).

Which of the following is most likely to uncover the etiology of her hypoglycemia and glycemic variability?

A. Abdominal CT
B. Cosyntropin-stimulation test
C. Gastric-emptying study
D. Psychiatric evaluation
E. Review of carbohydrate counting skills

24

An 18-year-old woman is seen for erratic blood glucose values. Type 1 diabetes mellitus was diagnosed 2 years ago, and a regimen of basal and mealtime insulins was initiated. Her glycemic control has always been adequate, with hemoglobin A_{1c} values around 7.0% (53 mmol/mol). However, a few weeks ago, she started to notice unpredictable blood glucose values with recurrent hypoglycemic episodes (blood glucose 45 to 60 mg/dL [2.5-3.3 mmol/L]). These episodes have occurred mainly after meals and have been accompanied by symptoms. Despite eating more snacks to prevent hypoglycemia, she has lost 4 lb (1.8 kg) in the past 2 weeks. She has no gastrointestinal concerns or dizziness. Her menses are regular. Her current medications are insulins glargine and lispro.

On physical examination, her blood pressure is 110/70 mm Hg and BMI is 22 kg/m². Examination findings are unremarkable.

Laboratory test results:
- Hemoglobin A_{1c} = 6.7% (4.0%-5.6%) (50 mmol/mol [20-38 mmol/mol])
- Serum cortisol (random) = 11 µg/dL (5-25 µg/dL) (303.5 nmol/L [137.9-689.7 nmol/L])
- Electrolytes, normal
- Creatinine, normal

Further workup is done.

An elevation of which of the following would most likely explain her hypoglycemia?

A. ACTH
B. Free T_4
C. Glutamic acid decarboxylase 65 antibodies
D. 21-Hydroxylase antibodies
E. Tissue transglutaminase IgA antibodies

25

A 59-year-old man with newly diagnosed type 2 diabetes mellitus presents to establish care. He has no concerns. He has hyperlipidemia and hypertension. He does not smoke cigarettes. He is taking benazepril, 20 mg daily, and atorvastatin, 40 mg daily.

On physical examination, his blood pressure is 128/78 mm Hg, pulse rate is 87 beats/min, and BMI is 30.8 kg/m².

Laboratory test results:
- Hemoglobin A_{1c} = 7.8% (4.0%-5.6%) (62 mmol/mol [20-38 mmol/mol])
- Plasma glucose (fasting) = 148 mg/dL (70-99 mg/dL) (SI: 8.2 mmol/L [3.9-5.5 mmol/L])
- Serum creatinine = 1.17 mg/dL (0.7-1.3 mg/dL) (SI: 103.4 µmol/L [61.9-114.9 µmol/L])
- Total cholesterol = 136 mg/dL (<200 mg/dL [optimal]) (SI: 3.52 mmol/L [<5.18 mmol/L])
- LDL cholesterol = 72 mg/dL (<100 mg/dL [optimal]) (SI: 1.86 mmol/L [<2.59 mmol/L])
- HDL cholesterol = 40 mg/dL (>60 mg/dL) (SI: 1.04 mmol/L [>1.55 mmol/L])
- Triglycerides = 180 mg/dL (<150 mg/dL [optimal]) (SI: 2.03 mmol/L [<1.70 mmol/L])
- Urinary albumin-to-creatinine ratio = 32 mg/g creat (<30 mg/g creat)
- Basic metabolic panel, normal
- Complete blood cell count, normal

According to the online risk estimator of the American College of Cardiology and the American Heart Association (available at: www.cvriskcalculator.com), his 10-year calculated cardiovascular disease risk (heart disease or stroke) is 14.1%.

On the basis of his clinical presentation, laboratory test results, and 10-year atherosclerotic cardiovascular disease risk score, which of the following medications should be recommended for initial glycemic control?

A. Empagliflozin
B. Liraglutide
C. Metformin
D. Sitagliptin

26 A 54-year-old man who has had type 2 diabetes mellitus and hypertension for 19 years presents for his annual diabetes examination. He is troubled by erectile dysfunction that has developed over the last 2 to 3 years. He has retinopathy and has had coronary artery bypass surgery. Medications include lisinopril, atorvastatin, metformin, insulin glargine, and metoprolol.

On physical examination, his BMI is 31.3 kg/m^2. Seated, his pulse rate is 92 beats/min and blood pressure is 140/92 mm Hg. Standing for 2 minutes, his pulse rate is 92 beats/min and blood pressure is 119/72 mm Hg. He has absent sensation to a 10-g monofilament to the mid-shin.

Electrocardiography shows sinus rhythm, with a fixed R-R interval and evidence of a previous myocardial infarction.

Recent laboratory test results:
   Hemoglobin A$_{1c}$ = 8.6% (4.0%-5.6%) (70 mmol/mol [20-38 mmol/mol])
   Estimated glomerular filtration rate = 55 mL/min per 1.73 m^2 (>60 mL/min per 1.73 m^2)
   Testosterone = 220 ng/dL (300-900 ng/dL) (SI: 7.6 nmol/L [10.4-31.2 nmol/L])

Which of the following is the best initial management of this patient's erectile dysfunction?
   A. Begin intracavernosal alprostadil injections
   B. Begin sildenafil
   C. Improve glycemic control
   D. Refer to urology for penile prosthesis implantation

Diabetes Mellitus, Section 2 Board Review

Marie E. McDonnell, MD

27 A 31-year-old woman with a 9-year history of type 1 diabetes mellitus comes to clinic for routine follow-up. She is well educated on carbohydrate counting and had been doing well on multiple daily insulin injections (hemoglobin A_{1c} = 6.8% [51 mmol/mol]). She started using a new insulin pump 1 month ago and returns for reevaluation. Her hybrid closed-loop insulin pump has a preset glucose target range of 112.5 to 160 mg/dL (6.2-8.9 mmol/L).

Her device is downloaded to show data from the last month. The dashboard shows a mean glucose value of 180 mg/dL (10.0 mmol/L) with 57% time in range (70-180 mg/dL [3.9-10.0 mmol/L]). The algorithm is in use 92% of the time. On average, she receives 137 units of insulin per day; 60% is basal insulin (including automated basal), 19% is food bolus insulin, 9% is self-administered correction insulin, and 12% is automated correction insulin.

Which of the following is the most likely reason she has not achieved a lower mean glucose concentration?
- A. Her insulin sensitivity factor must be adjusted
- B. Her total daily insulin dose programmed in her pump is too high
- C. One or more insulin-to-carbohydrate ratios must be adjusted
- D. The automated insulin delivery algorithm is not in use for enough time

28 A patient with longstanding insulin-requiring type 2 diabetes mellitus is concerned that her new glucose monitoring device is not accurate. Her insurance company recently required her to switch to a different device, which has a similar fingerstick blood glucose monitor although it uses unique testing strips. She had some leftover supplies from her old meter, and she decided to compare results between the 2 meters using blood from the same fingerstick. One reading was 142 mg/dL (7.9 mmol/L), while the other reading was 168 mg/dL (9.3 mmol/L). She is concerned because she would be inclined to administer a different insulin dose depending on which meter she uses since they seem to produce inconsistent results.

Approximately 2 years ago, a certified diabetes educator documented that her glucose monitoring technique was correct.

Which of the following is the best recommendation for this patient?
- A. Calibrate the new glucose meter
- B. Compare results from the new meter with blood glucose results from the laboratory (the glucose discrepancy is outside of the US FDA acceptable range)
- C. Continue with the new meter (the glucose discrepancy is within the US FDA acceptable range)
- D. Replace the battery in the old glucose meter

29 A 32-year-old woman identified a random fingerstick blood glucose value of 176 mg/dL (9.8 mmol/L) last month when she tested herself using her daughter's glucose meter. Her 4-year-old daughter was diagnosed with type 1 diabetes mellitus 15 months ago and is on insulin pump therapy.

Several family members have autoimmune disease, and she requested that her primary care physician screen her for diabetes.

On physical examination, her BMI is 22 kg/m². She is in good health.

Laboratory test results (1 week ago):

Random blood glucose = 162 mg/dL (SI: 9.0 mmol/L)

Glutamic acid decarboxylase-65 antibodies = 2.3 nmol/L

Insulin antibodies = 14 nmol/L

C-peptide = 3.6 ng/mL (1.1-4.4 ng/mL) (SI: 1.19 nmol/L [0.17-0.66 nmol/L])

TSH = 1.2 mIU/L (0.5-5.0 mIU/L)

Hemoglobin A_{1c} = 6.4% (4.0%-5.6%) (46 mmol/mol [20-38 mmol/mol])

Which of the following interventions has been found to delay the onset of diabetes in similar patients?

A. Anti-CD3 monoclonal antibody

B. Comprehensive lifestyle modification

C. Insulin glargine

D. Liraglutide

E. Verapamil

30 A 28-year-old G2P1 woman at 18 weeks' gestation presents with severe shortness of breath 4 days after testing positive for the SARS-COV2 virus. Her oxygenation is stable on 4 L oxygen delivered by nasal cannula. Before pregnancy, she had prediabetes with a hemoglobin A_{1c} value of 6.3% (45 mmol/mol) and no other medical conditions. Her medications prior to hospitalization included a prenatal vitamin.

On physical examination, she is afebrile, blood pressure is 98/62 mm Hg, and pulse rate is 102 beats/min. She is alert and able to complete short sentences.

Laboratory tests results:

Bicarbonate = 15 mEq/L (21-28 mEq/L) (SI: 15 mmol/L [21-28 mmol/L])

Venous pH = 7.36 (7.35-7.45)

Glucose = 175 mg/dL (70-99 mg/dL) (SI: 9.7 mmol/L [3.9-5.5 mmol/L])

Potassium = 4.2 mEq/L (3.5-5.0 mEq/L) (SI: 4.2 mmol/L [3.5-5.0 mmol/L])

Anion gap = 12 mEq/L (3-11 mEq/L) (SI: 12 mmol/L [3-11 mmol/L])

Serum β-hydroxybutyrate = 4 mg/dL (<3.0 mg/dL) (SI: 384.2 μmol/L [<288.2 μmol/L])

Intravenous infusion is started with normal saline.

Which of the following is the best next step in her management?

A. Change intravenous fluids to lactated Ringer's solution

B. Observe

C. Start bicarbonate infusion

D. Start insulin infusion and potassium repletion

31 A new patient with type 1 diabetes mellitus presents 8 weeks into her first pregnancy. She is currently using a hybrid closed-loop insulin pump with continuous glucose monitoring. Prior to pregnancy, her glycemic control was excellent, with a hemoglobin A_{1c} value of 6.2% (44 mmol/mol). Her data before pregnancy generally showed that she spent 70% to 80% of the time in the range of 70 to 180 mg/dL (3.9-10.0 mmol/L).

Today she reports frustration that in the past week she has had more episodes of hyperglycemia (>180 mg/dL [>10.0 mmol/L]) in the early morning and during the day that are difficult to correct once they occur. She also describes an increased occurrence of mild, asymptomatic hypoglycemia (56-69 mg/dL [3.1-3.8 mmol/L]), which she treats conservatively with no more than 15 g of carbohydrate often in the form of a small mixed meal. In addition, she has had a few glucose measurements between 48 and 55 mg/dL (2.7-3.1 mmol/L), which she has sensed (sweating and tremulousness) and treated with 4 to 8 oz of juice.

Data downloaded from her pump show that her time in range is now 58%, time spent above 180 mg/dL (>10.0 mmol/L) is 23%, and time spent below 70 mg/dL (<3.9 mmol/L) is 19%. Her continuous glucose monitor download shows a pattern of recurrent hypoglycemic episodes often occurring around 3 AM and between meals during the day. Her glucose levels are frequently elevated for at least 2 hours after these episodes.

Which of the following is the most appropriate adjustment to this patient's regimen?

A. Discontinue insulin pump therapy and switch to a basal-bolus insulin regimen
B. Discontinue use of continuous glucose monitoring and rely solely on fingerstick blood glucose monitoring
C. Increase daytime basal rates by 10% to 15%
D. Provide reassurance without setting changes
E. Reduce all basal rates by 10% to 15% and deactivate the hybrid closed-loop algorithm in her pump

32 A 68-year-old man is referred after he was found to have a low testosterone concentration on fasting bloodwork performed 3 months ago to evaluate general fatigue. He states that he is not bothered by his slightly reduced libido and is more concerned about the elevated fasting blood glucose concentration he noticed in his test results. He has a strong family history of type 2 diabetes and cared for his father with advanced diabetic kidney disease and severe foot pain at the end of his life. He would like to avoid these diabetes-related complications.

He has had stable Crohn disease for 20 years and rheumatoid arthritis for 10 years. Findings on a cardiac exercise stress test performed 2 years ago to evaluate atypical chest pain were normal. Despite a mostly sedentary lifestyle and relatively high-carbohydrate diet, he feels he is in good overall health.

His BMI is 29 kg/m², and blood pressure is 138/72 mm Hg. Examination findings are otherwise unremarkable.

Laboratory tests results (sample drawn at 8 AM):
Total testosterone = 220 ng/dL (300-900 ng/dL) (SI: 7.6 nmol/L [10.4-31.2 nmol/L])
Hemoglobin A_{1c} = 6.3% (4.0%-5.6%) (45 mmol/mol [20-38 mmol/mol])
HDL cholesterol = 36 mg/dL (>60 mg/dL [optimal]) (SI: 0.93 mmol/L [>1.55 mmol/L])
LDL cholesterol = 190 mg/dL (<100 mg/dL [optimal]) (SI: 4.92 mmol/L [<2.59 mmol/L])
PSA = 4.2 ng/mL (<5.3 ng/mL) (SI: 4.2 µg/L [<5.3 µg/L])

Which of the following is the best next step to improve this patient's overall health?

A. Prescribe acarbose
B. Prescribe atorvastatin
C. Prescribe metformin
D. Prescribe testosterone
E. Refer to a program for behavioral lifestyle change

33 A 74-year-old man who has had moderately well-controlled type 2 diabetes mellitus for 12 years presents for routine follow-up. He recently presented with new-onset angina and was found to have multivessel coronary artery disease. He had coronary artery bypass surgery 2 months ago. At his follow-up visit with his cardiologist yesterday, echocardiography determined his ejection fraction to be 42%. Prior to this event, his diabetes was complicated only by mild distal polyneuropathy.

On physical examination, his blood pressure is 132/78 mm Hg and pulse rate is 68 beats/min. He appears well overall and examination findings are unremarkable.

Laboratory test results:
Hemoglobin A_{1c} = 6.9% (4.0%-5.6%) (52 mmol/mol [20-38 mmol/mol])
Serum creatinine = 1.4 mg/dL (0.7-1.3 mg/dL) (SI: 123.8 µmol/L [61.9-114.9 µmol/L])
Estimated glomerular filtration rate = 52 mL/min per 1.73 m² (>60 mL/min per 1.73 m²)
Urinary albumin-to-creatinine ratio = 54 mg/g creat (<30 mg/g creat)

His current medications include metformin, 1500 mg daily in divided doses; atorvastatin, 80 mg daily; lisinopril, 5 mg daily; metoprolol, 50 mg daily; and aspirin, 325 mg daily.

Which of the following is the most appropriate next therapeutic step?

A. Increase the lisinopril dosage to 10 mg daily
B. Prescribe dapagliflozin, 5 mg daily
C. Prescribe finerenone, 10 mg daily
D. Prescribe oral semaglutide, 3 mg daily
E. Recommend no change

34 A 52-year-old woman presents for evaluation of type 2 diabetes mellitus. Diabetes was diagnosed at age 32 years in the setting of morbid obesity and approximately 5 years after having gestational diabetes. Since being diagnosed, she has struggled to maintain good disease control, with hemoglobin A_{1c} values between 9% and 10% and BMI between 38 and 42 kg/m². She has moderate to severe nonproliferative retinopathy in both eyes and distal polyneuropathy affecting her feet. Eight months ago, she underwent a gastric sleeve procedure and has lost 90 lb (40.8 kg). She feels well and bikes 30 minutes daily.

On physical examination, her BMI is 32 kg/m², blood pressure is 128/72 mm Hg, and pulse rate is 84 beats/min.

Laboratory test results:
Point-of-care hemoglobin A_{1c} = 6.7% (4.0%-5.6%) (50 mmol/mol [20-38 mmol/mol])
Sodium = 142 mEq/L (136-142 mEq/L) (SI: 142 mmol/L [136-142 mmol/L])
Potassium = 3.8 mEq/L (3.5-5.0 mEq/L) (SI: 3.8 mmol/L [3.5-5.0 mmol/L])
Creatinine = 1.68 mg/dL (0.6-1.1 mg/dL) (SI: 148.5 μmol/L [53.0-97.2 μmol/L])
Estimated glomerular filtration rate = 42 mL/min per 1.73 m² (>60 mL/min per 1.73 m²)
Glucose = 180 mg/dL (70-99 mg/dL) (SI: 10.0 mmol/L [3.9-5.5 mmol/L])
Urinary albumin-to-creatinine ratio = 280 mg/g creat (<30 mg/g creat)
LDL cholesterol = 72 mg/dL (<100 mg/dL [optimal]) (SI: 1.86 mmol/L [<2.59 mmol/L])
HDL cholesterol = 36 mg/dL (>60 mg/dL [optimal]) (SI: 0.93 mmol/L [>1.55 mmol/L])

Her current medications include dulaglutide, 1.5 mg weekly; losartan, 25 mg daily; and simvastatin, 20 mg daily. She reports that she is unable to tolerate SGLT-2 inhibitors because of recurrent, severe vaginal yeast infections.

Which of the following is the best next step in this patient's management?
   A. Add finerenone, 10 mg daily
   B. Add insulin glargine, 0.15 units/kg per day
   C. Increase the dulaglutide dosage to 3 mg weekly
   D. Increase the losartan dosage to 50 mg daily
   E. Increase the simvastatin dosage to 40 mg daily

35 A 48-year-old man with well-controlled cystic fibrosis–related diabetes returns to clinic for routine follow-up after starting to use a continuous glucose monitoring device 6 weeks ago. He finds it to be a useful tool and says that it has helped him achieve better glycemic control without frequent, painful fingersticks. However, his wife expresses concern that he is ignoring low-glucose alarms overnight. This first happened after the second week using the device, when he and his wife were awakened by the alarm that sounded for a glucose reading of 52 mg/dL (2.9 mmol/L). Despite being asymptomatic, he drank 4 oz of juice and ate 5 crackers. Upon waking 3 hours later, his glucose value was 256 mg/dL (14.2 mmol/L). After this event, he decided to respond to alarms by getting up and going to the bathroom, which seemed to resolve the alarm. In the last week, he moved the device receiver out of his bedroom so he would not hear alarms and has slept without disturbance.

He has had no changes in medications and his health has been stable. His medications include insulin glargine, 22 units; insulin lispro, 4 to 12 units prior to meals only; azithromycin; albuterol; calcium citrate; cholecalciferol; ciprofloxacin; elexacaftor/tezacaftor/ivacaftor; and gabapentin.

On physical examination, his weight is stable at 163 lb (74 kg) and his blood pressure is 124/72 mm Hg. The sensor site on his left arm is intact without erythema or discoloration.

His continuous glucose monitoring download documents the following similar pattern recurring every 2 to 3 nights, with the daytime pattern being relatively consistent on a daily basis (*see image at the top of the following page*).

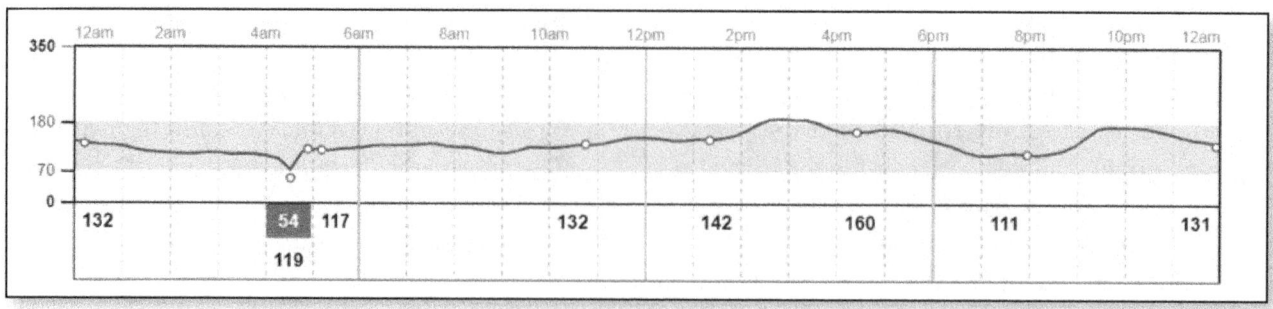

Which of the following is the best next step in this patient's management?
- A. Discuss replacing ciprofloxacin with his pulmonologist
- B. Relocate the glucose sensor
- C. Reduce the insulin glargine dosage
- D. Reduce the predinner lispro insulin dose

36 A 31-year-old man with type 1 diabetes mellitus diagnosed 2 months ago presents with episodes of recurrent hypoglycemia. He uses an insulin pump and recently started continuous glucose monitoring. His current hemoglobin A_{1c} value is 6.3% (45 mmol/mol), which has decreased from 9.2% (77 mmol/mol) at diagnosis. Over the past few weeks, his blood glucose values after meals have frequently been between 70 and 80 mg/dL (3.9-4.4 mmol/L). He also has fasting hypoglycemia (50-70 mg/dL [2.8-3.9 mmol/L]) once or twice weekly. Two nights in the last week he was awakened during sleep by a low alarm from his continuous glucose monitor.

How should this patient be advised regarding the best course of action now?
- A. Discontinue insulin pump therapy
- B. Increase carbohydrate intake to at least 50 g with each meal
- C. Reduce all insulin doses by 10% to 20%
- D. Reduce the basal insulin dose by 10% to 20%
- E. Start hybrid closed-loop insulin pump

37 A 57-year-old woman with primary polycythemia presents for management of type 2 diabetes mellitus, which she has had for 16 years. She currently takes metformin, 1000 mg twice daily, and insulin glargine, 20 units once daily. Her hemoglobin A_{1c} level is 6.7% (50 mmol/mol), and she has no signs or symptoms of hypoglycemia. She is a professional violinist and has consistently declined glucose monitoring using fingerstick blood glucose.

Professional continuous glucose monitoring is recommended. She wears the device for 10 days, and the numerical results of her ambulatory glucose profile are shown (*see image below*).

Which of the following is the correct interpretation of this patient's ambulatory glucose profile?
- A. Her overall glycemic control meets recommended targets
- B. She has acceptable glucose variability
- C. She has excessive hyperglycemia
- D. She has excessive hypoglycemia
- E. The mean glucose value is consistent with her hemoglobin A_{1c} value

38 A 46-year-old man with an 8-year history of diabetes mellitus returns for follow-up and reports blurry vision. Over several years, he has not achieved target glycemic control due to ineffectiveness of combination noninsulin therapy or inability to tolerate these therapies. Two

Avg Glucose mg/dL		Very Low	Low	In Target Range	High	Very High		Coefficient of Variation	SD mg/dL
		< 54 mg/dL	< 70 mg/dL	70 - 180 mg/dL	> 180 mg/dL	> 250 mg/dL			
162		0.2%	3.2%	62.3%	34.5%	11.4%		44.3%	72
Glucose Exposure				Glucose Ranges				Glucose Variability	

months ago, he started insulin following a virtual education visit and has been measuring fingerstick blood glucose 4 times daily. As advised, he discontinued glipizide and continued metformin. He has called his endocrinologist every 2 weeks for insulin dosage titration. Glucose readings have been ranging from 180 mg/dL (10.0 mmol/L) (fasting) to 400 mg/dL (22.2 mmol/L). He is now taking 95 units of insulin glargine twice daily and 30 units of insulin aspart with each meal (total daily insulin dose = 288 units). Other medications include metformin and simvastatin.

On physical examination, he is alert and appears mildly fatigued. His blood pressure is 158/76 mm Hg, and pulse rate is 88 beats/min. His weight is 185.2 lb (84 kg) (BMI = 32 kg/m^2). The rest of the examination findings are normal.

Laboratory test results:
Random blood glucose = 366 mg/dL (70-99 mg/dL) (SI: 20.3 mmol/L [3.9-5.5 mmol/L])
Hemoglobin A$_{1c}$ 4 months ago = 8.2% (4.0%-5.6%) (66 mmol/mol [20-38 mmol/mol])
Hemoglobin A$_{1c}$ now = 9.8% (84 mmol/mol)

Which of the following is the best next step in this patient's management?
   A. Admit him to the emergency department for administration of intravenous normal saline
   B. Ask him to demonstrate how he self-administers insulin injections
   C. Increase the dosages of insulin glargine and insulin aspart by 30% each
   D. Restart glipizide
   E. Stop both insulin glargine and insulin aspart and begin U500 regular insulin, 250 units in split doses

39 A 34-year-old woman who was followed for management of type 2 diabetes mellitus during pregnancy returns for follow-up after delivering a healthy baby 2 weeks ago. She asks about environmental factors that could affect her child's risk of developing diabetes.

Which of the following environmental interventions should be advised to reduce the risk of her child developing diabetes?
   A. Following a diet low in omega-3 fatty acids for 2 years
   B. Avoiding sugar-sweetened beverages
   C. Delaying routine childhood vaccines until 1 year of age
   D. Exposing to tree nuts within the first 6 months
   E. Switching to cow milk after 3 months of breastfeeding

40 A 26-year-old man with a 5-year history of type 1 diabetes mellitus is referred because he is interested in insulin pump therapy. He travels often for work, and he has an erratic eating schedule. However, he has good glycemic control, and he no longer wants to administer multiple daily insulin injections. His current insulin regimen consists of insulin glargine, 22 units at bedtime, and insulin lispro, 6 units with each meal (total daily insulin dose: 40 units).

Self-monitoring of blood glucose shows values ranging between 80 and 130 mg/dL (4.4-7.2 mmol/L). He rarely has hypoglycemic events.

On physical examination, his BMI is 24 kg/m^2. Examination findings are unremarkable.

A recent hemoglobin A$_{1c}$ measurement is 6.9% (4.0%-5.6%) (52 mmol/mol [20-38 mmol/mol]).

After he undergoes intensive education (basal-bolus concept, carbohydrate counting, etc), his current injection regimen should be switched to insulin pump therapy (with lispro) with which of the following parameters?

Answer	Basal rate (X units/h)	Carbohydrate ratio (1 unit/X g)	Sensitivity factor (1 unit/X mg/dL)
A.	0.9	20	60
B.	0.6	15	55
C.	1.2	15	45
D.	1.4	10	30
E.	0.6	10	25

41 An 18-year-old man is referred for management of type 1 diabetes mellitus, which was recently diagnosed during a hospital admission for diabetic ketoacidosis. He is taking basal and mealtime insulins. He is currently doing well, with most blood glucose measurements within range. He uses a continuous glucose monitor and reports no symptoms or concerns.

Which of the following should be measured as part of screening for other autoimmune diseases?

    A. 21-Hydroxylase antibodies

    B. Antinuclear antibodies

    C. Glutamic acid decarboxylase-65 antibodies

    D. Tissue transglutaminase antibodies

    E. TPO antibodies

42 A 25-year-old man with a 2-year history of type 1 diabetes mellitus has just started to play tennis recently and is preparing for a 1-hour tennis game to be played at 8 AM. The last time he played, he had a severe hypoglycemic episode that required his friend to assist him with finding his glucose tablets. His usual regimen is insulin glargine, 14 units every morning, and insulin lispro with an insulin-to-carbohydrate ratio of 1:10 for meals. He eats breakfast at 7 AM. His most recent hemoglobin A_{1c} value is 6.7% (4.0%-5.6%) (52 mmol/mol [20-38 mmol/mol]).

He asks for advice about his insulin regimen the morning of the tennis game, assuming on that day his fasting glucose is in the usual range of 120 to 140 mg/dL (6.7-7.8 mmol/L).

Which of the following is the best recommendation?

    A. Eat breakfast, take insulin glargine (14 units) and insulin lispro with an insulin-to-carbohydrate ratio of 1:20

    B. Eat breakfast, take insulin lispro with an insulin-to-carbohydrate ratio of 1:10 and delay the glargine dose to the evening

    C. Eat breakfast, take insulin lispro with an insulin-to-carbohydrate ratio of 1:10 and lower the glargine dose to 7 units

    D. Skip breakfast and insulin lispro; drink 8 oz of orange juice before the game

43 A 68-year-old man with a 22-year history of type 2 diabetes mellitus is admitted to the hospital with severe hyperglycemia and change in mental status. The patient lives alone and was found by his neighbor in a confused state.

On physical examination, the patient is lethargic and unable to answer any questions. His temperature is 100.5°F (38.1°C), blood pressure is 100/60 mm Hg, and pulse rate is 130 beats/min. His weight is 230 lb (104 kg) (BMI = 32 kg/m²). Skin and mucous membranes are dry. There is no focal neurologic deficit.

Laboratory test results:

    Hemoglobin A_{1c} = 10.5% (4.0%-5.6%)
      (91 mmol/mol [20-38 mmol/mol])

    Plasma glucose = 1300 mg/dL (70-99 mg/dL)
      (SI: 72.2 mmol/L [3.9-5.5 mmol/L])

    Serum sodium = 126 mEq/L (136-142 mEq/L)
      (SI: 126 mmol/L [136-142 mmol/L])

    Serum potassium = 4.5 mEq/L (3.5-5.0 mEq/L)
      (SI: 4.5 mmol/L [3.5-5.0 mmol/L])

    Serum bicarbonate = 21 mEq/L (21-28 mEq/L)
      (SI: 21 mmol/L [21-28 mmol/L])

    Serum chloride = 106 mEq/L (96-106 mEq/L)
      (SI: 106 mmol/L [96-106 mmol/L])

    Serum creatinine = 1.9 mg/dL (0.7-1.3 mg/dL)
      (SI: 168.0 µmol/L [61.9-114.9 µmol/L])

    Arterial pH = 7.35 (7.35-7.45)

    Serum β-hydroxybutyrate = 2.6 mg/dL
      (<3.0 mg/dL) (SI: 249.8 µmol/L [<288.2 µmol/L])

Which of the following is the best next step?

Answer	Fluids over the first hour	Intravenous insulin
A.	1.5 L of 0.9% NaCl	Bolus of 10 units, then 10 units per h
B.	1.5 L of 0.9% NaCl	Bolus of 20 units then 20 units per h
C.	1.5 L of 0.45% NaCl	Bolus of 10 units, then 10 units per h
D.	1.5 L of 0.45% NaCl	Bolus of 5 units, then 5 units per h
E.	1.5 L of 3.0% NaCl	Bolus of 10 units, then 10 units per h

44 A 47-year-old man with a 19-year history of type 1 diabetes mellitus has no diabetes-related complications and no specific concerns. He is treated with insulins degludec and aspart. His blood pressure is 129/68 mm Hg, and BMI is 28 kg/m^2.

Laboratory test results:
- Hemoglobin A$_{1c}$ = 7.2% (4.0%-5.6%) (55 mmol/mol [20-38 mmol/mol])
- Total cholesterol = 173 mg/dL (<200 mg/dL [optimal]) (SI: 4.48 mmol/L [<5.18 mmol/L])
- LDL cholesterol = 92 mg/dL (<100 mg/dL [optimal]) (SI: 2.38 mmol/L [<2.59 mmol/L])
- HDL cholesterol = 45 mg/dL (>60 mg/dL [optimal]) (SI: 1.17 mmol/L [>1.55 mmol/L])
- Triglycerides = 178 mg/dL (<150 mg/dL [optimal]) (SI: 2.01 mmol/L [<1.70 mmol/L])
- Serum creatinine = 0.86 mg/dL (0.7-1.3 mg/dL) (SI: 76.0 mmol/L [61.9-114.9 mmol/L])
- Urinary albumin-to-creatinine ratio = 19 mg/g creat (<30 mg/g creat)

How should this patient be advised regarding the best course of action to reduce his risk for cardiovascular disease?

- A. Intensify his treatment regimen to attain a target hemoglobin A$_{1c}$ value <7.0% (<53 mmol/mol)
- B. Refer to a nutritionist for dietary instruction for weight loss
- C. Start aspirin, 81 mg daily
- D. Start treatment with a statin
- E. Start treatment with an ACE inhibitor

45 A 58-year-old woman with a 4-year history of type 2 diabetes mellitus is concerned about her cardiovascular health. Her diabetes has been treated with metformin. She had gestational diabetes in her 30s and has hypertension and dyslipidemia. She is taking ramipril, 5 mg daily, and simvastatin, 20 mg daily. There is no known cardiovascular disease. Her family history, however, is notable for type 2 diabetes, hypertension, and death of myocardial infarction in several relatives before age 50 years. She has smoked cigarettes for 10 years and has attempted to quit 3 times unsuccessfully.

On physical examination, her blood pressure is 118/70 mm Hg and BMI is 30 kg/m^2. Examination findings are otherwise unremarkable.

Laboratory test results:
- Hemoglobin A$_{1c}$ = 7.2% (4.0%-5.6%) (55 mmol/mol [20-38 mmol/mol])
- Estimated glomerular filtration rate, normal
- Liver function, normal
- TSH, normal
- LDL cholesterol = 120 mg/dL (<100 mg/dL [optimal]) (SI: 3.11 mmol/L [<2.59 mmol/L])
- HDL cholesterol = 45 mg/dL (>60 mg/dL [optimal]) (SI: 1.67 mmol/L [>1.55 mmol/L])
- Triglycerides = 145 mg/dL (<150 mg/dL [optimal]) (SI: 1.64 mmol/L [<1.70 mmol/L])

Which of the following medications is most likely to lead to significantly lower rates of major vascular events in this patient?

- A. Aspirin, 100 mg daily
- B. Empagliflozin, 25 mg daily
- C. Lixisenatide, 20 mcg daily
- D. Rosuvastatin, 20 mg daily
- E. Sitagliptin, 100 mg daily

46 A 31-year-old woman with a 22-year history of type 1 diabetes mellitus was recently told by her ophthalmologist that she has early nonproliferative diabetic retinopathy. She is concerned about progression and losing her vision and asks what she can do to help prevent progression of this complication.

In addressing her concern, you explain that the amount of vision loss due to diabetic retinopathy that can be prevented at this early nonproliferative stage with targeted glycemic, blood pressure, and lipid control is expected to be:

- A. <10%
- B. 20%-30%
- C. 50%
- D. 75%
- E. >90%

47 A 35-year-old woman with a 5-year history of type 2 diabetes mellitus presents with new skin lesions. She reports nonpainful lesions on her upper chest that have grown splotchy red and pruritic over the past 2 months. She has not traveled recently and has had no unusual contacts, new skin creams or lotions, or systemic illness. On physical examination, the lesions are visible (*see image*).

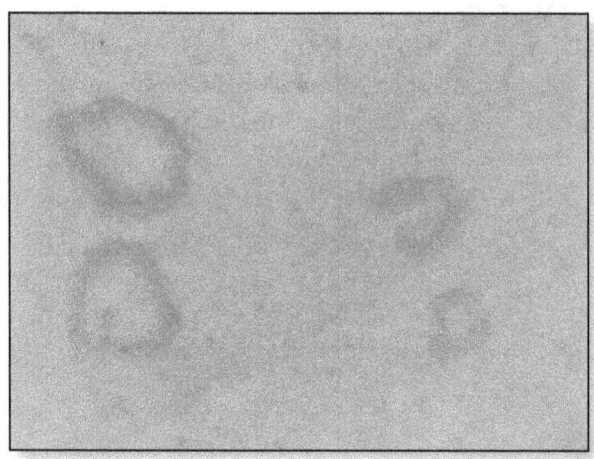

Which of the following is the most likely diagnosis?
  A. Disseminated granuloma annulare
  B. Lichen planus
  C. Necrobiosis lipoidica
  D. Tinea corporis

48 A 46-year-old woman returns for a second opinion regarding her diabetes care. She had gestational diabetes during the last 2 of her 4 pregnancies and was noted to have a blood glucose concentration of 231 mg/dL (12.8 mmol/L) 6 years ago (she was asymptomatic at the time). Initially, metformin was prescribed in combination with lifestyle modifications, and her hemoglobin A_{1c} level subsequently decreased from 8.6% to 6.8% (70 to 51 mmol/mol). Two years ago, she lost her health insurance and although she has continued metformin, 1000 mg twice daily, she has not seen a physician. When she recently obtained new health insurance, she returned to her primary care physician who noted her hemoglobin A_{1c} level to be 8.3% (67 mmol/mol). Her medical history is notable for hypertension, seasonal allergies, and recurrent urinary tract infections. Her primary care physician documented normal electrolytes and kidney function and no albuminuria. Retinal photography was interpreted to be unremarkable.

On physical examination, her blood pressure is 126/78 mm Hg and BMI is 30 kg/m². She has no evidence of peripheral neuropathy.

Her primary care physician gave her a prescription for sitagliptin, but the copay is much higher than she expected. She is wondering whether this is a good choice for her.

Besides cost, which of the following is the biggest concern with the use of sitagliptin in this patient?
  A. Increased risk for arthritis
  B. Increased risk for nasopharyngitis
  C. Increased risk for nephrotoxicity
  D. Increased risk for urinary tract infection
  E. Insufficient potency

49 A 29-year-old woman is referred for weight management. Schizophrenia was diagnosed 2 years ago. The patient reports a 15-lb (6.8-kg) weight gain since starting treatment with an antipsychotic medication.

On physical examination, her blood pressure is 130/70 mm Hg and BMI is 32 kg/m².

Laboratory test results:
  Hemoglobin A_{1c} = 6.3% (4.0%-5.6%) (45 mmol/mol [20-38 mmol/mol])
  Total cholesterol = 215 mg/dL (<200 mg/dL [optimal]) (SI: 5.57 mmol/L [<5.18 mmol/L])
  Triglycerides = 310 mg/dL (<150 mg/dL [optimal]) (SI: 3.50 mmol/L [<1.70 mmol/L])
  LDL cholesterol = 125 mg/dL (<100 mg/dL [optimal]) (SI: 3.24 mmol/L [<2.59 mmol/L])
  HDL cholesterol = 36 mg/dL (>60 mg/dL [optimal]) (SI: 0.93 mmol/L [>1.55 mmol/L])
  Creatinine = 0.9 mg/dL (0.6-1.1 mg/dL) (SI: 79.6 μmol/L [53.0-97.2 μmol/L])
  TSH = 1.6 mIU/L (0.5-5.0 mIU/L)

Which antipsychotic medication is this patient most likely taking?

    A. Aripiprazole

    B. Clozapine

    C. Quetiapine

    D. Risperidone

50

A 62-year-old woman with a 22-year history of type 2 diabetes mellitus presents for routine follow-up. She recently developed unstable angina for which she underwent coronary artery revascularization. She also has hyperlipidemia, hypertension, chronic kidney disease, and congestive heart failure.

She takes insulin degludec U100, 30 units once daily; insulin lispro, 15 units before meals; aspirin, 81 mg daily; clopidogrel; carvedilol; metolazone; and furosemide. She previously took atorvastatin, 80 mg daily, but experienced severe myalgias. The dosage was reduced to 40 mg daily and she is tolerating this well. She is concerned about her new diagnosis of coronary artery disease and asks whether she should be taking any other medications to reduce risk for heart attack or stroke.

On physical examination, her BMI is 31 kg/m². Her blood pressure is 124/81 mm Hg, and pulse rate is 86 beats/min. Lungs are clear on auscultation, and the rest of her examination findings are normal except for mild reduction in sensation bilaterally in the feet.

Laboratory test results:

    Hemoglobin A_{1c} = 9.7% (4.0%-5.6%) (83 mmol/mol [20-38 mmol/mol])

    AST, normal

    ALT, normal

    Estimated glomerular filtration rate = 32 mL/min per 1.73 m² (>60 mL/min per 1.73 m²)

    Total cholesterol = 135 mg/dL (<200 mg/dL [optimal]) (SI: 3.50 mmol/L [<5.18 mmol/L])

    HDL cholesterol = 37 mg/dL (>60 mg/dL [optimal]) (SI: 0.96 mmol/L [>1.55 mmol/L])

    LDL cholesterol = 78 mg/dL (<100 mg/dL [optimal]) (SI: 2.02 mmol/L [<2.59 mmol/L])

    Triglycerides = 100 mg/dL (<150 mg/dL [optimal]) (SI: 1.13 mmol/L [<1.70 mmol/L])

This woman is at very high risk for future atherosclerotic cardiovascular disease events.

Which agent should be added as the best next step to reduce this patient's risk of a future cardiovascular event?

    A. Coenzyme Q10

    B. Colchicine

    C. Evolocumab

    D. Ezetimibe

    E. Icosapent ethyl

51

A 48-year-old woman has new-onset type 2 diabetes mellitus. Nonalcoholic steatohepatitis was recently diagnosed after routine testing showed abnormal liver function. Subsequent workup, including a liver biopsy, revealed nonalcoholic steatohepatitis with pathologic evidence of steatosis, lobular inflammation, hepatocellular ballooning, and fibrosis. There is no evidence of cirrhosis. Her BMI is 32 kg/m².

Laboratory test results:

    Hemoglobin A_{1c} = 8.0% (4.0%-5.6%) (64 mmol/mol [20-38 mmol/mol])

    Creatinine = 0.8 mg/dL (0.6-1.1 mg/dL) (SI: 70.7 μmol/L [53.0-97.2 μmol/L])

    ALT = 89 U/L (10-40 U/L) (SI: 1.49 μkat/L [0.17-0.67 μkat/L])

    TSH = 2.5 mIU/L (0.5-5.0 mIU/L)

The hepatologist suggests prescribing an antidiabetes agent that would also improve her liver histology.

Which of the following medications would be the best choice given these concerns?

    A. Dapagliflozin

    B. Dulaglutide

    C. Metformin

    D. Pioglitazone

    E. Sitagliptin

52 A 49-year-old man with a history of morbid obesity, hypothyroidism, and type 2 diabetes mellitus had a gastric bypass operation 14 months ago. His preoperative BMI was 42 kg/m². After surgery, his diabetes resolved and his insulin therapy was discontinued. His weight fell and stabilized at a BMI of 29 kg/m². He was told to take a potent multivitamin and 1200 mg of calcium daily. He has not had any follow-up for the last 4 months. Over the previous month, he has had several episodes where he felt shaky, sweaty, and irritable. A family member brought him to the emergency department yesterday at 11:00 AM for confusion that had developed after eating a large breakfast at a buffet restaurant. His glucose concentration was documented to be 35 mg/dL (1.9 mmol/L).

After treating the acute hypoglycemia and stabilizing his condition, which of the following would be the most appropriate management to prevent a recurrent episode?

    A. Diazoxide

    B. Low-carbohydrate diet

    C. Octreotide

    D. Partial pancreatectomy

Female Reproduction Board Review

Kathryn A. Martin, MD

1 A 30-year-old woman with functional hypothalamic amenorrhea seeks management advice. She had menarche at age 14 years. She developed secondary amenorrhea at age 16 years, and this was attributed to low body weight and intensive exercise. After 2 years of amenorrhea and a decrease in her BMI to 17 kg/m², her pediatrician prescribed a combined oral contraceptive (20 mcg ethinyl estradiol/1 mg norethindrone acetate). She continued the oral contraceptive until age 28 years when she wanted to conceive. Her BMI at that time had increased to 19.2 kg/m², but amenorrhea persisted.

Laboratory test results:
> LH = 1.2 mIU/mL (1.0-18.0 mIU/mL)
> (SI: 1.2 IU/L [1.0-18.0 IU/L])
> FSH = 1.3 mIU/mL (2.0-12.0 mIU/mL)
> (SI: 1.3 IU/L [2.0-12.0 IU/L])
> Estradiol = 6 pg/mL (10-180 pg/mL)
> (SI: 22.0 pmol/L [36.7-660.8 pmol/L])
> Prolactin = 10 ng/mL (4-30 ng/mL)
> (SI: 0.43 nmol/L [0.17-1.30 nmol/L])
> TSH = 1.3 mIU/L (0.5-5.0 mIU/L)

She initially tried ovulation induction with clomiphene citrate followed by letrozole. She had no ovarian response to either medication (no follicular growth). She was then referred to an infertility center for gonadotropin therapy. She underwent 1 cycle of standard recombinant FSH injections. After 9 days of treatment, she had 2 dominant follicles on transvaginal ultrasonography (18 mm in the right ovary, 21 mm in the left ovary) with a serum estradiol concentration less than 20 pg/mL (<73.4 pmol/L). Given the lack of response, the cycle was canceled. However, she was offered another treatment cycle with gonadotropins.

Which of the following modifications is the best next step in this patient's fertility management?
- A. Add clomiphene citrate
- B. Add letrozole
- C. Add LH
- D. Increase the dosage of FSH
- E. Recommend in vitro fertilization

2 A 20-year-old woman with polycystic ovary syndrome is referred to discuss options for cycle management and treatment of hyperandrogenism. Menarche was at age 11 years, and she subsequently had 5 to 6 menstrual cycles per year. At age 14 years, an oral contraceptive was recommended for cycle management, but the patient's mother was not comfortable with this option. She has therefore prescribed medroxyprogesterone acetate, 10 mg daily for 12 days monthly, for cycle management/endometrial protection, and she has continued this regimen. However, she has gradually developed acne and facial hair growth that she finds bothersome. She has no comorbidities and no family history of myocardial infarction, stroke, or venous thromboembolism.

Her BMI is 30 kg/m² (increased from 25 kg/m² at age 14 years). Her blood pressure is 110/60 mm Hg. Hirsutism is evident on her upper lip, chin, upper and lower neck, midsternum, and upper abdomen, and her Ferriman-Gallwey score is 11. She also has noncystic but moderate facial acne.

Laboratory test results:

Lipid profile, normal

Hemoglobin A_{1c}, normal

Total testosterone = 40 ng/dL (8-60 ng/dL)
(SI: 1.39 nmol/L [0.3-2.1 nmol/L])

Serum 17-hydroxyprogesterone = 40 ng/dL
(<80 ng/dL) (SI: 1.21 nmol/L [<2.42 nmol/L])

A low-dosage combined estrogen (20 mcg ethinyl estradiol) progestin oral contraceptive is recommended for contraception and management of her hirsutism, acne, and irregular menstrual cycles.

If she starts a combined oral contraceptive, which of the following outcomes is she more likely to experience when compared with women without obesity?

A. Contraceptive failure
B. Impaired glucose tolerance
C. No differences
D. Unscheduled bleeding
E. Weight gain

3 A 26-year-old woman seeks consultation for hair loss. Menarche was at age 11 years, and her cycles have always been irregular. At age 17 years, she was started on a combined oral estrogen-progestin contraceptive for cycle control and management of acne and facial hair. She stopped the pill 18 months ago to see if her periods would be more regular. She has menses every 45 to 60 days. Acne and hirsutism have gradually worsened since stopping the combined oral contraceptive, and she has also noticed hair loss on the crown of her scalp. She has tried vitamins and biotin for hair loss with no obvious benefit. She is otherwise in good health.

On physical examination, she has short hair with visible thinning over the frontal scalp and vertex of the scalp and no evidence of scarring.

Laboratory test results (sample drawn on cycle day 3):

Serum total testosterone = 55 ng/dL (8-60 ng/dL)
(SI: 1.9 nmol/L [0.3-2.1 nmol/L])

LH = 7.2 mIU/mL (1.0-18.0 mIU/mL)
(SI: 7.2 IU/L [1.0-18.0 IU/L])

FSH = 4.1 mIU/mL (2.0-12.0 mIU/mL)
(SI: 4.1 IU/L [2.0-12.0 IU/L])

Estradiol = 28 pg/mL (10-180 pg/mL)
(SI: 102.7 pmol/L [36.7-660.8 pmol/L])

TSH = 1.8 mIU/L (0.5-5.0 mIU/L)

Which of the following is the most likely diagnosis regarding her hair loss?

A. Alopecia areata
B. Female-pattern hair loss
C. Frontal fibrosing alopecia
D. Telogen effluvium
E. Traction alopecia

4 A 52-year-old menopausal woman asks about testosterone therapy. She has been on a regimen of menopausal hormone therapy (transdermal estradiol [0.0375 mg twice weekly] with oral progesterone [100 mg daily]) since age 49 years for severe hot flashes and night sweats that interfered with her ability to sleep and function well at work. She has had complete resolution of her vasomotor symptoms. She notes some vaginal dryness, but her main concern is a gradual decline in libido over the past 20 years. A recent serum testosterone concentration is 22 ng/dL (0.76 nmol/L) compared with 31 ng/dL (1.08 nmol/L) when she was 30 years old. She has read that testosterone treatment would restore her libido to "normal."

Which of the following should be the first suggestion for this patient?

A. An increase in the transdermal estradiol dosage
B. Low-dosage vaginal estrogen
C. Oral DHEA therapy
D. Sex therapy
E. Testosterone therapy

5 A 48-year-old woman has been experiencing hot flashes and night sweats for the past 6 months. Her vasomotor symptoms disrupt her sleep, resulting in fatigue and difficulty functioning at work. She has also developed anxiety symptoms. She has had a levonorgestrel-releasing intrauterine device, so she does not have the biological marker of menses to help define the transition and final menstrual period. She has no personal or family history of venous thromboembolism.

On physical examination, her height is 64 in (162.6 cm) and weight is 135 lb (61.2 kg) (BMI = 23.2 kg/m^2).

Her primary care physician and gynecologist have recommended against menopausal hormone therapy because her grandmother had breast cancer at age 85 years.

Laboratory test results:
    FSH = 180.0 mIU/mL (SI: 180.0 IU/L)
    Estradiol = 10 pg/mL (SI: 36.7 pmol/L)

Which of the following additional evaluations is most important to determine whether she is a candidate for menopausal hormone therapy?
    A. Breast MRI
    B. Genetic testing for *BRCA1* and *BRCA2*
    C. Hemoglobin A$_{1c}$ measurement
    D. Hypercoagulability profile
    E. 5-Year breast cancer risk calculation

6 A 44-year-old perimenopausal woman is referred by her psychopharmacologist for consultation regarding perimenopausal symptoms. One year ago, she noted a change in her menstrual cycles (previously every 28 days, but now every 35 to 55 days with heavy bleeding). Other symptoms include night sweats, hot flashes, and new-onset depression. Citalopram was prescribed 6 months ago, and the dosage has been titrated to 30 mg daily, but she still has some mild symptoms of depression. She is otherwise in excellent health and has no personal or family history of hypertension, coronary disease, breast cancer, or venous thromboembolism.

Laboratory test results (sample drawn on cycle day 3):
    FSH = 40.0 mIU/L (2.0-12.0 mIU/mL [follicular])
        (SI: 40.0 IU/L [2.0-12.0 IU/L])
    Prolactin = 15 ng/mL (4-30 ng/mL)
        (SI: 0.65 nmol/L [0.17-1.30 nmol/L])
    TSH = 2.0 mIU/L (0.5-5.0 mIU/L)
    hCG, negative

On physical examination, her blood pressure is 105/70 mm Hg and BMI is 21 kg/m^2.

Which of the following is the best next step in this patient's management?
    A. Increase the citalopram dosage to 40 mg daily
    B. Refer for cognitive behavioral therapy
    C. Start a low-dosage continuous estrogen-progestin oral contraceptive (20 mcg ethinyl estradiol; 1 mg norethindrone acetate)
    D. Start oral estradiol, 2 mg daily, and micronized progesterone, 200 mg on days 1 to 12 of each calendar month

7 A 46-year-old woman seeks evaluation for irregular menses. Since menarche at age 12 years, she had regular 28- to 30-day cycles until age 43 years when her intermenstrual interval shortened to 24 to 25 days. For the past year, her cycles have become more unpredictable, occurring every 40 to 60 days. She experiences night sweats that interfere with sleep, particularly during the week prior to menses. Recent hCG measurement was negative, and her TSH concentration was normal. She would like to know what is causing her irregular periods and night sweats.

On physical examination, her blood pressure is 90/65 mm Hg and BMI is 22 kg/m^2.

Which of the following should be measured to determine the cause of this patient's problem?
    A. Antimullerian hormone
    B. FSH
    C. Prolactin
    D. Serum estradiol
    E. No testing required

8 A 38-year-old woman seeks evaluation of hormonal symptoms that are becoming increasingly difficult to manage. She has always had minor mood changes before her periods. However, for the past 2 years, she has experienced premenstrual anger, irritability, and tearfulness that start approximately 6 days before menses and continue until day 2 or 3 of menses. These symptoms are accompanied by bloating, night sweats, and fatigue, and she has difficulty functioning at work. The patient's menstrual cycles occur approximately once monthly.

On physical examination, her BMI is 24 kg/m², pulse rate is 88 beats/min, and blood pressure is 130/80 mm Hg.

Which of the following is the best next step to confirm her diagnosis?
- A. Daily prospective symptom diary for 2 cycles
- B. Day 3 serum FSH measurement
- C. Depression screening
- D. Serum antimullerian hormone measurement
- E. Serum TSH measurement

9 A 20-year-old woman with Turner syndrome is transitioning care from her pediatrician to an adult provider. She has a history of primary amenorrhea and short stature.

On physical examination, her blood pressure is 140/90 mm Hg. Her height is 56 in (142.2 cm) (BMI = 28 kg/m²). She has absent breast development and scant pubic and axillary hair. She is on a combined estrogen-progestin regimen and has been seeing her pediatrician yearly. Last year, cardiac MRI showed no evidence of aortic dilatation and no significant cardiovascular anomalies.

Past laboratory test results:
FSH = 35.0 mIU/mL (2.0-12.0 mIU/mL)
(SI: 35.0 IU/L [2.0-12.0 IU/L])
LH = 28.0 mIU/mL (1.0-18.0 mIU/mL)
(SI: 28.0 IU/L [1.0-18.0 IU/L])
Estradiol = <10 pg/mL (10-180 pg/mL)
(SI: <36.7 pmol/L [36.7-660.8 pmol/L])
Karyotype = 45,X

Which of the following tests should be ordered today (and at each yearly visit)?
- A. Antimullerian hormone measurement, transvaginal ultrasonography
- B. Celiac disease screening, electrocardiography, hemoglobin A_{1c} measurement
- C. Complete blood cell count, echocardiography, thyroid function tests
- D. Hemoglobin A_{1c} measurement, liver enzymes, thyroid function tests
- E. Hemoglobin A_{1c} measurement, kidney ultrasonography, liver enzymes

10 A 54-year-old woman presents with concerns of scalp hair loss and facial hair growth. Menarche was at age 12 years, and she had regular menses during her reproductive years. Her final menstrual period was 5 years ago. Over the past 4 to 5 years, she has gained weight and developed acne, hirsutism, and hair loss.

On physical examination, her BMI is 34 kg/m² (compared with 29 kg/m² 4 years ago). Blood pressure is 150/90 mm Hg. She has terminal hairs on her upper lip, chin, and neck, as well as hair on her upper abdomen, lower back, and midsternum with a Ferriman-Gallwey score of 12 (>8 considered to be abnormal). She has thinning hair over the frontal scalp and vertex of the scalp. She has acanthosis nigricans in the axillae and on the neck and elbows. Her clitoris measures 11 mm × 5 mm (upper normal limit for clitoral index is 35 mm²).

Laboratory test results:
Testosterone = 350 ng/dL (8-60 ng/dL)
(SI: 12.1 nmol/L [0.3-2.1 nmol/L])
DHEA-S = 120 µg/dL (15-200 µg/dL)
(SI: 3.25 µmol/L [0.41-5.42 µmol/L])
FSH = 19.0 mIU/mL (>30.0 mIU/mL
[postmenopausal]) (SI: 19.0 IU/L [>30.0 IU/L])
LH = 8.0 mIU/mL (>30.0 mIU/mL
[postmenopausal]) (SI: 8.0 IU/L [>30.0 IU/L])

Which of the following is the best next test to evaluate this patient?
- A. Adrenal CT
- B. 1-mg Dexamethasone-suppression test
- C. Serum 17-hydroxyprogesterone measurement
- D. Serum inhibin measurement
- E. Transvaginal ultrasonography

11 A 28-year-old woman seeks evaluation for polycystic ovary syndrome. She has oligomenorrhea, hirsutism, and acne. Transvaginal ultrasonography shows polycystic ovary morphology. She is eager to start treatment for her acne and hirsutism. An estrogen-progestin contraceptive (ethinyl estradiol, 20 mcg, with norethindrone acetate, 1 mg) is prescribed. Eight months later, the patient returns for follow-up evaluation. Her acne has improved, but she reports that she has not had any bleeding during the placebo week for the past 4 cycles. Several home pregnancy tests have been negative. She has not missed a single pill, and she takes no other medications. She wonders whether the pill has "stopped working."

On physical examination, her BMI is 22 kg/m^2.

Which of the following is the best next step in this patient's management?
   A. Endometrial biopsy
   B. Monthly serum hCG measurements
   C. Reassurance; no evaluation needed
   D. Serum estradiol measurement
   E. Serum prolactin measurement

12 A 22-year-old woman with a 4-year history of functional hypothalamic amenorrhea comes to clinic for follow-up. She has a history of excessive exercise and restricted eating. BMI at her initial visit was 17 kg/m^2, and she had low bone mineral density (Z-score at femoral neck = −2.2). She understands that her low bone mineral density is related to her nutrition and excessive exercise, as evaluation for secondary causes has been negative. Eighteen months ago, she decided to implement lifestyle changes by moderating her exercise and improving her nutrition. Her weight has increased, and her BMI is now 18.5 kg/m^2. She is pleased that she has been able to make these changes but is disappointed that her periods have not returned. She wonders whether something else is wrong.

Laboratory test results:
   hCG = <3.0 mIU/mL (<3.0 mIU/mL)
      (SI: <3.0 IU/L [<3.0 IU/L])
   TSH = 1.9 mIU/L (0.5-5.0 mIU/L)
   Prolactin = 15 ng/mL (4-30 ng/mL)
      (SI: 0.65 nmol/L [0.17-1.30 nmol/L])
   Estradiol = 110 pg/mL (10-180 pg/mL)
      (SI: 403.8 pmol/L [36.7-660.8 pmol/L])
   LH = 6.0 mIU/mL (1.0-18.0 mIU/mL)
      (SI: 6.0 IU/L [1.0-18.0 IU/L])
   FSH = 8.0 mIU/mL (2.0-12.0 mIU/mL)
      (SI: 8.0 IU/L [2.0-12.0 IU/L])

Progesterone = 7.0 ng/mL (≤1.0 ng/mL)
   (SI: 22.3 nmol/L [≤3.2 nmol/L])

Which of the following should be recommended now?
   A. No treatment
   B. Isoflavone supplements
   C. Start alendronate, 70 mg weekly
   D. Start a low-dosage combined estrogen-progestin oral contraceptive
   E. Start transdermal 0.1 mg 17β-estradiol patch with cyclic micronized progesterone, 200 mg

13 A 46-year-old woman (G3, P2, Ab1) presents to discuss hormonal contraception. Menarche was at age 13 years and her menstrual cycles were always regular (every 28 to 32 days). For the past 9 to 12 months, her cycles have become both irregular (occurring every 2 to 3 months) and heavy. At a recent visit to her primary care physician, her hematocrit level was 32% (0.32) and iron supplementation was initiated.

On physical examination, her BMI is 35 kg/m^2, blood pressure is 140/90 mm Hg, and pulse rate is 80 beats/min.

Which of the following methods of contraception would be best for this patient?
   A. Combined estrogen-progestin oral contraceptive with ethinyl estradiol, 35 mcg, with levonorgestrel
   B. Copper intrauterine device
   C. Cyclic medroxyprogesterone, 10 days/month
   D. Depo-medroxyprogesterone injections
   E. Levonorgestrel-releasing intrauterine device

14 A 19-year-old patient is referred to discuss transgender hormone therapy. Sex assigned at birth was male. Preferred pronouns are female (she/her/hers). She has disclosed her gender dysphoria to family and close friends and is seeing a therapist. For the past year, she has experimented with wearing make-up and dressing in feminine clothes on the weekends. She uses gender-neutral bathrooms at work. Her medical history is notable for heterozygosity for a factor V Leiden pathogenic variant identified on screening after her mother had an unprovoked pulmonary embolism. She does not smoke cigarettes and takes no medications. Her BMI is 22 kg/m², and blood pressure is 110/70 mm Hg. Her therapist is supportive of her decision to start hormone therapy to alleviate dysphoria.

Which of the following would be the most appropriate initial hormone regimen for this patient?
- A. Leuprolide (GnRH agonist), 3.75 mg intramuscularly, plus estradiol, 2 mg orally
- B. Leuprolide (GnRH agonist), 3.75 mg intramuscularly, plus estradiol, 50 mcg by transdermal patch
- C. Low-dosage birth control pill containing 20 mcg of ethinyl estradiol and drospirenone plus spironolactone, 100 mg orally
- D. Spironolactone, 100 mg, and finasteride, 5 mg orally

15 An 18-year-old woman requests evaluation for primary amenorrhea. She was a healthy baby and experienced normal growth and development during early childhood. Pubic hair appeared at age 9 years and breast development started at age 11 years, but she has never menstruated. She is not sexually active.

On physical examination, her height is 65 in (165 cm) and weight is 132 lb (60 kg) (BMI = 22 kg/m²). Mild acne is noted on her face and back. Several dark hairs are present on her upper lip and chest. The patient has Tanner stage 5 breasts and stage 5 pubic hair.

Laboratory test results:
   Serum LH = 8.0 mIU/L (1.0-18.0 mIU/L)
      (SI: 8.0 IU/L [1.0-18.0 IU/L])
   FSH = 6.0 mIU/mL (2.0-12.0 mIU/mL)
      (SI: 6.0 IU/L [2.0-12.0 IU/L])
   Serum prolactin = 8 ng/mL (4-23 ng/mL)
      (SI: 0.35 nmol/L [0.17-1.00 nmol/L])
   Serum estradiol = 60 pg/mL (10-180 pg/mL)
      (SI: 220.3 pmol/L [36.7-660.8 pmol/L])
   Serum testosterone = 29 ng/dL (8-60 ng/dL)
      (SI: 1.0 nmol/L [0.3-2.1 nmol/L])

Pelvic ultrasonography reveals absence of a uterus.

Which of the following is this patient's most likely karyotype?
- A. 45,X
- B. 46,XX
- C. 46,XY
- D. 45,X/46,XX
- E. 47,XXY

16 A 24-year-old woman presents with a change in her intermenstrual interval. Menarche was at age 13 years, and she had regular menses during high school and college. She took an oral contraceptive pill from age 20 to 22 years. After stopping the oral contraceptive, she initially had 28- to 30-day cycles, but more recently she has been having menses every 22 to 23 days. She has autoimmune hypothyroidism and takes a stable levothyroxine dosage. She exercises for 1 hour 3 times weekly. She has mild acne, no hot flashes, and no galactorrhea. Her BMI is 20 kg/m².

Laboratory test results (samples drawn on cycle day 3):
   FSH = 20.0 mIU/mL (2.0-12.0 mIU/mL [follicular])
      (SI: 20.0 IU/L [2.0-12.0 IU/L])
   LH = 60.0 mIU/mL (1.0-18.0 mIU/mL [follicular])
      (SI: 60.0 IU/L [1.0-18.0 IU/L])
   Estradiol = 28 pg/mL (10-180 pg/mL [follicular])
      (SI: 102.8 pmol/L [36.7-660.8 pmol/L])
   Antimullerian hormone = 0.9 ng/mL
      (0.9-9.5 ng/mL) (SI: 6.4 pmol/L
      [6.4-67.9 pmol/L])
   TSH = 2.1 mIU/L (0.5-5.0 mIU/L)
   Karyotype = 46,XX
   FMR1 gene testing, no premutation detected

Which of the following is most important to measure next?
- A. GAD-65 antibodies
- B. 21-Hydroxylase antibodies
- C. IGF-1
- D. Inhibin B
- E. Serum ovarian antibodies

Male Reproduction Board Review

Stephanie Page, MD, PhD

1 A 38-year-old man with Klinefelter syndrome is referred for ongoing care. He has been on intramuscular testosterone cypionate, 150 mg every 2 weeks, for 5 years to treat hypogonadism. He takes lisinopril, 10 mg daily, for hypertension and oxycodone, 30 mg daily, for chronic back pain following a car accident. He is married and has no children.

He has had diminished libido over the last 2 years and has developed unwanted breast tissue over the last 2 months.

On physical examination, he is a tall, slender man with mild central adiposity. His blood pressure is 145/90 mm Hg, pulse rate is 80 beats/min, and BMI is 28 kg/m². His skin is clear except for mild acne on his back, and he has normal male-pattern facial hair with a thin beard. He has scant chest hair and nontender 2-cm gynecomastia on the right side that is firm and immobile and nontender 1-cm gynecomastia on the left side. Testicular volume is 10 cc bilaterally.

Fasting laboratory test results (sample drawn midway between his scheduled testosterone injections):

Testosterone = 400 ng/dL (300-900 ng/dL)
    (SI: 13.9 nmol/L [10.4-31.2 nmol/L])
Estradiol = 50 pg/mL (10-40 pg/mL)
    (SI: 183.2 pmol/L [36.7-146.8 pmol/L])
LH = 3.0 mIU/mL (1.0-9.0 mIU/mL)
    (SI: 3.0 IU/L [1.0-9.0 IU/L])
FSH = 4.5 mIU/mL (1.0-13.0 mIU/mL)
    (SI: 4.5 IU/L [1.0-13.0 IU/L])
Hematocrit = 48% (41%-51%) (SI: 0.48 [0.41-.050])

Which of the following is the most appropriate next step in the management of patient's gynecomastia?

A. Add anastrozole, 1 mg daily
B. Increase the intramuscular testosterone dosage to 200 mg every 2 weeks
C. Refer for mammography
D. Switch to transdermal 1% testosterone therapy, 50 mg daily
E. Work with his pain specialist to decrease his oxycodone dosage

2 A 54-year-old man who has been HIV positive for 15 years is referred by his primary care provider for unintentional weight loss. He has had considerable difficulty maintaining his weight over the last year and has lost approximately 4 lb (1.81 kg) in the last 6 months despite a robust appetite.

CD4 cell count has been within the normal range for more than 10 years while on highly active antiretroviral therapy (dolutegravir, abacavir, and lamivudine). He has hypertension treated with 2 medications. He has no concerns regarding sexual function and shaves daily. He has had no febrile illnesses, and findings from gastrointestinal workup, including evaluation for celiac sprue, are normal.

Laboratory test results (sample drawn at 8 AM while fasting):

Hematocrit = 39% (41%-51%) (SI: 0.39 [0.41-0.51])
TSH = 2.0 mIU/L (0.5-5.0 mIU/L)
Hemoglobin A$_{1c}$ = 5.7% (4.0%-5.6%) (39 mmol/mol [20-38 mmol/mol])
Total testosterone = 390 ng/dL (300-900 ng/dL)
    (SI: 13.5 nmol/L [10.4-31.2 nmol/L])
Free testosterone = 7.9 ng/dL (9-30 ng/dL)
    (SI: 0.27 nmol/L [0.31-1.04 nmol/L])

On physical examination, he is a thin man with normal male-pattern body hair. His weight is 165 lb (74.8 kg) (BMI = 18 kg/m²). His blood pressure is 155/92 mm Hg, and pulse rate is 75 beats/min. Testicular volume is 20 cc bilaterally.

Additional laboratory test results (ordered 1 week later, sample drawn at 8 AM):

Total testosterone: 370 ng/dL (300-900 ng/dL) (SI: 12.8 nmol/L [10.4-31.2 nmol/L])

Free testosterone = 7.7 ng/dL (9-30 ng/dL) (SI: 0.27 nmol/L [0.31-1.04 nmol/L])

LH = 5.2 mIU/mL (1.0-9.0 mIU/mL) (SI: 5.2 IU/L [1.0-9.0 IU/L])

PSA = 2.0 ng/mL (<2.8 ng/mL) (SI: 2.0 µg/L [<2.8 µg/L])

Cortisol = 24 µg/dL (5-25 µg/dL) (SI: 662.1 nmol/L [137.9-689.7 nmol/L])

Which of the following is the best recommendation to address this patient's weight loss?

A. Initiate finasteride, 5 mg daily

B. Initiate intramuscular testosterone enanthate injections, 200 mg every 2 weeks

C. Initiate megestrol acetate therapy, 800 mg daily

D. Initiate oral testosterone undecanoate therapy, 237 mg twice daily

E. Refer to nutritionist for counseling and instructions on keeping a food diary

3 A 25-year-old man is referred for concerns about future fertility. Type 2 diabetes mellitus was recently diagnosed with an initial hemoglobin A_{1c} value of 8.7% (72 mmol/mol). Three months ago, metformin was initiated at a dosage of 500 mg twice daily, and his hemoglobin A_{1c} value is now 8.1% (65 mmol/mol).

He has a sedentary job and does not exercise. He has recently married and has no concerns regarding sexual function and libido. The couple does not desire children for a few years, but the patient did a home sperm kit and his sperm count was "below normal." He is concerned about future fertility.

Laboratory test results:

Total testosterone = 290 ng/dL (300-900 ng/dL) (SI: nmol/L [10.4-31.2 nmol/L])

LH = 3.0 mIU/mL (1.0-9.0 mIU/mL) (SI: 3.0 IU/L [1.0-9.0 IU/L])

FSH = 5.0 mIU/mL (1.0-13.0 mIU/mL) (SI: 5.0 IU/L [1.0-13.0 IU/L])

Semen analysis = 14 million sperm/mL

On physical examination, his blood pressure is 132/86 mm Hg and BMI is 34 kg/m². He has normal male-pattern body hair. He has central adiposity. Testicular volume is 20 cc bilaterally, and his testes have no palpable nodules. There is a small, 4-mm, left-sided grade 2 varicocele (palpable without Valsalva).

Additional laboratory test results (sample drawn at 8 AM while fasting):

Total testosterone = 280 ng/dL (300-900 ng/dL) (SI: 9.7 nmol/L [10.4-31.2 nmol/L])

Free testosterone (calculated) = 16 ng/dL (9-30 ng/dL) (SI: 0.56 nmol/L [0.31-1.04 nmol/L])

Semen analysis = 20 million sperm/mL; motility and morphology are normal

Which of the following is the best next step in this patient's management to optimize his future fertility?

A. Increase the metformin dosage to 1000 mg twice daily, refer to nutritionist, and encourage lifestyle modifications including weight-loss goals

B. Refer to urology for varicocele repair

C. Start clomiphene citrate, 25 mg daily

D. Start hCG therapy, 1500 IU 3 times weekly

E. Start testosterone enanthate, 200 mg intramuscularly every 2 weeks

4 A 34-year-old transgender man who initiated testosterone therapy 6 months ago is concerned about acne and a lack of voice deepening. Menses ceased 4 months ago, and he states that he consistently administers biweekly testosterone injections (150 mg testosterone cypionate every 2 weeks).

Laboratory test results obtained midway through his testosterone dosing interval:

Hemoglobin = 16.8 g/dL (13.8-17.2 g/dL)
(SI: 168 g/L [138-172 g/L])
Hematocrit = 48% (41%-51%) (SI: 0.48 [0.41-0.51])
Total testosterone = 450 ng/dL (300-900 ng/dL)
(SI: 15.6 nmol/L [10.4-31.2 nmol/L])
Free testosterone = 16.0 ng/dL (9.0-30.0 ng/dL)
(SI: 0.56 nmol/L [0.31-1.04 nmol/L])

On physical examination, he has mild acne on his forehead at the midline and over his back, modest facial hair at the chin line and above his upper lip, and acne at the midline of his anterior chest. His voice seems unchanged.

Which of the following is the most appropriate next step to address his concerns?

A. Add cetrorelix, a GnRH antagonist
B. Decrease testosterone dosage to 125 mg every 2 weeks
C. Increase testosterone dosage to 200 mg every 2 weeks
D. Maintain testosterone dosage as is and counsel the patient regarding the expected timeline for masculinizing effects
E. Refer the patient to otolaryngology for consideration of surgical thyroplasty

5 A 26-year-old man presents for evaluation of infertility. His wife has had normal findings on fertility evaluation, has normal menstrual cycles, and had a previous pregnancy. They are having regular intercourse. The patient completed normal spontaneous puberty at age 13 years and reports normal libido and erectile function. He had a pituitary macroadenoma removed at age 24 years and is treated with daily transdermal testosterone gel, hydrocortisone, and levothyroxine. He takes methadone, 30 mg daily, as part of his recovery from opioid addiction.

On physical examination, he is normally virilized. He has some central adiposity (BMI 31 kg/m²). His blood pressure is 135/88 mm Hg, and pulse rate is 80 beats/min. He has normal male-pattern hair, including a beard. Testicular volume is 15 cc bilaterally.

Initial laboratory test results:

LH = 0.7 mIU/mL (1.0-9.0 mIU/mL)
(SI: 0.7 IU/L [1.0-9.0 IU/L])
FSH = 0.8 IU/mL (1.0-13.0 mIU/mL)
(SI: 0.8 IU/L [1.0-13.0 IU/L])
Total testosterone = 450 ng/dL (300-900 ng/dL)
(SI: 15.6 nmol/L [10.4-31.2 nmol/L])
Free T_4 = 1.0 ng/dL (0.8-1.8 ng/dL)
(SI: 12.9 pmol/L [10.3-23.17 pmol/L])
Semen analyses = 0.0 million sperm/mL

Transdermal testosterone gel is discontinued and hCG injections, 750 IU 3 times weekly, are initiated.

He returns for follow-up in 2 months and reports that he and his wife have not achieved fertility. He has not been ill and reports some decrease in libido.

Laboratory test results:

LH = 0.3 mIU/mL (1.0-9.0 mIU/mL)
(SI: 0.3 IU/L [1.0-9.0 IU/L])
FSH = 1.0 IU/mL (1.0-13.0 mIU/mL)
(SI: 1.0 IU/L [1.0-13.0 IU/L])
Testosterone = 200 ng/dL (300-900 ng/dL)
(SI: 6.9 nmol/L [10.4-31.2 nmol/L])
Semen analysis = 0.0 million sperm/mL

Which of the following is the most appropriate next step?

A. Add daily testosterone gel
B. Add recombinant FSH, 75 IU daily
C. In conjunction with his pain doctor, work to gradually decrease his methadone dosage to 10 mg daily
D. Increase the hCG dosage to 1500 IU 3 times weekly
E. Wait another 3 months before altering the current regimen

6 A 28-year-old man is concerned about recent-onset breast tenderness and swelling associated with weight loss, irritability, and insomnia. His only medication is extended-release methylphenidate, 50 mg daily, which he takes for attention-deficit disorder. He reports no use of anabolic steroids or recreational drugs.

On physical examination, his BMI is 23 kg/m² and pulse rate is 100 beats/min. He has normal facial, axillary, and pubic hair. He has 1-cm bilateral breast enlargement that is tender to palpation. Testicular volume is 20 cc bilaterally, and there are no palpable masses.

Laboratory test results:
    TSH = <0.01 mIU/L (0.5-5.0 mIU/L)
    Free T₄ = 4.6 ng/dL (0.8-1.8 ng/dL)
      (SI: 57.2 pmol/L [10.30-23.17 pmol/L])
    Total T₃ = 410 ng/dL (70-200 ng/dL)
      (SI: 6.31 nmol/L [1.08-3.08 nmol/L])

Which of the following hormone profiles would be expected in this patient with gynecomastia?

	Total testosterone	Free testosterone	Estradiol	LH
A.	Low	Low	High	Low
B.	High or high-normal	Low or low-normal	High	Normal
C.	Normal	Normal	High	Low
D.	High	High	High	High

7 A 19-year-old man is referred by his oncologist to discuss options for fertility preservation after a recent diagnosis of Hodgkin lymphoma, which will require treatment with alkylating agents. The patient is currently single but may wish to have children in the future.

On physical examination, testicular volume is 25 cc bilaterally.

Laboratory test results:
    Total testosterone = 280 ng/dL (300-900 ng/dL)
      (SI: 9.7 nmol/L [10.4-31.2 nmol/L])
    LH = 2.0 mIU/mL (1.0-9.0 mIU/mL)
      (SI: 2.0 IU/L [1.0-9.0 IU/L])
    Semen analysis = 11 million sperm/mL

Which of the following is the most reliable option for optimizing his potential to father children in the future?
  A. Combination of testosterone and progestin to suppress spermatogenesis during chemotherapy
  B. Cryopreservation of spermatogonial stem cells before chemotherapy for future transplant
  C. Sperm cryopreservation before chemotherapy
  D. Treatment with a GnRH agonist to suppress spermatogenesis during chemotherapy
  E. Treatment with hCG prior to cryopreservation

8 A 62-year-old man with a 10-year history of type 2 diabetes mellitus seeks help for erectile dysfunction. He reports a normal libido. He has hypertension and dyslipidemia. He takes lisinopril, 20 mg; atorvastatin, 40 mg daily; and metformin, 1000 mg twice daily. He checks his blood glucose once daily and reports fasting glucose values of 160 to 220 mg/dL (8.9-12.2 mmol/L). He has a sedentary desk job but is active, walking his dog 60 minutes daily without chest discomfort. He skis and hikes on the weekends. He has no family history of heart disease.

On physical examination, his blood pressure is 128/72 mm Hg, pulse rate is 68 beats/min, and BMI is 34 kg/m². He is well virilized, and testicular volume is 20 cc bilaterally. Findings on cardiopulmonary, abdominal, and neurologic examinations are normal.

Laboratory test results (sample drawn at 8 AM while fasting):
    Total testosterone = 420 ng/dL (300-900 ng/dL)
      (SI: 14.6 nmol/L [10.4-31.2 nmol/L])
    Total cholesterol = 215 mg/dL (<200 mg/dL [optimal]) (SI: 5.57 nmol/L [<5.18 mmol/L])
    HDL cholesterol = 42 mg/dL (>60 mg/dL [optimal]) (SI: 1.09 nmol/L [>1.55 mmol/L])
    LDL cholesterol = 115 mg/dL (<100 mg/dL [optimal]) (SI: 2.98 nmol/L [<2.59 mmol/L])
    Triglycerides = 190 mg/dL (<150 mmol/L [optimal]) (SI: 2.15 nmol/L [<1.70 mmol/L])
    Hemoglobin A₁c = 8.5% (4.0%-5.6%) (69 mmol/mol [20-38 mmol/mol])

Which of the following is the best next step for the management of this patient's erectile dysfunction?

  A. Addition of a second drug to treat his dyslipidemia
  B. Cardiac stress echocardiography
  C. Intensification of his glucose-lowering regimen
  D. Measurement of calculated free testosterone
  E. Trial of an oral phosphodiesterase inhibitor

9 A 60-year-old man is referred for consideration of hormone therapy for erectile dysfunction. He has been married for 1 year, and he and his wife, age 35 years, would like to conceive. He has 2 children from a previous marriage. He has type 2 diabetes mellitus, hypertension, and hyperlipidemia. He takes metformin, 500 mg twice daily; lisinopril, 10 mg daily; and atorvastatin, 20 mg daily. He reports normal libido. He has never smoked cigarettes, and he exercises on a treadmill 30 minutes daily. His current BMI is 29 kg/m². Prior to his second marriage, he reports that he lost 50 lb (22.7 kg) and markedly improved his glycemic control (hemoglobin A_{1c} 2 years ago was 8.9% [74 mmol/mol]). He has maintained this weight loss.

He was recently prescribed sildenafil, a phosphodiesterase inhibitor, and he started with half a pill and then increased to a full tablet with no notable improvement in erectile function over the next several months. His primary care physician measured his total testosterone (292 ng/dL [10.1 nmol/L]). He is eager to initiate additional therapies to improve his sexual function. His blood pressure is 132/76 mm Hg, and pulse rate is 74 beats/min.

Laboratory test results:
  Total testosterone = 320 ng/dL (300-900 ng/dL) (SI: 11.1 nmol/L [10.4-31.2 nmol/L])
  Free testosterone (calculated) = 11 ng/dL (9-30 ng/dL) (SI: 0.38 nmol/L [0.31-1.04 nmol/L])
  FSH = 3.0 mIU/mL (1.0-13.0 mIU/mL) (SI: 3.0 IU/L [1.0-13.0 IU/L])
  LH = 4.0 mIU/mL (1.0-9.0 mIU/mL) (SI: 4.0 IU/L [1.0-9.0 IU/L])

Hemoglobin A_{1c} = 6.8% (4.0%-5.6%) (51 mmol/mol [20-38 mmol/mol])
Total cholesterol = 195 mg/dL (<200 mg/dL [optimal]) (SI: 5.05 mmol/L [<5.18 mmol/L])
LDL cholesterol = 96 mg/dL (<100 mg/dL [optimal]) (SI: 2.49 mmol/L [<2.59 mmol/L])

Which of the following is the best next step in this patient's management?

  A. Increase his metformin dosage to 500 mg 3 times daily
  B. Start alprostadil injections
  C. Start finasteride
  D. Start subcutaneous hCG, 1000 IU 3 times weekly
  E. Start testosterone gel

10 A 72-year-old man is referred by his primary care physician for further management of hypogonadism diagnosed when he presented with decreased energy and libido. At baseline, he had 2 morning testosterone values in the hypogonadal range (190 and 215 ng/dL [6.6 and 7.5 nmol/L]) and a hematocrit measurement of 50% (0.50). He has received intramuscular injections of testosterone cypionate, 200 mg every 2 weeks, for the past 6 months. His libido has improved on this regimen, but he continues to feel tired and sometimes takes an afternoon nap. He does not smoke cigarettes.

On physical examination, his BMI is 36 kg/m². He is well virilized, he has normal findings on testicular examination, and his lungs are clear to auscultation. A trough testosterone level drawn before his next injection is 310 ng/dL (10.8 nmol/L), and his hematocrit is now 54% (0.54).

Which of the following is the best next step in this patient's management?

  A. Arrange for monthly phlebotomy
  B. Decrease his intramuscular testosterone dosage to 100 mg every 2 weeks
  C. Increase his intramuscular testosterone dosage to 250 mg every 2 weeks
  D. Schedule a sleep study
  E. Switch from testosterone cypionate to enanthate at the current dosage

11 A 73-year-old man wishes to discuss treatment options for newly diagnosed hypogonadism. He is not keen on the idea of having to apply a testosterone gel or patch daily and expresses a preference for injections. He has a history of depression and hypertension, which are both well-controlled on citalopram and lisinopril. He has no history of cardiovascular disease. He has read about the long-acting depot formulation of testosterone undecanoate. He likes the fact that the injection must only be administered every 10 weeks and asks for additional information about its safety profile.

Which of the following is a potential adverse effect that this patient might experience as a result of this regimen?
- A. Cough and shortness of breath following the injection
- B. Flu-like illness
- C. Jaundice
- D. Significant fluctuations in energy levels and mood
- E. Significant increase in blood pressure

12 A 38-year-old man is found to have a low testosterone concentration during an extensive laboratory evaluation performed as part of a health insurance screening with his new employer. He reports normal energy levels and sexual function and has no history of headaches or vision problems. He reports decreased sense of smell that he attributes to a recent viral infection. He goes to the gym regularly, drinks 1 to 2 cocktails per night, and follows a ketogenic diet.

On physical examination, his BMI is 28 kg/m². He has no gynecomastia. He has normal facial, axillary, and pubic hair. Testicular volume is 10 cc bilaterally, and he has a normal phallus.

Laboratory test results:
    Testosterone = 51 ng/dL (300-900 ng/dL)
        (SI: 1.8 nmol/L [10.4-31.2 nmol/L])
    LH = <1.0 mIU/mL (1.0-9.0 mIU/mL)
        (SI: <1.0 IU/L [1.0-9.0 IU/L])
    FSH = <1.0 mIU/mL (1.0-13.0 mIU/mL)
        (SI: <1.0 IU/L [1.0-13.0 IU/L])
    Hematocrit = 52% (41%-51%) (SI: 0.52 [0.41-0.51])

    Prolactin = 24 ng/mL (4-23 ng/mL)
        (SI: 1.04 nmol/L [0.17-1.00 nmol/L])

Pituitary MRI shows a 5-mm hypoenhancing lesion.

Which of the following is this patient's most likely diagnosis?
- A. Anabolic steroid use
- B. Hereditary hemochromatosis
- C. Kallmann syndrome
- D. Opioid use
- E. Prolactinoma

13 A primary care physician asks for help in interpreting the hormone profile of a male patient whom she suspects is taking anabolic steroids or supplements.

Laboratory test results:
    TSH= 0.8 mIU/L (0.5-5.0 mIU/L)
    Total testosterone = 950 ng/dL (300-900 ng/dL)
        (SI: 33.0 nmol/L [10.4-31.2 nmol/L])
    Estradiol = 15 pg/mL (4-40 pg/mL)
        (SI: 55.1 pmol/L [36.7-146.8 pmol/L])
    LH = 2.0 mIU/mL (1.0-9.0 mIU/mL)
        (SI: 2.0 IU/L [1.0-9.0 IU/L])
    FSH = 2.0 mIU/mL (1.0-13.0 mIU/mL)
        (SI: 2.0 IU/L [1.0-13.0 IU/L])
    HDL cholesterol = 30 mg/dL (>60 mg/dL
        [optimal]) (SI: 0.78 mmol/L [>1.55 mmol/L])

Which of the following regimens best explains this patient's hormone profile?
- A. Androgenic anabolic steroid plus an aromatase inhibitor
- B. Desiccated thyroid and DHEA
- C. Exogenous hCG
- D. 5α-reductase inhibitor
- E. Testosterone plus an aromatase inhibitor

14 A 67-year-old man seeks evaluation for inability to ejaculate. He reports a normal libido and is sexually active with his wife. He has noticed that it takes a little longer to get an erection than in the past, but he can still get and maintain one that is adequate for intercourse. He generally reaches orgasm but is concerned that there is no longer an ejaculate. His history is notable for hypertension and benign prostatic hyperplasia for which he takes hydrochlorothiazide, 12.5 mg daily, and tamsulosin, 0.4 mg daily.

On physical examination, his BMI is 31 kg/m^2 and blood pressure is 125/80 mm Hg. He is well virilized, and testicular volume is 15 cc bilaterally. Rectal examination reveals mild prostate enlargement. His morning testosterone concentration is 325 ng/dL (11.3 nmol/L).

Which of the following strategies is most likely to help his ejaculatory dysfunction?
- A. Initiate testosterone replacement
- B. Refer him to urology for transurethral resection of the prostate
- C. Start a phosphodiesterase-5 inhibitor
- D. Substitute dutasteride for tamsulosin
- E. Substitute spironolactone for hydrochlorothiazide

15 A 29-year-old man is referred for evaluation of hypogonadism 2 months after sustaining a head injury after being knocked off his motorcycle. Brain MRI findings are normal. He has made good progress since his accident but still has some problems with short-term memory and strength. His libido, which had been quite low when he was discharged from hospital, has begun to improve and he gets spontaneous erections a few times per week. He is married and would like to start a family in the next 1 to 2 years.

On physical examination, his BMI is 23 kg/m^2. He has normal secondary sexual characteristics and normal testicular size. His neurologic examination reveals no focal deficits.

Laboratory test results:
Total testosterone = 180 ng/dL (300-900 ng/dL)
(SI: 6.2 nmol/L [10.4-31.2 nmol/L])
LH = 3.9 mIU/mL (1.0-9.0 mIU/mL) (SI: 3.9 IU/L [1.0-9.0 IU/L])

Which of the following is the most appropriate next step in this patient's management?
- A. Reevaluate his hypothalamic-pituitary-gonadal axis in 6 months
- B. Start a phosphodiesterase-5 inhibitor
- C. Start testosterone replacement
- D. Start treatment with hCG

16 An 18-year-old man is referred for further evaluation of congenital hypogonadotropic hypogonadism. He has no sense of smell, which was confirmed by quantitative smell testing. There is no history of deafness. There is no family history of anosmia, delayed puberty, or hypogonadism.

On physical examination, his height is 67 in (170.2 cm) (BMI = 22 kg/m^2), and arm span is 70 in (177.8 cm). He has slight axillary hair and Tanner stage 2 pubic hair but no facial or chest hair. He has a normal phallus, and his testes measure 2 cc bilaterally. There is no evidence of synkinesia. Musculoskeletal examination shows syndactyly of the fingers and toes.

Laboratory test results:
Total testosterone = 52 ng/dL (300-900 ng/dL)
(SI: 1.8 nmol/L [10.4-31.2 nmol/L]
Gonadotropins, undetectable
IGF-1, low
Prolactin, normal
TSH, normal
Free T$_4$, normal
ACTH, normal

Pituitary MRI shows no structural abnormality.

A pathogenic variant in which of the following genes most likely underlies his presentation?
- A. *ANOS1*
- B. *CHD7*
- C. *GNRHR*
- D. *FGFR1*
- E. *NR0B1*

Obesity and Lipids Board Review

Sangeeta R. Kashyap, MD

1 A 42-year-old well-appearing woman with a history of type 2 diabetes mellitus controlled with diet and metformin (hemoglobin A_{1c} = 7.2% [55 mmol/mol]) underwent a Roux-en-Y gastric bypass 3 years ago. Her BMI was 45 kg/m2 prior to surgery. She had an uneventful recovery and lost 130 lb (60 kg) in 6 months. Her diabetes resolved immediately after surgery. Her current hemoglobin A_{1c} level is 5.3% (34 mmol/mol). She no longer takes metformin.

One year ago, she started having episodes of diaphoresis, heart pounding, and shakiness. She has not lost consciousness but recently began having difficulty speaking and thinking, which has been interfering with her professional life. These episodes occur 2 to 3 times per week during the day. She does not recall having any symptoms at night. She has gained 30 lb (13.6 kg) over the last year, as her carbohydrate intake increased.

Findings on physical examination are normal.

She undergoes a mixed-meal study following unrestricted carbohydrate ingestion for 3 days. Ninety minutes into the study, she develops palpitations, weakness, drowsiness, and blurred vision. Her plasma glucose concentration is 50 mg/dL (2.8 mmol/L).

Her symptoms improve several minutes after glucose ingestion.

Which of the following initial treatment options should be offered before discharge?
  A. Dietary modification and acarbose
  B. Ketogenic diet
  C. Liraglutide
  D. Propranolol
  E. Reversal of gastric bypass

2 A 40-year-old woman with a history of hyperlipidemia, prediabetes, and obesity (BMI = 33 kg/m²) comes for a follow-up appointment. Several months ago, she had a bout of major depression after the anniversary of her son's death. Despite engaging in psychotherapy, she began having suicidal thoughts and was referred to psychiatry. Her psychiatrist prescribed a medication, but after 8 weeks she noted a 12-lb (5.4-kg) weight gain and increased hunger. She is concerned that she will become diabetic if she continues to gain weight at this pace. She takes atorvastatin for hyperlipidemia.

Which of the following antidepressant drugs is most likely responsible for her initial weight gain?
  A. Amitriptyline
  B. Bupropion
  C. Fluoxetine
  D. Paroxetine
  E. Venlafaxine

3 A 22-year-old woman with class 3 obesity complicated by obstructive sleep apnea, impaired glucose tolerance, and polycystic ovary syndrome underwent gastric bypass surgery 9 months ago. She is able to tolerate small low-carbohydrate meals and has lost more than 50 lb (22.6 kg). Her current BMI is 36 kg/m², which is down from 45 kg/m2 prior to surgery. Her menses are now regular, and she and her husband are interested in pregnancy. She is adherent to her regimen of daily replacement supplements, including a chewable multivitamin, sublingual vitamin B_{12}, calcium citrate, vitamin D_3, and iron daily.

Which of the following is the most appropriate clinical advice for this patient regarding pregnancy planning?

A. Avoid pregnancy until she is weight stable (use a nonoral contraceptive agent)
B. Proceed with pregnancy as long as her hemoglobin A_{1c} level is in the normal range (ie, <5.7% [<39 mmol/mol])
C. Proceed with pregnancy as long as she increases vitamin supplementation dosages to those recommended during pregnancy
D. Proceed with pregnancy but advise her that breastfeeding after gastric bypass is contraindicated
E. Proceed with pregnancy with no need to monitor nutritional or micronutrient status as long as she is weight stable following bariatric surgery

4 A 64-year-old man with no clinical atherosclerotic cardiovascular disease seeks evaluation regarding his lipid panel. He has chronic atrial fibrillation, hyperlipidemia, and hypertension. Medications include metoprolol and atorvastatin, 80 mg daily. He drinks 10 to 12 alcoholic beverages per week and does not follow any specific meal plan. He eats at fast-food restaurants once or twice weekly.

His BMI is 33 kg/m², and blood pressure is 135/80 mm Hg.

Laboratory test results (8 AM, fasting):
Hemoglobin A_{1c} = 5.7% (4.0%-5.6%) (39 mmol/mol [20-38 mmol/mol])
Total cholesterol = 170 mg/dL (SI: 5.90 mmol/L)
Triglycerides = 385 mg/dL (SI: 4.35 mmol/L)
HDL cholesterol = 36 mg/dL (SI: 1.25 mmol/L)
LDL cholesterol = 57 mg/dL (SI: 1.98 mmol/L)
Non-HDL cholesterol = 134 mg/dL (SI: 4.65 mmol/L)
TSH = 1.7 mIU/L (0.5-5.0 mIU/L)

Which of the following is the best next step in the treatment of this patient's hyperlipidemia?

A. Change atorvastatin, 80 mg daily, to rosuvastatin, 40 mg daily, after measurement of apolipoprotein B
B. Refer him for nutritional counseling to reduce his intake of saturated fat and alcohol
C. Start fenofibrate, 145 mg once daily
D. Start niacin, 1000 mg twice daily

5 A 52-year-old man with a history of coronary artery disease status post stent of the right coronary artery seeks consultation for lipid management. His father had coronary artery disease in his late 40s. He has a history of atrial fibrillation, hypertension, and prediabetes and quit cigarette smoking 10 years ago. Following stent placement, he was prescribed atorvastatin, 80 mg daily, but was only able to tolerate 40 mg daily because of myalgias. Ezetimibe was subsequently prescribed to achieve target LDL-cholesterol levels.

His 6-month follow-up LDL-cholesterol measurement is 120 mg/dL (3.11 mmol/L). He has not been tolerant of either evolocumab or alirocumab due to severe injection site inflammation/swelling.

Which of the following steps would be expected to lower this patient's LDL cholesterol to target for secondary prevention?

A. Change atorvastatin to rosuvastatin, 20 mg daily
B. Start bempedoic acid
C. Start fenofibrate
D. Start niacin
E. Start omega-3 fatty acids, 4 g daily

6 A 35-year-old White woman with history of gastroesophageal reflux disease, dyslipidemia, mild liver steatosis, and polycystic ovary syndrome presents for weight management. Her BMI is 42 kg/m². She lost 15 lb (6.8 kg) with protein-sparing modified fasting and an aerobic exercise program, but she regained the weight within 2 years. She is interested in taking a medication that would help reduce weight, cardiovascular risk, and liver fat levels. She currently takes atorvastatin. She has a strong family history of coronary artery disease; her father had a myocardial infarction at age 55 years.

Which of the following agents would be most effective in achieving this patient's goals?

  A. Bupropion
  B. Orlistat
  C. Phentermine
  D. Semaglutide

7 A 44-year-old man with a history of type 2 diabetes mellitus, dyslipidemia, hypertension, and BMI of 38 kg/m2 presents for counseling regarding his weight and related conditions. He reports reduced energy and low back pain but is otherwise asymptomatic. He does not use tobacco or drink alcohol. His medications include metformin; atorvastatin, 40 mg daily; and lisinopril, 10 mg daily.

Laboratory test results:
  Hemoglobin A_{1c} = 7.2% (4.0%-5.6%) (55 mmol/mol [20-38 mmol/mol])
  LDL cholesterol = 95 mg/dL (SI: 2.46 mmol/L)
  Triglycerides = 320 mg/dL (SI: 3.62 mmol/L)
  ALT, normal
  AST, normal

Which of the following is the best initial approach to evaluate for nonalcoholic steatohepatitis in this patient?

  A. Assess for secondary causes of liver fibrosis, including alcohol history, hepatitis, and medications that can cause liver steatosis
  B. Calculate FIB-4 score and consider liver elastography
  C. No need to evaluate liver for nonalcoholic steatohepatitis, as his transaminase levels are normal
  D. Perform liver ultrasonography and prescribe vitamin E, as he is at high risk for nonalcoholic steatohepatitis

8 A 60-year-old woman with class 1 obesity and a history of prediabetes, ulcerative colitis, osteoarthritis, uncontrolled hypertension managed with 2 medications, and gout seeks advice regarding a healthy diet. She would like to lose 10 lb (4.5 kg) and better control her blood pressure. She has a positive family history of colorectal cancer in her mother and diabetes and coronary artery disease in her father.

She is provided with instructions to start a new meal plan. After 3 months of diligently following the plan, she has reduced her body weight by 12 lb (5.4 kg) and overall feels her quality of life has improved. Her blood pressure is better controlled, and she is now taking only 1 antihypertensive medication.

Which of the following meal plans did this patient most likely follow based on data from clinical trials?

  A. DASH diet
  B. Gluten-free diet
  C. Ketogenic diet
  D. Meal replacement shake plan
  E. Vegan diet

9 A 23-year-old man seeks help addressing high cholesterol. He was seen at a local health fair where he was told that his cholesterol was extremely high and that he should seek care.

On physical examination, he has small yellowish papules on his abdomen, lower back, and the extensor surfaces of his arms.

  Fasting lipid panel:
  Total cholesterol = 325 mg/dL (SI: 8.42 mmol/L)
  Triglycerides = 3450 mg/dL (SI: 38.99 mmol/L)
  HDL cholesterol = 30 mg/dL (SI: 0.78 mmol/L)
  LDL cholesterol, cannot be calculated

Which of the following abnormalities does this patient most likely have?

  A. Apolipoprotein *E2/E2*
  B. ATP-binding cassette A1 (ABCA1) deficiency
  C. LDL receptor deficiency
  D. Lipoprotein lipase deficiency
  E. Overproduction of apolipoprotein B

10 A new drug acting by which of the following mechanisms would be predicted to be an effective weight-loss medication?

  A. Ghrelin receptor antagonist
  B. GLP-1 receptor antagonist
  C. Leptin antagonist
  D. Melanocortin 4 receptor (MC4R) antagonist
  E. Neuropeptide Y (NPY) receptor agonist

11 An 18-year-old man is referred by an ophthalmologist after documentation of abnormal cholesterol levels. The patient describes progressive fatigue over the last 4 years. When his parents noticed clouding of his corneas, they took him to see an ophthalmologist who ordered the following laboratory tests (fasting):

HDL cholesterol = 6 mg/dL (SI: 0.16 mmol/L)
LDL cholesterol = 190 mg/dL (SI: 4.92 mmol/L)
Triglycerides = 290 mg/dL (SI: 3.28 mmol/L)

On physical examination, he is a thin, ill-appearing young man. His tonsils are normal color and size, and he has no tendinous xanthomas. Additional laboratory testing documents 3+ proteinuria and a serum creatinine concentration of 2.8 mg/dL (247.5 μmol/L).

Which of the following abnormalities does this patient most likely have?

A. ATP-binding cassette A1 (ABCA1) deficiency
B. Defective apolipoprotein B
C. Lecithin-cholesterol acyltransferase deficiency
D. Lipoprotein lipase deficiency
E. Surreptitious testosterone abuse

12 A 23-year-old Japanese woman seeks consultation after a high cholesterol level was documented during screening at a health fair. She is healthy, takes oral contraceptives and no other medications, and drinks 1 to 3 alcoholic beverages each week.

Fasting lipid levels:
Total cholesterol = 230 mg/dL (SI: 5.96 mmol/L)
HDL cholesterol = 110 mg/dL (SI: 2.85 mmol/L)
Triglycerides = 78 mg/dL (SI: 0.88 mmol/L)
LDL cholesterol = 104 mg/dL (SI: 2.69 mmol/L)

Which of the following is the most likely explanation for her lipid levels?

A. Apolipoprotein A1 deficiency
B. Cholesteryl ester transfer protein deficiency
C. Interference with lipid assays
D. Lipoprotein lipase deficiency
E. Oral contraceptive use

13 A 50-year-old woman comes to see you for help losing weight. She wants to start a diet, and her friend told her that a high-protein diet has been shown to be more effective than a low-fat diet in producing sustained weight loss. She does not care for meat and other high-fat foods but is willing to try a low-carbohydrate diet if that is the best way to lose weight. She asks your opinion at today's appointment.

Which of the following is the best recommendation to help this patient produce sustained weight loss?

A. High-protein diet
B. Intermittent fasting
C. Low-carbohydrate diet
D. Mediterranean diet
E. Any diet to which the patient can adhere

14 A 25-year-old woman is referred for evaluation of increased cholesterol levels. She is under the care of several other physicians for progressive ataxia, a seizure disorder, and behavioral problems. She developed cataracts as an adolescent. Her family history includes a maternal uncle with premature coronary artery disease.

On physical examination, she has bilateral Achilles tendon thickening.

Fasting lipid profile:
Total cholesterol = 301 mg/dL (SI: 7.80 mmol/L)
Triglycerides = 130 mg/dL (SI: 1.47 mmol/L)
HDL cholesterol = 51 mg/dL (SI: 1.32 mmol/L)
LDL cholesterol = 130 mg/dL (SI: 3.37 mmol/L)

Which of the following is the most likely cause of her lipid profile?

A. Cerebrotendinous xanthomatosis
B. Familial combined heterozygous hyperlipidemia
C. Familial defective apolipoprotein B_{100}
D. Familial hypercholesterolemia
E. Sitosterolemia

15 A 45-year-old woman is concerned about her weight. She says that her mother had obesity but her father was thin. She wonders whether her genetic risk could be determined.

On the basis of available evidence, how much of the variance of BMI in unselected populations of adults can be explained by genetic polymorphisms identified to date in genome-wide association studies?

A. 2% to 4%

B. 10% to 30%

C. 40% to 60%

D. 70% to 85%

16 A 55-year-old woman is concerned about high cholesterol. Menopause occurred 3 years ago. She does not have diabetes or cardiovascular disease. However, she is concerned because her father had a myocardial infarction at age 45 years. He was treated aggressively with atorvastatin, 80 mg daily, and ezetimibe, 10 mg daily, and is doing well at age 85 years.

Fasting lipid profile:

Analyte	Baseline	After change to vegan diet	Reference ranges
Total cholesterol	252 mg/dL (SI: 6.53 mmol/L)	239 mg/dL (SI: 6.19 mmol/L)	<200 mg/dL (SI: <5.18 mmol/L)
LDL cholesterol	169 mg/dL (SI: 4.38 mmol/L)	123 mg/dL (SI: 3.19 mmol/L)	<100 mg/dL (SI: <2.59 mmol/L)
HDL cholesterol	47 mg/dL (SI: 1.22 mmol/L)	41 mg/dL (SI: 1.06 mmol/L)	>60 mg/dL (SI: >1.55 mmol/L)
Triglycerides	214 mg/dL (SI: 2.42 mmol/L)	374 mg/dL (SI: 4.23 mmol/L)	<150 mg/dL (SI: <1.70 mmol/L)

Measurements of TSH and fasting glucose are normal. Her 10-year cardiovascular disease risk is estimated to be 6.3%. She does not want to take a statin. She undergoes CT to determine her coronary artery calcium score, which returns as "0." She elects to follow a vegan diet rich in olive oil and low in saturated fat. Six months later, her LDL-cholesterol value is 123 mg/dL (3.19 mmol/L).

Which of the following is the best next test to assess her risk of cardiovascular disease?

A. Apolipoprotein B measurement

B. Chylomicron measurement

C. Lipoprotein (a) measurement

D. Non–HDL-cholesterol measurement

E. Nuclear magnetic resonance spectroscopy

17 A 37-year-old man seeks evaluation for hyperlipidemia. A cholesterol panel was done 1 year ago, and a repeated panel was done last week.

Measurement	Last year	Current
Total cholesterol	190 mg/dL (SI: 4.92 mmol/L)	220 mg/dL (SI: 5.70 mmol/L)
Triglycerides	115 mg/dL (SI: 1.30 mmol/L)	130 mg/dL (SI: 1.47 mmol/L)
LDL cholesterol	123 mg/dL (SI: 3.19 mmol/L)	150 mg/dL (SI: 3.89 mmol/L)
HDL cholesterol	43 mg/dL (SI: 1.11 mmol/L)	44 mg/dL (SI: 1.14 mmol/L)

He is concerned about the increase in his cholesterol. Since his cholesterol was checked 1 year ago, he has gained 6 lb (2.7 kg) (BMI 28 kg/m²). He reports working longer hours (sedentary desk job), sleeping less, and feeling quite fatigued. He has changed his diet and eliminated fried foods and sweets but struggles with constipation. He drinks 2 glasses of red wine daily. He has been exercising regularly to lose weight. His wife states that he has been snoring a lot lately. He has a family history of type 2 diabetes, but his hemoglobin A_{1c} value last year was 5.2% (33 mmol/mol).

Which of the following is the most likely cause of this patient's increased cholesterol?

A. Alcohol intake

B. Hypothyroidism

C. Sleep apnea

D. Undiagnosed diabetes mellitus

18 A 45-year-old woman seeks help losing weight. She has a seizure disorder and was prescribed increasing dosages of gabapentin 2 years ago for this problem. She now takes gabapentin, 600 mg 3 times daily. Since starting this medication, she has gained 30 lb (13.6 kg); her current BMI is 39 kg/m². She has depression, for which her neurologist prescribed fluoxetine, 20 mg daily. Her hemoglobin A_{1c} level is 6.2% (44 mmol/mol), but she is not being treated for diabetes.

Which of the following is most likely to produce and sustain the most weight loss over the next 12 months in this patient?
   A. Begin a low-carbohydrate diet
   B. Change from fluoxetine to bupropion
   C. Change from gabapentin to topiramate
   D. Initiate treatment with metformin

19 A 36-year-old woman with a peak lifetime BMI of 46 kg/m² had a laparoscopic gastric bypass operation in another state 8 weeks ago. She initially did well, but over the last 3 weeks she has had episodes of vomiting. Over the last 5 days, she has been vomiting almost everything she eats. Over the last 2 days, her husband says that she has become increasingly confused, dysarthric, and unsteady on her feet. On neurologic examination, she is clearly confused, has nystagmus, is unsteady on standing, has decreased sensation in her lower extremities, and has a right third nerve palsy.

This patient most likely has a deficiency of which of the following?
   A. Folate
   B. Thiamine
   C. Vitamin B_{12}
   D. Zinc

20 A 44-year-old man recently presented with new-onset angina and a positive exercise stress test. He reports no history of hypertension, diabetes mellitus, or cigarette smoking. He follows no specific diet but exercises regularly. His father died of a myocardial infarction at age 45 years, and his brother underwent a revascularization procedure at age 46 years. His father and brother had lipid abnormalities characterized by high triglycerides and low HDL cholesterol. The patient's physical examination findings are normal.

Fasting lipid levels:
   Total cholesterol = 270 mg/dL (SI: 6.99 mmol/L)
   Triglycerides = 300 mg/dL (SI: 3.39 mmol/L)
   HDL cholesterol = 30 mg/dL (SI: 0.78 mmol/L)
   LDL cholesterol = 180 mg/dL (SI: 4.66 mmol/L)

Which of the following best explains his lipid profile?
   A. Apolipoprotein A1 deficiency
   B. Familial combined hyperlipidemia
   C. Familial defective apolipoprotein B
   D. Familial hypercholesterolemia
   E. Lipoprotein lipase deficiency

21 A 27-year-old woman with a history of hypertriglyceridemia and pancreatitis has controlled her hypertriglyceridemia reasonably well with diet and fenofibrate. Her triglyceride concentrations on this program have ranged from 595 to 880 mg/dL (6.72 to 9.94 mmol/L). She has 2 children, aged 4 and 7 years, and she developed gestational diabetes during her last pregnancy. She was not prescribed oral contraceptive pills because of hypertriglyceridemia. She now returns 8 months after her last visit and states that she is 26 weeks pregnant and stopped taking fenofibrate.

Laboratory test results:
   Total cholesterol = 300 mg/dL (SI: 7.77 mmol/L)
   Triglycerides = 815 mg/dL (SI: 9.21 mmol/L)
   HDL cholesterol = 31 mg/dL (SI: 0.80 mmol/L)
   Fasting glucose = 105 mg/dL (SI: 5.8 mmol/L)
   Hemoglobin A_{1c} = 7.0% (53 mmol/mol)

Which of the following is the most reasonable strategy now?
   A. Resume fenofibrate
   B. Substitute atorvastatin for fenofibrate
   C. Substitute nicotinic acid for fenofibrate
   D. Substitute omega-3 fatty acids for fenofibrate

22 A 53-year-old woman has an abnormal lipid profile that was documented as part of routine testing ordered by her primary care physician after menopause. Her total cholesterol concentration is greater than 600 mg/dL (>15.54 mmol/L) with an equal increase in triglycerides. She has been in good health and has no personal or family history of vascular disease. After menopause, she gained 20 lb (9.1 kg), and during the past year she has attempted to reduce her weight with a high-fat, low-carbohydrate diet. On this diet, her BMI has decreased from 35 to 29 kg/m^2. Thyroid function is normal. She has palmar xanthomas.

Which of the following would determine the underlying pathophysiology for this patient's disorder?

   A. Apolipoprotein A1 measurement
   B. Apolipoprotein E genotyping
   C. Assessment of LDL particle size
   D. Lipoprotein (a) genotyping

23 A 27-year-old man is referred because of low blood cholesterol levels.

Laboratory test results:
   Total cholesterol = 56 mg/dL (SI: 1.45 mmol/L)
   HDL cholesterol = 24 mg/dL (SI: 0.62 mmol/L)
   LDL cholesterol = 24 mg/dL (SI: 0.62 mmol/L)
   Triglycerides = 38 mg/dL (SI: 0.43 mmol/L)

BMI is 24 kg/m^2. He has no obvious medical conditions.

He is advised regarding lifestyle modifications. Which of the following is one possible complication from this patient's condition?

   A. Coronary artery disease
   B. Kidney failure
   C. Myositis
   D. Nonalcoholic fatty liver disease
   E. Tonsillitis

24 A patient with prediabetes and hypertension presents for ongoing care. When her weight is mentioned during the consultation, she becomes frustrated, saying health care providers always focus on her weight but that there is no evidence that she will live longer if she loses weight.

On physical examination, her height is 66 in (167.6 cm) and weight is 234 lb (106.4 kg) (BMI = 37.8 kg/m^2). Her blood pressure is 138/76 mm Hg, pulse rate is 86 beats/min, and respiratory rate is 16 breaths/min. Examination findings are otherwise unremarkable.

Laboratory test results:
   Hemoglobin A$_{1c}$ = 6.4% (4.0%-5.6%) (46 mmol/mol [20-38 mmol/mol])
   Total cholesterol = 220 mg/dL (SI: 5.70 mmol/L)
   Triglycerides = 380 mg/dL (SI: 4.29 mmol/L)
   HDL cholesterol = 36 mg/dL (SI: 0.93 mmol/L)
   LDL cholesterol = 108 mg/dL (SI: 2.80 mmol/L)

In which of the following groups has weight loss been shown to reduce mortality in randomized controlled trials?

   A. Persons with obesity treated with gastric bypass surgery
   B. Persons with obesity who are treated with weight-loss medications
   C. Persons with prediabetes treated with lifestyle intervention
   D. Persons with type 2 diabetes treated with lifestyle intervention

25 A 42-year-old woman with polycystic ovary syndrome is referred for weight management. Polycystic ovary syndrome was diagnosed at age 15 years. She gained weight through college and during her first job, which was very sedentary. She had a baby at age 36 years with the assistance of clomiphene but had difficulty losing weight after delivery. She has lost 18 lb (8.2 kg) over the last 6 months by participating in a commercial weight-loss program and exercising regularly, but her weight has plateaued. She has a history of migraines, prediabetes, fatty liver, and depression. Current medications include metformin and a selective serotonin reuptake inhibitor. She also has gallstones, which were noted on abdominal ultrasonography 6 months ago. Her BMI is 38 kg/m².

Which of the following should be recommended for continued weight loss?

A. Liraglutide, 3.0 mg daily
B. Naltrexone/bupropion
C. Orlistat
D. Phentermine/topiramate

26 A 36-year-old woman has been working to lose weight and improve her health. Her height is 67 in (170.2 cm), and weight is 245 lb (111.4 kg) (BMI = 38.4 kg/m²). She has type 2 diabetes mellitus and dyslipidemia. A low–glycemic index, reduced-calorie diet (–500 kcal daily) is recommended in addition to a regimen of aerobic exercise (walking on a treadmill for an hour) 5 days a week and resistance training 3 days a week. She keeps a daily food diary with an app on her phone. She has lost 40 lb (18.2 kg) over 2 years, but over the last 3 months, she regained 8 lb (3.6 kg). Her phone app food diary shows that she is consuming 1200 to 1400 kcal daily. She states she has maintained her exercise regimen, which is confirmed by her pedometer. She is frustrated and very concerned about the weight regain.

Which of the following is the main cause of her weight regain?

A. Decreased energy expenditure
B. Decreased satiety
C. Increased appetite
D. Increased energy expenditure

Pituitary Board Review

Laurence Katznelson, MD

1 A 42-year-old man with headaches is evaluated with MRI and is found to have a 2.6-cm sellar mass that extends into the left cavernous sinus. His headaches have been worsening over the past 2 months. He describes normal vision. In retrospect, he has had reduced libido over the preceding 6 months, along with progressive erectile dysfunction. He has also noted more fatigue and reduced short-term memory.

On physical examination, he is a tired-appearing man. His blood pressure is 96/66 mm Hg, pulse rate is 96 beats/min, and BMI is 31.1 kg/m². Examination findings are unremarkable except for increased abdominal girth.

Laboratory test results:

Random cortisol (midafternoon) = 7.8 µg/dL (SI: 215.2 nmol/L)

Testosterone = 121 ng/dL (300-900 ng/dL) (SI: 4.2 nmol/L [10.4-31.2 nmol/L])

LH = 0.4 mIU/mL (1.0-9.0 mIU/mL) (SI: 0.4 IU/L [1.0-9.0 IU/L])

FSH = 2.1 mIU/mL (1.0-13.0 mIU/mL) (SI: 2.1 IU/L [1.0-13.0 IU/L])

IGF-1 = 45 ng/mL (98-261 ng/mL) (SI: 5.9 nmol/L [12.8-34.2 nmol/L])

Prolactin = 142 ng/mL (4-23 ng/mL) (SI: 6.17 nmol/L [0.17-1.00 nmol/L])

TSH = 0.3 mIU/L (0.5-5.0 mIU/L)

Free T₄ = 0.9 ng/dL (0.8-1.8 ng/dL) (SI: 11.58 pmol/L [10.30-23.17 pmol/L])

Transsphenoidal surgery with an experienced neurosurgeon reveals an SF-1 staining pituitary adenoma. Postoperative MRI scan shows residual tumor in the left cavernous sinus. Repeated MRI 6 months later shows growth of the cavernous sinus tumor.

Which of the following treatments is the best choice now to manage the residual tumor and control tumor growth?
  A. Another surgery
  B. Bromocriptine
  C. Cabergoline
  D. Octreotide long-acting release
  E. Stereotactic radiotherapy

2 A 41-year-old woman presents with acromegaly. She previously underwent transsphenoidal surgery for a macroadenoma, and she has residual disease in the left cavernous sinus. Her postoperative IGF-1 concentration was 932 ng/mL (98-261 ng/mL) (SI: 122.1 nmol/L [12.8-34.2 nmol/L]). Octreotide long-acting release, 20 mg monthly, was initiated, which lowered her IGF-1 concentration to 850 ng/mL (111.4 nmol/L). The octreotide dosage was increased to 30 mg monthly, but her IGF-1 concentration remains unchanged and the tumor is slightly larger on MRI.

Which of the following interventions would best reduce this patient's tumor size and IGF-1 levels in the next 6 months?
  A. Add cabergoline
  B. Add pegvisomant
  C. Perform stereotactic radiotherapy
  D. Switch to pasireotide
  E. Switch to the oral octreotide capsule

3 A 35-year-old man is interested in fertility. He has history of a clinically nonfunctioning pituitary macroadenoma with surgical removal at age 31 years. Following the surgery, he had panhypopituitarism and he currently takes hormone replacement with levothyroxine, hydrocortisone, GH, and transdermal testosterone. He has good energy and states he has normal libido and erectile function.

On physical examination, he is well virilized, with 10-mL testes bilaterally that have normal consistency. Semen analysis documents azoospermia.

Which of the following is the best next step in this patient's management?

A. Add an aromatase inhibitor
B. Refer for microdissection testicular sperm extraction
C. Switch from transdermal testosterone to clomiphene citrate
D. Switch from transdermal testosterone to hCG injections, 3 times weekly
E. Switch from transdermal testosterone to hCG injections, 3 times weekly, and FSH injections, twice weekly

4 A 45-year-old man underwent surgery for Cushing disease 3 years ago. He was prescribed glucocorticoids postoperatively, but these were discontinued 3 months later. His hypertension and hyperglycemia resolved. Recently, he has noticed facial rounding, plethora, and increased abdominal fat. He has again become hyperglycemic with a hemoglobin A_{1c} level of 7.3% (56 mmol/mol). A late-night salivary cortisol measurement is elevated. MRI shows no clear evidence of tumor. He decides to start medical treatment for Cushing disease, which reduces his signs and symptoms and improves his blood pressure.

Analytes and clinical findings	Before medical therapy	After 2 weeks of medical therapy
Urinary free cortisol	89 µg/24 h (SI: 246 nmol/d)	112 µg/24 h (SI: 309 nmol/d)
ACTH	48 pg/mL (SI: 10.6 pmol/L)	63 pg/mL (SI: 13.9 pmol/L)
Fasting glucose	113 mg/dL (SI: 6.3 mmol/L)	92 mg/dL (SI: 5.1 mmol/L)
Blood pressure	135/84 mm Hg	128/84 mm Hg

Reference ranges: urinary free cortisol, 4-50 µg/24 h (SI: 11-138 nmol/d); ACTH, 10-60 pg/mL (SI: 2.2-13.2 pmol/L); fasting glucose, 70-99 mg/dL (SI: 3.9-5.5 mmol/L).

Which of the following medications did this patient receive?

A. Cabergoline
B. Levoketoconazole
C. Mifepristone
D. Osilodrostat
E. Pasireotide long-acting release

5 A 41-year-old man presents with fatigue. His history is notable for a severe frontal, throbbing headache 8 months earlier that came on suddenly and lasted 4 days. He decided not to go to a hospital at that time. Since then, he has noted progressive fatigue. He has a distant history of renal cell carcinoma and underwent total resection and is currently in remission. He has no polyuria or polydipsia.

On physical examination, he appears fatigued but comfortable. His blood pressure is 96/68 mm Hg, and pulse rate is 74 beats/min. He has increased abdominal girth.

Laboratory test results:
Fasting blood glucose = 109 mg/dL (70-99 mg/dL) (SI: 6.0 mmol/L [3.9-5.5 mmol/L])
TSH = 1.2 mIU/L (0.5-5.0 mIU/L)
Free T_4 = 1.3 ng/dL (0.8-1.8 ng/dL) (SI: 16.73 pmol/L [10.30-23.17 pmol/L])
Cortisol (8 AM) = 15 µg/dL (5-25 µg/dL) (SI: 413.8 nmol/L [137.9-689.7 nmol/L])
Total testosterone (8 AM) = 250 ng/dL (300-900 ng/dL) (SI: 8.7 nmol/L [10.4-31.2 nmol/L])
IGF-1 = 82 ng/mL (98-261 ng/mL) (SI: 10.7 nmol/L [12.8-34.2 nmol/L])

MRI shows empty sella with irregularity of soft tissue along the left side of the sellar floor.

Which of the following is this patient's most likely diagnosis?

A. Craniopharyngioma
B. Lymphocytic hypophysitis
C. Metastasis to the sella
D. Neurosarcoidosis
E. Pituitary apoplexy

6 A 27-year-old woman (G0) presents for evaluation after her gynecologist noted hyperprolactinemia. She had menarche at age 12 years and has always had normal menses. In the past 8 months, she noted scant, bilateral nipple discharge, but this does not bother her. She is considering fertility although not for a few years. Her gynecologist measured a cycle day 21 serum progesterone concentration, which was low. She has no headaches, hirsutism, or acne.

On physical examination, she appears comfortable. Her blood pressure is 96/68 mm Hg, and pulse rate is 74 beats/min. There are no physical stigmata of acromegaly or Cushing disease. She has scant bilateral nipple discharge on palpation. Her breast examination findings are otherwise normal.

Laboratory test results:
Prolactin = 54 ng/mL (4-30 ng/mL)
(SI: 2.35 nmol/L [0.17-1.30 nmol/L])
IGF-1 = 185 ng/mL (117-321 ng/mL)
(SI: 24.2 nmol/L [15.3-42.1 nmol/L])
TSH = 2.5 mIU/L (0.5-5.0 mIU/L)
Free T_4 = 1.3 ng/dL (0.8-1.8 ng/dL)
(SI:16.73 pmol/L [10.30-23.17 pmol/L])

MRI reveals a 7-mm hypoenhancing abnormality in the left side of the sella, with mild deviation of the stalk to the right.

Which of the following is the most appropriate next step in this patient's management?
A. Another pituitary MRI in 6 months
B. Cabergoline therapy
C. Prolactin measurement with serial dilution
D. Repeated clinical assessment and laboratory monitoring in 6 months
E. Stereotactic radiotherapy

7 A 24-year-old woman is referred for endocrine evaluation. Her parents report that she received GH injections since age 1 year for growth failure and GH deficiency. Her growth rate was appropriate while on treatment. At age 9 years, she developed fatigue and weight gain, and laboratory tests revealed the following:

TSH = 0.2 mIU/L (0.5-5.0 mIU/L)
Free T_4 = 0.3 ng/dL (0.8-1.8 ng/dL) (SI: 3.9 pmol/L [10.30-23.17 pmol/L])

Levothyroxine was initiated at that time. Menarche occurred at age 11 years, and her periods have always been regular. At age 15 years, she was in a bike accident and had brief loss of consciousness. Concussion was subsequently diagnosed. She stopped taking GH when she completed growth at age 18 years. She has no polyuria or polydipsia.

Laboratory test results (ordered by the referring physician):
Prolactin = 2 ng/mL (4-30 ng/mL) (SI: 0.09 nmol/L [0.17-1.30 nmol/L])
Free T_4 = 1.3 ng/dL (0.8-1.8 ng/dL) (SI: 16.7 pmol/L [10.30-23.17 pmol/L])
LH = 13.0 mIU/mL (1.0-18.0 mIU/L [follicular]) (SI: 13.0 IU/L [1.0-18.0 IU/L])
FSH = 9.0 mIU/mL (2.0-12.0 mIU/L [follicular]) (SI: 9.0 IU/L [1.0-13.0 IU/L])

A 250-mcg intravenous cosyntropin-stimulation test results in a 60-minute serum cortisol value of 23 μg/dL (635 nmol/L). Brain MRI reveals a slight reduction in sellar contents.

On physical examination, she has normal vital signs and appears euthyroid.

Which of the following is the most likely cause of these biochemical findings?
A. Langerhans cell histiocytosis
B. Hypopituitarism following brain injury
C. Pathogenic variant in the *POU1F1* gene
D. Pathogenic variant in the *PROP1* gene
E. Pathogenic variant in the *TBX19 (TPIT)* gene

8 A 65-year-old man has a history of renal cell cancer with metastases to the lung. He has been undergoing chemotherapy, including treatment with nivolumab. Approximately 5 months earlier, he complained of headache, and findings on brain MRI were normal. Over the past 3 weeks, he has noted abrupt onset of frequent urination and increased thirst, along with new headaches. MRI is performed, which documents a 1.5-cm hypoenhancing sellar mass.

On physical examination, he is a tired-appearing man. His blood pressure is 98/66 mm Hg, pulse rate is 92 beats/min, and BMI is 21.1 kg/m².

Laboratory test results:
    Serum sodium = 152 mEq/L (136-142 mEq/L)
        (SI: 152 mmol/L [136-142 mmol/L])
    Prolactin = 53 ng/mL (4-30 ng/mL)
        (SI: 2.3 nmol/L [0.17-1.30 nmol/L])
    Plasma glucose = 89 mg/dL (70-99 mg/dL)
        (SI: 4.9 mmol/L [3.9-5.5 mmol/L])
    Free T$_4$ = 0.9 ng/dL (0.8-1.8 ng/dL)
        (SI: 11.6 pmol/L [10.30-23.17 pmol/L])
    TSH = 0.8 mIU/L (0.5-5.0 mIU/L)

Which of the following is the most likely diagnosis?
    A. Clinically nonfunctioning pituitary adenoma
    B. Histiocytosis
    C. Metastasis
    D. Nivolumab-induced hypophysitis
    E. Prolactinoma

9 A 42-year-old man reports fatigue, weight gain, and decreased strength. He describes worsening short-term memory recall, and he has felt slightly more depressed than usual. He has a known history of a pituitary adenoma, and he underwent transsphenoidal surgery 3 years ago. Since the operation, he has had normal thyroid and adrenal function. He has normal libido but has had some difficulty maintaining an erection over the past year. On physical examination, he is overweight, with increased abdominal girth.

Laboratory test results:
    Complete blood cell count, normal
    Fasting blood glucose = 123 mg/dL (70-99 mg/dL)
        (SI: 6.8 mmol/L [3.9-5.5 mmol/L])
    TSH = 1.2 mIU/L (0.5-5.0 mIU/L)
    Free T$_4$ = 1.5 ng/dL (0.8-1.8 ng/dL)
        (SI: 19.3 pmol/L [10.30-23.17 pmol/L])
    Cortisol (8 AM) = 16 μg/dL (5-25 μg/dL)
        (SI: 441.4 nmol/L [137.9-689.7 nmol/L])

Total testosterone (8 AM) = 250 ng/dL
    (300-900 ng/dL) (SI: 8.7 nmol/L
    [10.4-31.2 nmol/L])
IGF-1 = 95 ng/mL (98-261 ng/mL)
    (SI: 12.4 nmol/L [12.8-34.2 nmol/L])

Which of the following tests should be performed to determine the cause of this patient's signs and symptoms?
    A. Cosyntropin-stimulation test
    B. Glucagon-stimulation test with measurement of GH
    C. Gonadotropin measurement
    D. IGFBP-3 measurement
    E. Morning GH measurement

10 A 38-year-old woman presents with symptoms of weight loss, tremor, palpitations, and sweating that have been progressive over the past 4 months. She has had mild frontal headaches, and her menses are irregular.

On physical examination, her blood pressure is 150/95 mm Hg and pulse rate is 96 beats/min. She has no proptosis. She has an enlarged, nontender thyroid gland. Her skin is moist and warm.

Laboratory test results:
    Free T$_4$ = 2.8 ng/dL (0.8-1.8 ng/dL)
        (SI: 36.0 pmol/L [10.30-23.17 pmol/L])
    Total T$_3$ = 413 ng/dL (70-200 ng/dL)
        (SI: 6.36 nmol/L [1.08-3.08 nmol/L])
    TSH = 1.9 mIU/L (0.5-5.0 mIU/L)
    Prolactin = 28 ng/mL (4-30 ng/mL)
        (SI: 1.21 nmol/L [0.17-1.30 nmol/L])

A radioiodine scan reveals 50% uptake in a homogeneous pattern in the thyroid gland.

Which of the following is the best next step to confirm this patient's diagnosis?
    A. Assessment for a pathogenic variant in the thyroid hormone receptor gene
    B. Assessment of TSH response to a trial of cabergoline
    C. Diagnostic trial of thyroid hormone
    D. α-Subunit measurement
    E. Thyroid-stimulating immunoglobulin measurement

11 A 33-year-old woman has had partial hypopituitarism for 10 years after successful resection of a corticotroph pituitary adenoma. She has been treated with hydrocortisone, levothyroxine, and a low-dosage oral contraceptive pill. Given progressive fatigue, she undergoes testing for GH reserve, and she is found to have GH deficiency. She opts to start GH replacement.

Which of the following may occur after initiation of GH replacement in this patient?
- A. A decrease in blood glucose
- B. A need to increase the hydrocortisone dosage
- C. A need to reduce the oral contraceptive pill dosage
- D. A need to reduce the levothyroxine dosage
- E. An increase in serum prolactin

12 A 44-year-old woman undergoes transsphenoidal surgery for a clinically nonfunctioning pituitary macroadenoma. Immediately following surgery, she is found to have normal adrenal function, and she is discharged home on day 3 without evidence of diabetes insipidus. On day 7, she calls the clinic and describes nausea and fatigue. On day 8, she has laboratory tests and is admitted to the intensive care unit after the following results are documented:

Serum sodium = 118 mEq/L (136-142 mEq/L) (SI: 118 mmol/L [136-142 mmol/L])

Urine osmolality = 373 mOsm/kg (150-1150 mOsm/kg) (SI: 373 mmol/kg [150-1150 mmol/kg])

On physical examination, her blood pressure is 125/84 mm Hg and pulse rate is 84 beats/min. Her weight is 130 lb (59 kg). She is fatigued but answers questions appropriately. Her volume status appears normal.

Which of the following is the most rapid and effective method to correct her serum sodium?
- A. Restrict free water intake to less than 1500 mL/24 h
- B. Start demeclocycline
- C. Start hypertonic saline at a rate of 5 mL/h
- D. Start intravenous normal saline at a rate of 200 mL/h
- E. Start tolvaptan

13 Acromegaly is diagnosed in a 63-year-old woman. Initial MRI shows a 1.3-cm pituitary tumor with minimal extension superiorly and laterally. After transsphenoidal surgery with an experienced neurosurgeon, she still has some residual tumor in the left cavernous sinus. She has persistent, unremitting frontal headaches, and her arthralgias are painful. Hypertension persists following surgery. Her postoperative GH level is 3.0 ng/mL (3.0 μg/L) and it does not suppress with hyperglycemia after a glucose load. Her IGF-1 level is 624 ng/mL (72-207 ng/mL) (SI: 81.7 nmol/L [9.4-27.1 nmol/L]).

Which of the following treatment options should be recommended now as the next step?
- A. Another transsphenoidal surgery
- B. Cabergoline
- C. Lanreotide depot monthly
- D. Pegvisomant weekly
- E. Stereotactic radiosurgery to address the residual tumor

14 A 41-year-old woman presents with amenorrhea and galactorrhea and is found to have a prolactin concentration of 152 ng/mL (4-30 ng/mL) (SI: 6.61 nmol/L [0.17-1.30 nmol/L]). MRI documents a 2.4-cm pituitary adenoma that abuts the optic chiasm. While taking bromocriptine, 2.5 mg daily, her prolactin level decreases to 18 ng/mL (0.78 nmol/L), menses return but are irregular, and galactorrhea improves. Follow-up MRI in 3 months shows no change in adenoma size. She asks whether this management is sufficient for long-term care.

Which of the following should be the next management step?
- A. Administer octreotide long-acting release
- B. Discuss surgery
- C. Increase the bromocriptine dosage
- D. Perform pituitary-directed MRI in 6 months
- E. Switch bromocriptine to cabergoline

15 A 37-year-old woman with amenorrhea and galactorrhea is found to have a prolactin concentration of 1593 ng/mL (69.3 nmol/L) and a 2.6-cm pituitary macroadenoma on MRI. With cabergoline, 0.5 mg twice weekly, prolactin levels normalize and the tumor size decreases to 7 mm. Over the next 18 months (while taking her medication regularly), her prolactin level increases to 284 ng/mL (12.3 nmol/L) and her tumor grows to 1.4 cm. Despite a gradual increase in the cabergoline dosage to 2 mg daily over the next year, her prolactin concentration rises to 4513 ng/mL (196.2 nmol/L) and her tumor grows to 3.2 cm and involves the local parenchyma. She subsequently undergoes a 2-stage transsphenoidal/transcranial near-total resection and stereotactic radiosurgery. Over the ensuing 8 months, the tumor continues to grow into the temporal and frontal lobes.

Which of the following treatments is the best choice now?

   A. Another craniotomy
   B. Conventional radiotherapy
   C. Octreotide long-acting release
   D. Pasireotide
   E. Temozolomide

16 A 28-year-old woman has had amenorrhea for 4 years and is found to have a serum prolactin concentration of 48.3 ng/mL (2.1 nmol/L). Evaluation documents normal thyroid, kidney, and hepatic function and a negative pregnancy test. MRI reveals a 4-mm hypointense area in the pituitary gland compatible with a microadenoma. Although she is sexually active, she is not planning to get pregnant for at least 4 to 5 years. She has poor health insurance and is concerned about the cost of medications.

Which of the following is the best treatment plan for this patient?

   A. Bromocriptine
   B. Cabergoline
   C. Oral contraceptives
   D. Reassurance and observation
   E. Transsphenoidal surgery

17 Cushing disease is diagnosed in a 48-year-old woman.

Preoperative laboratory test results:
   Cortisol (8 AM) = 26.7 µg/dL (5-25 µg/dL)
      (SI: 736.6 nmol/L [137.9-689.7 nmol/L])
   ACTH (8 AM) = 109 pg/mL (10-60 pg/mL)
      (SI: 24.0 pmol/L [2.2-13.2 pmol/L])

MRI shows a 4-mm pituitary lesion. Glucocorticoids are withheld after surgery. Twenty-four hours after transsphenoidal surgery, her morning cortisol concentration is 11 µg/dL (303.5 nmol/L). Seventy-two hours after surgery, her morning cortisol and ACTH concentrations are 10.2 µg/dL (281.4 nmol/L) and 31 pg/mL (6.8 pmol/L), respectively, and she is discharged home. Two weeks postoperatively, her morning cortisol concentration is 13 µg/dL (358.6 nmol/L). She feels weak and tired.

Which of the following is the best management recommendation?

   A. Another transsphenoidal surgery
   B. Cosyntropin-stimulation test to determine whether maintenance hydrocortisone treatment is needed
   C. Hydrocortisone daily
   D. Medical therapy with mitotane
   E. Stereotactic radiosurgery

18 A 64-year-old man is found to have a 2.3-cm sellar mass abutting the optic chiasm after his ophthalmologist identified a left eye visual field defect. MRI shows a relatively normal-sized sella with a large cystic mass extending in a suprasellar fashion. In retrospect, he has had headaches, poor energy, frequent urination, increased thirst, and a 46-lb (20.9-kg) weight gain over the past 2 years.

Laboratory test results:
   Complete blood cell count, normal
   Hematocrit = 32% (41%-51%) (SI: 0.32 [0.41-0.51])
   Fasting blood glucose = 78 mg/dL (70-99 mg/dL)
      (SI: 7.3 mmol/L [3.9-5.5 mmol/L])
   TSH = 0.5 mIU/L (0.5-5.0 mIU/L)

Free T_4 = 0.6 ng/dL (0.8-1.8 ng/dL)
(SI: 7.72 pmol/L [10.30-23.17 pmol/L])
Prolactin = 42.7 ng/mL (4-23 ng/mL)
(SI: 1.86 nmol/L [0.17-1.00 nmol/L])
Cortisol (8 AM) = 6 µg/dL (5-25 µg/dL)
(SI: 165.5 nmol/L [137.9-689.7 nmol/L])
Total testosterone (8 AM) = 115 ng/dL
(300-900 ng/dL) (SI: 4.0 nmol/L
[10.4-31.2 nmol/L])
IGF-1 = 76 ng/mL (72-207 ng/mL)
(SI: 10.0 nmol/L [9.4-27.1 nmol/L])
Sodium = 154 mEq/L (136-142 mEq/L)
(SI: 154 mmol/L [136-142 mmol/L])
Potassium = 3.9 mEq/L (3.5-5.0 mEq/L)
(SI: 3.9 mmol/L [3.5-5.0 mmol/L])

Which of the following is the most likely diagnosis?
A. Craniopharyngioma
B. Gonadotroph adenoma
C. Langerhans cell histiocytosis
D. Prolactinoma
E. Silent corticotroph adenoma

19 A 30-year-old woman develops progressive, severe headaches, nausea, vomiting, and fatigue during her 33rd week of pregnancy. She has no notable medical history and was able to become pregnant within 2 months of trying. Her pregnancy course has been smooth until now.

Physical examination findings are normal for 33 weeks' gestation. Her obstetrician persuades the radiologist to perform a noncontrast MRI of her head, and she is found to have a diffusely enlarged pituitary gland with suprasellar extension to the optic chiasm, but without compression of the chiasm.

Laboratory test results:
Total T_4 = 13.0 µg/dL (5.5-12.5 µg/dL)
(SI: 167.3 nmol/L [70.8-160.9 nmol/L])
TSH = 1.3 mIU/L (0.5-5.0 mIU/L)
Cortisol (8 AM) = 6.0 µg/dL (5-25 µg/dL)
(SI: 165.5 nmol/L [137.9-689.7 nmol/L])
ACTH (8 AM) = 9.3 pg/mL (10-60 pg/mL)
(SI: 2.0 pmol/L [2.2-13.2 pmol/L])

Prolactin = 137 ng/mL (4-30 ng/mL)
(SI: 5.96 nmol/L [0.17-1.30 nmol/L])

Which of the following is the most likely diagnosis of the mass?
A. Histiocytosis
B. Lymphocytic hypophysitis
C. Normal pregnancy
D. Pituitary adenoma
E. Rathke cyst

20 A 43-year-old woman presents with weight loss, tremor, palpitations, and sweating. She has mild frontal headaches, irregular menses, and atrial fibrillation.

Laboratory test results:
Free T_4 = 2.3 ng/dL (0.8-1.8 ng/dL)
(SI: 29.60 pmol/L [10.30-23.17 pmol/L])
Total T_3 = 386 ng/dL (70-200 ng/dL)
(SI: 5.94 nmol/L [1.08-3.08 nmol/L])
TSH = 2.8 mIU/L (0.5-5.0 mIU/L)
Prolactin = 33 ng/mL (4-30 ng/mL)
(SI: 1.43 nmol/L [0.17-1.30 nmol/L])

A radioiodine scan reveals 55% uptake in a homogeneous pattern in the thyroid gland. Brain MRI reveals a 2.1-cm pituitary adenoma invading the cavernous sinus. She is caring for her elderly parent and cannot take time off for surgery.

Which of the following is the best next step for managing both the hyperthyroidism and the pituitary adenoma?
A. Cabergoline
B. Methimazole
C. Octreotide long-acting release
D. Radiation therapy
E. Radioactive iodine

21 A 19-year-old man is evaluated because of headaches, decreased libido, and progressive fatigue and is found to have what appears to be an 11-mm Rathke cleft cyst on MRI. He recalls having some problems with increased urinary frequency and thirst several years ago, but he no longer has these symptoms.

On physical examination, he has a sallow complexion, a normal-sized phallus and testes, and a sparse beard.

Laboratory test results (8 AM):
Serum sodium = 144 mEq/L (136-142 mEq/L)
(SI: 144 mmol/L [136-142 mmol/L])
Urine specific gravity = 1.004
Serum cortisol (8 AM) = 7.0 µg/dL (5-25 µg/dL)
(SI: 193.1 nmol/L [137-39-689.7 nmol/L])
Free T_4 = 0.5 ng/dL (0.8-1.8 ng/dL)
(SI: 6.43 pmol/L [10.3-23.2 pmol/L])
TSH = 1.4 mIU/L (0.5-5.0 mIU/L)
Testosterone = 293 ng/dL (300-900 ng/dL)
(SI: 10.2 nmol/L [10.4-31.2 nmol/L])

Which of the following might be expected with initiation of hydrocortisone and levothyroxine in this patient?
A. Increase in polyuria and polydipsia
B. Marked decrease in libido
C. Orthostatic hypotension
D. Rapid development of hyponatremia

22 A 29-year-old man underwent surgical removal of a nonfunctioning pituitary macroadenoma 3 years ago. He has hypopituitarism and is currently taking hormone replacement with levothyroxine, hydrocortisone, GH, and injectable testosterone ester. He has normal libido and erectile function. He is interested in fertility.

On physical examination, he is well virilized with 18-mL testes bilaterally that have normal consistency.

Which of the following should be the next step in this patient's management?
A. Obtain a semen analysis
B. Switch from testosterone to clomiphene citrate
C. Switch from testosterone to hCG injections, 3 times weekly
D. Switch from testosterone to hCG injections, 3 times weekly, and FSH injections, twice weekly
E. Suggest he consider adoption

Thyroid Board Review

Jacqueline Jonklaas, MD, PhD, MPH

1 A 35-year-old primigravida woman is referred by her obstetrician at 11 weeks' gestation. She feels well except for recent-onset fatigue, and her pregnancy appears to be progressing normally. She has no chronic medical conditions and there is no family history of thyroid disorders. She is not currently taking any medications except for an iodine-containing prenatal vitamin. Prior to conceiving this pregnancy, the patient had 2 screening TSH values of 4.6 and 4.8 mIU/L (ordered by her primary care physician 1 and 5 years ago, respectively). A TSH value 1 week ago was 5.1 mIU/L. There is no pregnancy-specific reference range provided by the laboratory, but the nonpregnant reference interval is 0.4 to 4.5 mIU/L. A free T_4 value is also within the normal nonpregnancy reference range at 1.1 ng/dL (14.2 pmol/L).

Findings on physical examination are unremarkable. On palpation, her thyroid gland is at the upper limit of normal size.

Which of the following is the best next step in this patient's evaluation and/or treatment?
- A. Measure total T_4
- B. Measure TPO antibodies
- C. Measure TSH at a laboratory that provides a pregnancy-specific reference range
- D. Repeat TSH measurement at the same laboratory
- E. Start levothyroxine therapy immediately

2 A 71-year-old woman undergoes thyroidectomy for papillary thyroid cancer, and pathology shows a 4-cm tumor with extrathyroidal extension and bilateral nodal disease. Subsequent workup documents numerous bilateral pulmonary nodules. The patient is referred for dosimetric calculation for her initial radioactive iodine therapy using rhTSH stimulation. The dosimetric protocol shows iodine-avid disease remaining in the neck and also in the bilateral lung fields. Results of baseline pulmonary function tests, complete blood count, and comprehensive metabolic panel are all normal. Based on the dosimetry, an activity of 260 mCi is selected and administered in an inpatient setting. The patient is educated about the adverse effects of radioactive iodine and follows the advised precautions. A posttherapy scan also shows substantial neck and lung uptake, but no other areas of iodine avidity. Initially the patient does well after her therapy with some mild salivary gland swelling and discomfort, along with xerostomia, all of which improve. Approximately 3 weeks after her therapy, the patient notes a dry nose and then experiences epistaxis. This first episode initially resolves, but then she has recurrent episodes of nasal bleeding over a 4-week period.

Which of the following is most likely to be found in this patient following her radioactive iodine treatment?
- A. Bone marrow suppression
- B. Elevated serum creatinine
- C. Intranasal metastases from papillary thyroid cancer
- D. Maxillary sinus metastases from papillary thyroid cancer
- E. Skeletal metastases from papillary thyroid cancer

3 A 57-year-old man was diagnosed with Graves disease 24 months ago. At the time of diagnosis, his free T_4 and total T_3 levels were approximately 3-fold elevated (6.1 ng/dL [78.5 pmol/L] and 635 ng/dL [9.8 nmol/L], respectively), and his TRAb levels were significantly elevated at 5.1 IU/L. The patient was initially treated with methimazole, 30 mg daily, with subsequent resolution of his hyperthyroid symptoms and shrinkage of his goiter. He tolerated the methimazole without significant adverse effects and without worsening of mild Graves orbitopathy. He was able to continue his job as the host of a morning news show without any problems. Six months ago, he was taking methimazole, 5 mg daily, and remained euthyroid. His TRAb concentration was minimally elevated at 2.2 IU/L. He elected to discontinue methimazole. Today, he returns for follow-up and reports that his hyperthyroid symptoms have returned.

Recurrent hyperthyroidism is confirmed by laboratory test results:
    TSH = <0.02 mIU/L (0.5-5.0 mIU/L)
    Free T$_4$ = 3.5 ng/dL (0.8-1.8 ng/dL)
        (SI: 45.05 pmol/L [10.30-23.17 pmol/L])
    Total T$_3$ = 460 ng/dL (70-200 ng/dL)
        (SI: 7.08 nmol/L [1.08-3.08 nmol/L])
    TRAb = 3.5 IU/L (≤1.75 IU/L)

Treatment options, including radioactive iodine therapy, resumption of methimazole, and thyroidectomy, are discussed with the patient. He patient states that he is willing to consider each of these choices. His greatest concerns are protecting his quality of life, ensuring his professional activities are not affected, and preventing further hyperthyroid symptoms.

Which of the following treatment options is the best recommendation?
    A. A 1-year retrial of methimazole
    B. Long-term methimazole therapy
    C. Radioactive iodine therapy
    D. Thyroidectomy
    E. Thyroid lobectomy

4 A 53-year-old man presents with signs and symptoms of hyperthyroidism with accompanying moderately severe thyroid eye disease. He reports dry, itching eyes and significant protrusion of both eyes.

On physical examination, he has mild soft-tissue involvement, mild eye dysmotility, and significant proptosis. He does not have diplopia. His initial clinical activity score is 4.

The patient's thyroid function tests show an undetectable TSH value, significant elevation of both thyroid hormone concentrations, and an elevated TRAb concentration of 4.7 IU/L.

He responds well to methimazole therapy with a downward trend in thyroid hormone levels. However, proptosis worsens, yielding a clinical activity score of 5.

The patient's medical history is notable for a mild creatinine elevation thought to be secondary to previously uncontrolled hypertension. Currently his blood pressure is well controlled and he has no diabetes mellitus or cardiovascular disease. He presents for ophthalmology consultation regarding treatment of thyroid eye disease.

Based on this patient's presentation and progression, which of the following would be a reasonable primary therapy?
    A. Azathioprine
    B. High-dosage intravenous glucocorticoids
    C. Orbital decompression surgery
    D. Selenium
    E. Teprotumumab

5 A 21-year-old asymptomatic woman is found to have a right thyroid nodule on routine physical examination. She is then referred by her primary care physician to an endocrinologist. The thyroid nodule is mobile and firm and no cervical adenopathy is palpated. Her serum TSH concentration is normal. Thyroid ultrasonography shows a 3-cm nodule with moderately suspicious features (hypoechoic and solid; TI-RADS 4), with no abnormalities noted in the left thyroid lobe. The patient undergoes FNA biopsy of the nodule. Cytology from this biopsy is interpreted to be Bethesda IV (suspicious for follicular neoplasm). The biopsy specimen is sent for testing with a pathogenic variant panel and a microRNA classifier. Genetic testing does not detect any pathogenic variants, and the microRNA panel result is designated as level 1 (negative). The patient subsequently consults with a surgeon and expresses a desire to avoid surgery if her cancer risk is low.

Which of the following is the best approach to this patient's management?

- A. No further follow-up for her nodule
- B. Follow-up thyroid ultrasonography in approximately 1 year
- C. Right lobectomy
- D. Total thyroidectomy
- E. Ultrasonography to assess for cervical adenopathy

6 A 32-year-old woman with obesity is found to have a slightly elevated serum TSH concentration during her evaluation prior to considering bariatric surgery. Her BMI is 44 kg/m². She has made longstanding efforts to reduce her weight, including dietary restriction, exercise, and medical therapy. She has been judged to be a good candidate for bariatric surgery by the health professionals in the weight-loss center she attends. Review of her medical records shows that she also had an elevated TSH value documented 2 years ago but had a normal TSH value 10 years ago. She has no personal history of thyroid disease, has never taken thyroid hormone therapy, and has no family history of obesity or thyroid disease.

Findings on thyroid examination are unremarkable.

The patient is ready to proceed with surgery, but she has been referred because of her elevated serum TSH value.

Laboratory test result:
 TSH = 6.1 mIU/L (0.5-5.0 mIU/L) (prior TSH values: 5.7 mIU/L [2 years ago] and 3.4 mIU/L [10 years ago])
 Free T_4 = 1.1 ng/dL (0.8-1.8 ng/dL) (SI: 14.16 pmol/L [10.30-23.17 pmol/L])
 Total T_3 = 137 ng/dL (70-200 ng/dL) (SI: 2.11 nmol/L [1.08-3.08 nmol/L])
 TPO antibodies, negative

Which of the following is the best advice for this patient?

- A. Hold surgery and begin levothyroxine therapy
- B. Hold surgery and measure serum leptin
- C. Hold surgery pending measurement of reverse T_3
- D. Proceed with surgery
- E. Recommend sleeve gastrectomy instead of Roux-en-Y gastric bypass

7 A 79-year-old man is referred by his primary care physician for persistent iatrogenic hyperthyroidism despite progressive reduction in his thyroid hormone dosage. The primary care physician supplies the additional information that she first saw the patient about a year ago and has been unable to locate his medical records. The patient himself has been unable to supply additional medical history, other than stating that he suffers from gout. He lives independently but does have assistance from his family in taking his medications.

During the visit, the patient has no symptoms suggestive of hyperthyroidism except for some anxiety. He notes that he feels very tired and that his longstanding cold intolerance has worsened.

On physical examination, his thyroid gland is nonpalpable and he has a mild tremor of his outstretched hands.

Laboratory test results:
 TSH = 0.2 mIU/L (0.5-5.0 mIU/L)
 Comprehensive metabolic panel, normal
 Hematocrit = 32% (41%-51%) (SI: 0.32 [0.41-0.51])

His current medications are prednisone, 5 mg daily, and levothyroxine, 25 mcg daily (reduced from 88 mcg daily).

Which of the following would be the best initial step in assessing this patient's endocrine status?

- A. Measure free T_4
- B. Measure testosterone
- C. Measure total T_3
- D. Perform a cosyntropin-stimulation test
- E. Perform pituitary MRI

8 A 45-year-old woman is being monitored for a goiter and undergoes thyroidectomy for mild compressive symptoms. Three days after surgery, levothyroxine is started for postsurgical hypothyroidism. She maintains a regular schedule for taking levothyroxine, and her serum TSH level is consistently normal. She walks daily for exercise. Her menstrual periods are regular. During follow-up, she notes concerns about weight gain, which she dates to the time of her thyroidectomy.

When she returns for her 12-month follow-up appointment, she weighs 8.8 lb (4 kg) more than she had prior to thyroidectomy. Her only other medical condition is prediabetes. Her weight and TSH values are shown.

Assessment	Prethyroid-ectomy	3 Months after thyroidectomy	12 Months after thyroidectomy
Weight	158.3 lb (71.8 kg)	162.3 lb (73.6 kg)	167.1 lb (75.8 kg)
TSH	0.9 mIU/L	1.6 mIU/L	1.1 mIU/L

Which of the following most likely underlies this patient's weight gain?
- A. Failure to use combination therapy with levothyroxine and liothyronine
- B. Menopause
- C. Suboptimally treated hypothyroidism after thyroidectomy
- D. TSH value not at goal
- E. Thyroidectomy

9 A 27-year-old woman with Hashimoto hypothyroidism is diagnosed with a pT2, pN1b papillary thyroid cancer after total thyroidectomy and central neck and left lateral neck lymph node dissection. Her tumor is multifocal, with the largest focus being 2.9 cm; 31 of 72 lymph nodes are positive. Lymphocytic infiltration of the thyroid parenchyma is noted. The patient is treated with 150 mCi of radioactive iodine and placed on TSH-suppression therapy. Her posttherapy scan shows neck uptake consistent with lymph node metastases. She initially does well and has undetectable thyroglobulin, as measured by both immunochemiluminometric assay and radioimmunoassay, while maintaining a subnormal serum TSH concentration. However, thyroglobulin antibodies remained mildly positive at 10 IU/mL (normal <4 IU/mL). Cervical ultrasonography does not show any abnormal lymph nodes. A 1-year diagnostic iodine scan is negative and rhTSH does not stimulate an increase in thyroglobulin. During her second year of follow-up, thyroglobulin remains undetectable (measured by immunochemiluminometric assay), thyroglobulin antibodies remain relatively stable, and findings on surveillance cervical ultrasonography remain negative. However, the following year the patient is noted to have an upward trend in thyroglobulin antibodies, and the trend continues (*see table*).

Measurement	Year of follow-up				
	1	2	3	4	5
Thyroglobulin antibodies (normal <4 IU/mL)	10 IU/mL	14.6 IU/mL	17.7 IU/mL	130 IU/mL	393 IU/mL
	10.6 IU/mL	17.2 IU/mL	36.1 IU/mL	156 IU/mL	434 IU/mL

Which of the following is the most likely cause of the patient's rising thyroglobulin antibodies?
- A. Advancing Hashimoto thyroiditis affecting the patient's remnant thyroid
- B. Development of a second autoimmune disease
- C. Development of radioactive iodine–refractory disease
- D. Interference due to failure to use a mass spectrometry assay to measure thyroglobulin
- E. Recurrent papillary thyroid cancer

10 A 72-year-old man is referred by his pulmonologist prior to planned surgery for stage IIIa non–small cell lung cancer. As part of his workup for his lung cancer, a fluorodeoxyglucose PET scan is performed, which shows focal fluorodeoxyglucose uptake in the left lobe of the thyroid. No other uptake is seen in the surrounding neck area. The patient subsequently has thyroid ultrasonography, which shows a 1.5-cm thyroid nodule that is TI-RADS level 5. Suspicious features include punctate echogenic foci, irregular margins, and hypoechogenicity. No extrathyroidal extension or cervical adenopathy is appreciated. His serum TSH concentration is normal. The patient has hypertension and diabetes mellitus.

At his appointment, he states that immune checkpoint inhibitors, chemotherapy, and radiation are all being considered following his surgery. The pulmonologist has requested an opinion regarding further workup for the incidentally found thyroid nodule.

Which of the following is the best initial approach regarding the patient's thyroid nodule?

    A. Defer assessment of the thyroid nodule until initial treatment for lung cancer has been completed

    B. Measure free T_4

    C. Measure serum thyroglobulin

    D. Perform FNA biopsy of the thyroid nodule now

    E. Stain his lung biopsy specimen for thyroglobulin

11 A 59-year-old woman with postsurgical hypothyroidism presents for routine follow-up care. She has been on a stable levothyroxine dosage for many years. In addition to hypothyroidism, her medical history is notable only for newly diagnosed osteopenia, for which she has started calcium carbonate (taken separately from her levothyroxine at bedtime) and vitamin She has also recently been prescribed raloxifene for breast cancer chemoprevention. She feels depressed about the diagnosis of osteopenia and the recommendation to take raloxifene. She describes feeling fatigued, which is new since her last visit. Her serum TSH concentration is 11.3 mIU/L.

Which of the following is the most likely reason for her serum TSH elevation?

    A. Calcium supplementation

    B. Celiac sprue

    C. Medication nonadherence

    D. Raloxifene

    E. Vitamin D supplementation

12 A patient who had undergone thyroidectomy for papillary thyroid cancer is noted to have an enlarged lateral neck lymph node on routine examination approximately 3 years after initial treatment.

Which of the following is the most sensitive and specific indicator of metastatic disease within the enlarged lymph node?

    A. FNA cytology

    B. Neck ultrasonography

    C. PET-CT

    D. Stimulated serum thyroglobulin measurement

    E. Thyroglobulin measurement in the FNA rinse

13 A 42-year-old man is noted to have a serum TSH value of 12.1 mIU/L. He is asymptomatic and findings on physical examination are normal. Further testing reveals a free T_4 concentration of 1.3 ng/dL (16.7 pmol/L), with negative TPO and thyroglobulin antibodies. Findings on thyroid ultrasonography are normal. One of the patient's 2 children has similar laboratory test results.

Which of the following is the most likely cause of this patient's thyroid abnormality?

    A. Adrenal insufficiency

    B. Excess selenium exposure

    C. Hashimoto thyroiditis

    D. Resistance to thyroid hormone

    E. TSH resistance

14 A 66-year-old woman with follicular thyroid cancer and known distant metastases reports rib pain. She initially underwent thyroidectomy 8 year ago, and she has received multiple doses of radioiodine therapy, the last of which was 1 year ago. Her posttreatment scans have been negative.

Laboratory test results:
    TSH = 0.03 mIU/L
    Thyroglobulin = 3600 ng/mL (3600 µg/L)
    Thyroglobulin antibodies, negative

PET-CT demonstrates diffuse bone metastases in the ribs and spine.

Which of the following is most likely to reduce the risk of skeletal complications for her thyroid cancer?

    A. Dosimetry-based radioiodine

    B. Systemic chemotherapy with alkylating agents

    C. Teriparatide

    D. Total-body irradiation

    E. Zoledronic acid

15 A 32-year-old woman undergoes thyroidectomy with central neck dissection for a 4.5-cm papillary thyroid cancer. The tumor shows microscopic local invasion but no aggressive histology; 2 of 11 central lymph nodes contain tumor. The patient undergoes radioiodine remnant ablation using 100 mCi of ^{131}I, and a posttreatment scan shows no uptake outside of the thyroid bed. Surveillance testing at 6 months reveals a suppressed thyroglobulin concentration of 1.6 ng/mL (1.6 µg/L) with negative thyroglobulin antibodies and no adenopathy on neck ultrasonography. No additional therapy is given. Six months later, a suppressed thyroglobulin concentration is 0.6 ng/mL (0.6 µg/L), thyroglobulin antibodies remain negative, and neck ultrasonography is unchanged with no abnormal lymph nodes visualized. An rhTSH-assisted radioiodine whole-body scan 1 year after her initial treatment shows no areas of abnormal iodine uptake, and a stimulated thyroglobulin measurement is 5 ng/mL (5 µg/L).

Which of the following should be the next step in this patient's management?

A. CT of the chest
B. MRI of the neck
C. PET-CT
D. Repeated surveillance testing in 1 year
E. Thyroglobulin testing using a different assay

16 A 69-year-old man is admitted to the intensive care unit with hypotension due to sepsis. Despite aggressive therapy, the patient's condition continues to deteriorate. One month earlier, the patient had a normal thyroid laboratory panel.

Which of the following patterns is expected in this patient?

Answer	TSH	Total T₄	Total T₃	Free T₄
A.	10.0 mIU/L	7.0 µg/dL (SI: 90.1 nmol/L)	70 ng/dL (SI: 1.1 nmol/L)	0.7 ng/dL (SI: 9.0 pmol/L)
B.	7.5 mIU/L	5.5 µg/dL (SI: 70.8 nmol/L)	55 ng/dL (SI: 0.8 nmol/L)	0.8 ng/dL (SI: 10.3 pmol/L)
C.	0.2 mIU/L	2.5 µg/dL (SI: 32.2 nmol/L)	25 ng/dL (SI: 0.4 nmol/L)	0.5 ng/dL (SI: 6.4 pmol/L)
D.	5.0 mIU/L	12.0 µg/dL (SI: 154.4 nmol/L)	70 ng/dL (SI: 1.1 nmol/L)	2.2 ng/dL (SI: 28.3 pmol/L)
E.	0.01 mIU/L	12.0 µg/dL (SI: 154.4 nmol/L)	360 ng/dL (SI: 5.5 nmol/L)	2.2 ng/dL (SI: 28.3 pmol/L)

Reference ranges: TSH, 0.5-5.0 mIU/L; total T₄, 5.5-12.5 µg/dL (SI: 70.8-160.9 nmol/L); total T₃, 70-200 ng/dL (SI: 1.1-3.1 nmol/L); free T₄, 0.8-1.8 ng/dL (SI: 10.3-23.2 pmol/L).

17 A 34-year-old woman presents with symptoms of tachycardia, tremor, heat intolerance, and irregular menses.

On physical examination, her blood pressure is 128/77 mm Hg and pulse rate is 96 beats/min. She has a palpable, nontender, 3-cm, right-sided thyroid nodule.

Laboratory test results:
TSH = <0.01 mIU/L (0.5-5.0 mIU/L)
Free T₄ = 2.9 ng/dL (0.8-1.8 ng/dL) (SI: 37.3 pmol/L [10.30-23.17 pmol/L])
Total T₃ = 320 ng/dL (70-200 ng/dL) (SI: 4.9 nmol/L [1.08-3.08 nmol/L])
TPO antibodies = <2.0 IU/mL (<2.0 IU/mL) (SI: 37.0 kIU/L [<2.0 kIU/L])
Thyroid stimulating immunoglobulin = <120% (≤120% of basal activity)

Her radioactive iodine uptake is 26% at 24 hours (*see image*). In discussing therapeutic options, she makes it clear that her primary concern is to avoid the need for lifelong medication.

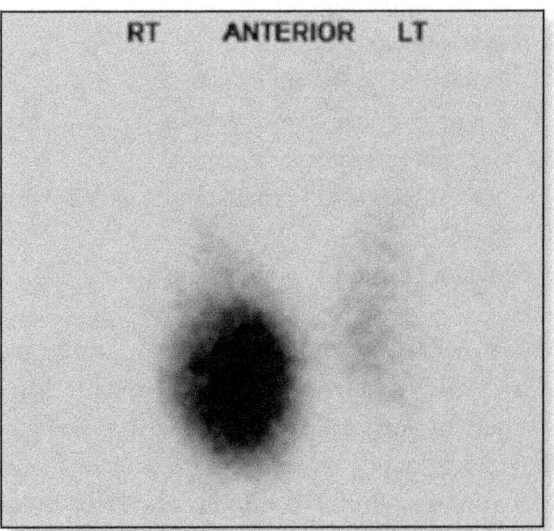

Which of the following therapeutic options would be most appropriate for this patient?

A. Ethanol injection
B. Methimazole
C. Radioactive iodine treatment
D. Radiofrequency ablation
E. Thyroid lobectomy

18 A 46-year-old woman with a history of postsurgical hypothyroidism is referred for evaluation of a high thyroid hormone dosage requirement. She takes levothyroxine on an empty stomach each morning, with no food or other medications for at least 1 hour. Her weight has been stable, but she has been increasingly fatigued. Her medical history is notable for Roux-en-Y gastric bypass surgery for obesity at age 40 years.

On physical examination, she has a thyroidectomy scar and trace pedal edema bilaterally. Her weight is 176 lb (79.8 kg), and BMI is 32 kg/m².

Her current medications include levothyroxine, 400 mcg daily, and a fish oil supplement twice daily.

Laboratory test results:
Free T_4 = 0.6 ng/dL (0.8-1.8 ng/dL)
  (SI: 7.72 pmol/L [10.30-23.17 pmol/L])
TSH = 18.2 mIU/L (0.5-5.0 mIU/L)
Screen for celiac disease, negative

Which of the following is the best next step in this patient's management?
  A. Change to liothyronine
  B. Change to once-weekly levothyroxine, 3 mg
  C. Give parenteral levothyroxine
  D. Increase the levothyroxine dosage to 500 mcg daily
  E. Switch brands of levothyroxine

19 A 74-year-old woman with fatigue and weight gain is referred for evaluation of subclinical hypothyroidism. The patient has gained 10 lb (4.5 kg) over the past 2 years since retirement, and frequently requires a midday nap. Her medical history is notable for hyperlipidemia, which has been managed by diet alone.

On physical examination, she has a normal-sized thyroid gland without palpable nodules. The rest of her examination findings are normal.

Laboratory test results:
Serum TSH = 8.9 mIU/L (0.5-5.0 mIU/L)
Free T_4 = 1.3 ng/dL (0.8-1.8 ng/dL)
  (SI: 16.7 pmol/L [10.30-23.17 pmol/L])

LDL cholesterol = 160 mg/dL (<100 mg/dL [optimal]) (SI: 4.14 mmol/L [<2.59 mmol/L])
HDL cholesterol = 38 mg/dL (>60 mg/dL [optimal]) (SI: 0.98 mmol/L [>1.55 mmol/L])
TPO antibodies, elevated

On repeated testing 3 months later, her TSH value is essentially unchanged.

Which potential effect of initiating levothyroxine treatment for this patient is most strongly supported by current evidence?
  A. Iatrogenic subclinical hyperthyroidism
  B. Improved cognitive function
  C. Increased HDL cholesterol
  D. Less fatigue
  E. Weight loss

20 A 32-year-old woman is found to have a TSH concentration of 0.14 mIU/L on laboratory tests performed as part of routine physical examination. She has no hyperthyroid symptoms. She is otherwise healthy and is not currently taking any medications or supplements. There is a small goiter on examination with no bruit and no palpable nodules. She has no signs of Graves eye disease. Her resting pulse rate is 78 beats/min.

Laboratory test results 4 months later:
TSH = 0.19 mIU/L (0.5-5.0 mIU/L)
Free T_4 = 1.6 ng/dL (0.8-1.8 ng/dL)
  (SI: 20.59 pmol/L [10.30-23.17 pmol/L])
Total T_3 = 166 ng/dL (70-200 ng/dL)
  (SI: 2.56 nmol/L [1.08-3.08 nmol/L])
Thyroid-stimulating immunoglobulin = 137%
  (≤120% of basal activity)

She has 2 children and is not planning additional pregnancies.

Which of the following is the best option?
  A. Repeat thyroid function tests in 3 to 6 months
  B. Schedule radioactive iodine treatment
  C. Schedule thyroid ultrasonography
  D. Start atenolol, 25 mg daily
  E. Start methimazole, 5 mg daily

21 A 55-year-old man presents with new-onset fatigue. He has a history of atrial fibrillation for which he had been taking amiodarone for 14 months. The amiodarone treatment was discontinued 2 months ago. Serum TSH was normal (1.47 mIU/L) at the time that the amiodarone was stopped.

He has a minimally enlarged thyroid gland on physical examination, without palpable nodules. His pulse rate is 92 beats/min. He has a fine tremor of his outstretched hands.

Laboratory test results:
TSH = <0.01 mIU/L (0.5-5.0 mIU/L)
Total T_3 = 263 ng/dL (70-200 ng/dL)
(SI: 4.1 nmol/L [1.08-3.08 nmol/L])
Free T_4 = 4.7 ng/dL (0.8-1.8 ng/dL)
(SI: 60.5 pmol/L [10.30-23.17 pmol/L])

Which of the following is the best test for establishing this patient's underlying thyroid pathophysiology? Radioactive iodine uptake

A. Serum IL-6 measurement
B. Serum TPO antibody measurement
C. Thyroid ultrasonography with color Doppler
D. Urine iodine measurement

22 A 76-year-old man is referred for evaluation of a neck mass. The patient notes dysphagia with solid foods and positional dyspnea when lying on his right side. On physical examination, he has a large goiter extending below the clavicle on the left side. His serum TSH concentration is 2.3 mIU/L, and radioiodine uptake is 8% at 24 hours. CT of the neck is shown (*see image*). The patient has a nonthyroid malignancy and is not considered to be a candidate for surgery.

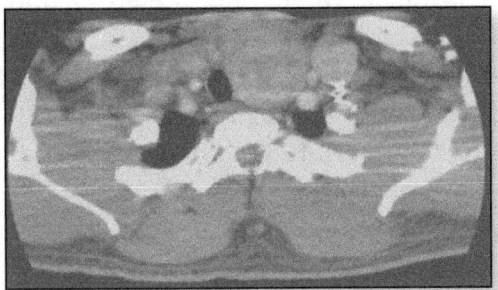

Which of the following should be the next step in this patient's management?

A. Levothyroxine suppressive therapy
B. No intervention until symptoms progress
C. Radioiodine therapy with rhTSH
D. Radioiodine therapy without rhTSH
E. Thermal ablation therapy

23 A 39-year-old woman presents with a 2.0-cm nodule at the lower pole of the left thyroid lobe (*see image*). FNA biopsy reveals watery, clear, colorless fluid.

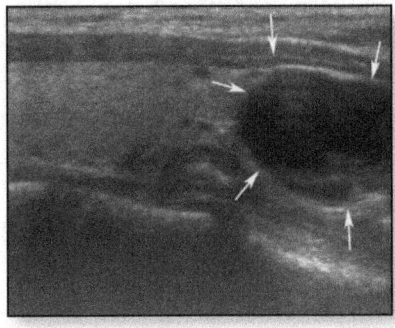

Which of the following is the most likely diagnosis?

A. Aberrant salivary gland cyst
B. Branchial cleft cyst
C. Follicular thyroid carcinoma
D. Parathyroid cyst
E. Thyroglossal duct cyst

24 A 56-year-old woman is found to have a thyroid nodule by her gynecologist. She has been in excellent health and takes no medications. Her family history is negative for thyroid cancer. Her serum TSH concentration is 1.8 mIU/L (0.5-5.0 mIU/L). The patient undergoes thyroid FNA biopsy, which shows a predominance of normal-appearing groups of follicular cells and colloid, as well as occasional focal groups of cells with enlarged nuclei and nuclear grooves.

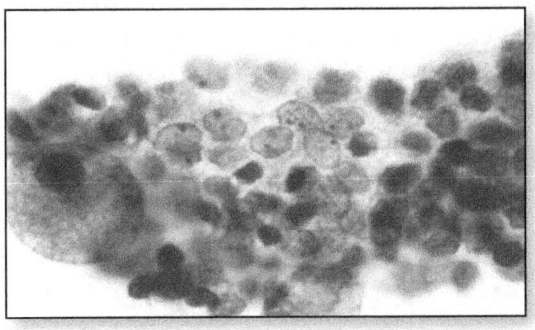

According to the Bethesda System for Reporting Thyroid Cytopathology, which of the following is the correct classification for this FNA biopsy result?

- A. Atypia of undetermined significance
- B. Benign
- C. Malignant
- D. Nondiagnostic
- E. Suspicious for malignancy

25 A 26-year-old woman presents for follow-up of hypothyroidism, which was diagnosed several years ago. She is currently being treated with levothyroxine, 88 mcg daily, and liothyronine, 10 mcg daily. Her regimen was changed to levothyroxine/liothyronine combination therapy 2 years ago because of persistent fatigue on levothyroxine alone; she reports that symptoms improved with this change and she is currently feeling well. Her most recent serum TSH value, measured 3 weeks ago, was 1.23 mIU/L. She reports that her period is 2 weeks late, and an in-office urine pregnancy test is positive.

Which of the following is the best option for this patient's thyroid hormone therapy now?

- A. Change to desiccated thyroid extract
- B. Continue current treatment
- C. Increase both the levothyroxine and liothyronine dosages by 25%
- D. Increase the levothyroxine dosage to 112 mcg daily and continue the current liothyronine dosage
- E. Stop liothyronine and increase the levothyroxine dosage to 150 mcg daily

26 A 49-year-old woman presents with a 3-month history of palpitations, tremor, irregular menses, and weight loss. She had previously been healthy and is not taking any medications. She does not have ophthalmopathy. Her thyroid gland is nontender and is not enlarged.

Laboratory test results:

Serum TSH = <0.01 mIU/L (0.5-5.0 mIU/L)

Total T_3 = 385 ng/dL (70-200 ng/dL)
(SI: 5.93 nmol/L [1.08-3.08 nmol/L])

Free T_4 = 2.4 ng/dL (0.8-1.8 ng/dL)
(SI: 30.9 pmol/L [10.30-23.17 pmol/L])

Serum thyroglobulin = 76 ng/mL (3-42 ng/mL)
(SI: 76 µg/L [3-42 µg/L])

TPO antibodies = <2.0 IU/mL (<2.0 kIU/L)

Urinary iodine = 112 µg/L (>100 µg/L)

Thyroid scan is performed, and radioactive iodine uptake is undetectable. A β-adrenergic blocker is started. She returns in 4 months and reports that palpitations are improved. However, she describes weight loss, irregular and frequent menses, frequent stools, and abdominal bloating. Laboratory test results are essentially unchanged.

Which of the following is the best next step?

- A. Inquire about exogenous sources of thyroid hormone
- B. Measure erythrocyte sedimentation rate
- C. Perform a whole-body radioactive iodine scan
- D. Perform thyroidectomy
- E. Start methimazole

27 A 32-year-old woman in her 16th week of pregnancy is referred for evaluation of thyrotoxicosis. She initially presented with palpitations and tremor. She has no nausea, vomiting, or abdominal pain. On physical examination, her pulse rate is 109 beats/min, and she has no ophthalmopathy. The thyroid gland is at the upper limit of normal size without tenderness, bruit, or nodules. Results from serial thyroid function tests are shown in the Table (*next page*).

Serum thyroglobulin is in the mid-normal range. The quantitative β-hCG reference range for 12 weeks' gestation is 22,846 to 114,774 mIU/mL (22,846-114,774 IU/L); reference range for 16 weeks' gestation is approximately 11,159 to 80,656 mIU/mL (11,159 to 80,656 IU/L).

Measurement	Time of testing			
	Prepregnancy	8 Weeks' gestation	12 Weeks' gestation	16 Weeks' gestation
TSH	0.51 mIU/L	0.012 mIU/L	<0.008 mIU/L	<0.008 mIU/L
Free T$_4$	0.9 ng/dL (SI: 11.6 pmol/L)	1.61 ng/dL (SI: 20.7 pmol/L)	1.98 ng/dL (SI: 25.5 pmol/L)	2.10 ng/dL (SI: 27.0 pmol/L)
Total T$_3$	...	...	301 ng/dL (SI: 4.64 nmol/L)	296 ng/dL (SI: 4.56 nmol/L)
β-hCG			56,450 mIU/mL	30,400 mIU/mL

Reference ranges: TSH, 0.5-5.0 mIU/L; free T$_4$, 0.8-1.8 ng/dL (10.3-23.2 pmol/L); total T$_3$, 70-200 ng/dL (1.1-3.1 nmol/L).

Which of the following is the most likely etiology of this patient's thyrotoxicosis?

A. Gestational thyrotoxicosis

B. Graves disease

C. Molar pregnancy

D. Subacute thyroiditis

E. Surreptitious use of thyroid extract

28 A 44-year-old woman is incidentally found to have a right thyroid nodule on cervical spine MRI, which was performed to evaluate posterior neck pain. She had been in good health previously and takes no medications. There is no history of radiation exposure or family history of thyroid cancer.

On physical examination, the nodule is not palpable and no adenopathy is noted. Ultrasonography confirms a 1.5-cm nodule with microcalcifications. FNA biopsy findings are suspicious for cancer, and the patient undergoes right thyroid lobectomy. A 1.4-cm classic papillary thyroid cancer is documented and lymphocytic infiltration of the thyroid lobe is also noted. No lymph nodes are removed. The postoperative serum TSH concentration is 5.0 mIU/L.

Which of the following is the best next step in this patient's management?

A. Completion thyroidectomy followed by radioiodine remnant ablation

B. Completion thyroidectomy without radioiodine remnant ablation

C. Radioiodine ablation of the left lobe of the thyroid

D. Thyroid hormone therapy with a target TSH level between 0.5 and 2.0 mIU/L

E. Thyroid hormone therapy with a target TSH of less than 0.5 mIU/L

29 A 37-year-old woman is noted to have a 3.2-cm right thyroid nodule. She is in good health and takes no medications. Family history is negative for thyroid cancer.

On physical examination, her blood pressure is 118/78 mm Hg and pulse rate is 80 beats/min. She has no palpable lymph nodes in the neck.

Findings on FNA biopsy are suggestive of medullary thyroid cancer.

Laboratory test results:
Serum calcitonin = 390 pg/mL (<8 pg/mL) (SI: 113.9 pmol/L [<2.34 pmol/L])
Serum calcium = 8.9 mg/dL (8.2-10.2 mg/dL) (SI: 2.2 mmol/L [2.1-2.6 mmol/L])
PTH = 33 pg/mL (10-65 pg/mL) (SI: 33 ng/L [10-65 ng/L])
Plasma metanephrines, normal
Genetic testing for *RET* germline pathogenic variants, negative

This patient should not undergo thyroidectomy until she has had which of the following assessments?

A. Adrenal CT

B. Fluorodeoxyglucose-PET scan

C. MRI liver

D. Neck ultrasonography

E. Sestamibi scan

30 A 67-year-man presents with signs and symptoms of thyrotoxicosis, including weight loss and palpitations.

On physical examination, a 3-cm right-sided throid nodule is palpated and a tremor of his outstretched hands is noted. Biochemical evaluation confirms hyperthyroidism. A diagnostic ^{123}I thyroid scan is performed (*see image*).

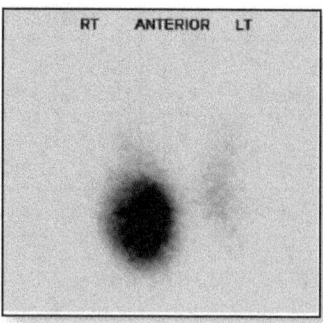

RT ANTERIOR LT

Which of the following is the most likely etiology of the patient's thyrotoxicosis?

A. Activating variant in the gene encoding the sodium-iodide symporter
B. Germline activating variant in the gene encoding the TSH receptor
C. Inactivating variant in the gene encoding the G_s alpha subunit
D. Somatic activating variant in the gene encoding the TSH receptor
E. Thyroid hemiagenesis and Graves disease

31 A 48-year-old woman presents after a thyroid nodule is noted incidentally on CT. She is not aware of anterior neck changes. Her serum TSH concentration is 2.37 mIU/L. She has no history of head or neck radiation and no family history of thyroid cancer. Thyroid ultrasonography demonstrates the following in the right thyroid lobe (*see image*).

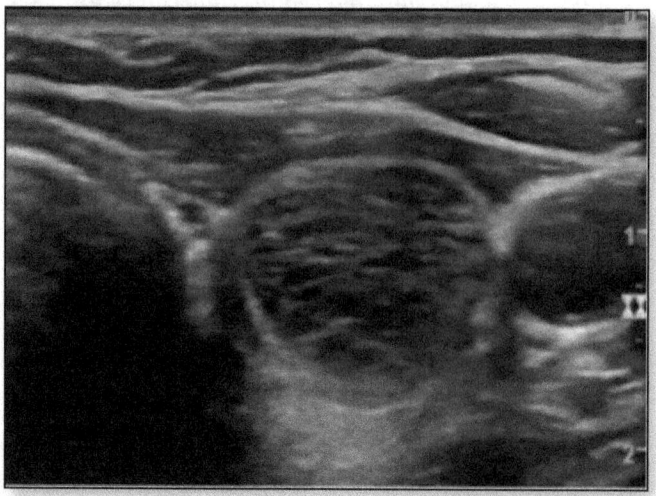

On the basis of the ultrasonographic pattern, which of the following best approximates her risk for malignancy?

A. <1%
B. <3%
C. 5%-10%
D. 10%-20%
E. 70%-90%

32 A 36-year-old man presents with a 2.6-cm left-sided thyroid nodule. This was first noted 18 months ago when it was palpated during a routine physical examination. On ultrasonography, the nodule is solid and hypoechoic, with irregular margins. There are no microcalcifications. There is no cervical lymphadenopathy. The right lobe has a normal echotexture, without any discrete nodules. The nodule was initially biopsied 6 months ago, and a repeated FNA biopsy was performed 3 months ago. Both biopsies were performed with ultrasound guidance, and the second time the biopsy was performed with on-site cytopathologic evaluation. A third attempt was made at the patient's request last week with no follicular cells being present in the aspirate. In each instance, the cytopathology was interpreted as Bethesda I (nondiagnostic/unsatisfactory), with an inadequate number of cells. The nodule has increased 7 to 9 mm in each dimension since initial ultrasonography 18 months ago. The patient has no compressive symptoms.

Laboratory test result:
    Serum TSH = 1.74 mIU/L (0.5-5.0 mIU/L)

Which of the following is the best next step in this patient's management?

A. Measure serum calcitonin
B. Perform ^{18}F-fluorodeoxyglucose PET/CT imaging
C. Perform thyroid lobectomy
D. Repeat ultrasonography in 6 to 12 months
E. Repeat ultrasound-guided FNA biopsy with molecular markers

33   A 59-year-old man presented 5 months ago with a palpable left-sided thyroid nodule. Thyroid ultrasonography demonstrated a solitary hypoechoic nodule with regular margins. FNA biopsy of the nodule was interpreted as Bethesda III (atypia of uncertain significance/ follicular lesion of uncertain significance), and he subsequently underwent left thyroid lobectomy 6 weeks ago. Surgical pathology revealed a 3.2-cm fully encapsulated tumor. This had a follicular growth pattern with no well-formed papillae and no psammoma bodies. No vascular or capsular invasion was detected after complete examination of the capsule. Nuclear enlargement, overlapping, and grooves were noted. There was no tumor necrosis.

Laboratory test results:
   Serum TSH = 2.54 mIU/L (0.5-53.0 mIU/L)
   Thyroglobulin antibodies = <4.0 IU/mL
      (≤4.0 IU/mL) (SI: <4.0 kIU/L [≤4.0 kIU/L])
   Thyroglobulin = 6 ng/mL (3-42 ng/mL) (SI: 6 μg/L
      [3-42 μg/L])

He returns today to discuss the surgical pathology and next steps for management.

Which of the following is the best next step in this patient's management?
   A. Completion thyroidectomy
   B. Completion thyroidectomy followed by radioiodine remnant ablation
   C. Levothyroxine therapy to keep TSH suppressed to less than 0.1 mIU/L
   D. Levothyroxine therapy with a goal TSH between 0.5 and 2.0 mIU/L
   E. Measurement of serum calcitonin

ENDOCRINE
BOARD
REVIEW

Adrenal Board Review

Tobias Else, MD

1 **ANSWER: B) Perform 1-mg dexamethasone-suppression test with next morning aldosterone measurement**

This patient has primary aldosteronism with hypertension, low-normal potassium levels, and positive screening (renin suppressed and an aldosterone-to-renin ratio >20). The plasma aldosterone concentration is greater than 20 ng/dL (>554.8 pmol/L) and confirmatory testing is not necessary. He is young and has a longstanding history of hypertension and likely primary aldosteronism, suggesting a hereditary cause of primary aldosteronism. Familial hyperaldosteronism (FH) has several subtypes:

- FH type 1: glucocorticoid-remediable aldoste-ronism with a chimeric *CYP11B1/CYP11B2* gene
- FH type 2: germline *CLCN2* variants
- FH type 3: germline *KCNJ5* pathogenic variants
- FH type 4: germline *CACNA1H* germline vari-ants and primary aldosteronism with seizure syndromes (PASNA) syndrome; germline *CACNA1D* variants.

While most of types of FH require genetic testing, FH type 1, glucocorticoid-remediable aldosteronism (GRA), can be detected by dexamethasone-suppression testing (Answer B). The genetic basis of GRA is a chimeric gene, in which *CYP11B2*, aldosterone synthase, harbors the *CYP11B1* promotor and becomes ACTH responsive. As in this case, there is an exaggerated response to cosyntropin stimulation, as seen with cosyntropin infusion during adrenal venous sampling. Suppressing the ACTH drive with dexamethasone suppression significantly reduces aldosterone levels, increasing the suspicion for GRA, which can then be confirmed by genetic testing. Patients with GRA often have a family history of primary aldosteronism and stroke (usually hemorrhagic). GRA can be treated with low-dosage dexamethasone suppression or spironolactone. However, dosages needed are much larger than 12.5 mg daily (Answer D). In a young male patient, eplerenone would be a better therapeutic option.

Bilateral adrenalectomy would cure GRA, but it would cause adrenal insufficiency, which confers greater morbidity than medical therapy. Left adrenalectomy (Answer C) would not cure the patient. Nodular adrenal glands are a common finding in GRA but are not the major source of aldosterone production. In general, only mineralocorticoid antagonists interfere with screening for primary aldosteronism.

Metoprolol has a minor effect on renin levels, but it does not need to be stopped (Answer E) for screening.

The imaging characteristics of the adrenal nodules and the patient's history are not suggestive of a clinically significant pheochromocytoma. Therefore, measuring metanephrines (Answer A) is incorrect. Clinically significant pheochromocytomas are usually 3 cm or larger.

EDUCATIONAL OBJECTIVE

Construct the differential diagnosis of primary aldosteronism, including genetic causes.

REFERENCE(S)

Seidel E, Schewe J, Scholl UI. Genetic causes of primary aldosteronism. *Exp Mol Med.* 2019;51(11):1-12. PMID: 31695023

Funder JW, Carey RM, Mantero F, et al. The management of primary aldosteronism: case detection, diagnosis, and treatment: an Endocrine Society clinical practice guideline. *J Clin Endocrinol Metab.* 2016;101(5):1889-1916. PMID: 26934393

McMahon GT, Dluhy RG. Glucocorticoid-remediable aldosteronism. *Cardiol Rev.* 2004;12(1):44-48. PMID: 14667264

2 ANSWER: E) Recommend further clinical observation and imaging as indicated

This patient has a large, heterogeneous adrenal incidentaloma that almost entirely consists of macroscopic fat on imaging (low Hounsfield units on CT, no signal drop-out on MRI), consistent with a myelolipoma. On microscopic examination, myelolipomas often have elements of predominantly fat, extramedullary hematopoiesis, and bone or calcifications. These tumors are invariably benign, and surgery is only indicated for compressive symptoms, such as abdominal discomfort, early satiety, bloating, or pain. The patient should be educated about these symptoms. Clinical monitoring (Answer E) is the mainstay of management.

Bilateral myelolipomas can be seen with longstanding, usually suboptimally treated congenital adrenal hyperplasia. They always are hormonally inactive. In addition, this patient does not have any features of hypercortisolism and screening for primary aldosteronism is negative. Therefore, no further biochemical screening or confirmation (Answers A and B) needs to be done.

An ^{18}FDG-PET scan (Answer D) can be helpful in distinguishing benign from malignant adrenal masses. Myelolipomas are not ^{18}FDG-PET positive; this diagnostic procedure is unnecessary, as the diagnosis can be made without it. Ten to 20 percent of benign adenomas are positive on ^{18}FDG-PET, and 10% of adrenal cancers and metastasis are negative on ^{18}FDG-PET. While ^{18}FDG-PET is generally helpful to distinguish between benign and malignant masses, it is not perfect and must be interpreted cautiously, with consideration of information from other imaging, biochemical testing, and clinical characteristics.

Biopsy (Answer C) is not needed to establish the diagnosis of myelolipoma.

EDUCATIONAL OBJECTIVE
Identify an incidentally discovered myelolipoma based on imaging characteristics and guide management.

REFERENCE(S)

Fassnacht M, Arlt W, Bancos I, et al. Management of adrenal incidentalomas: European Society of Endocrinology clinical practice guideline in collaboration with the European Network for the Study of Adrenal Tumors. *Eur J Endocrinol.* 2016;175(2):G1-G34. PMID: 27390021

Calissendorff J, Juhlin CC, Sundin A, Bancos I, Falhammar H. Adrenal myelolipomas. *Lancet Diabetes Endocrinol.* 2021;9(11):767-775. PMID: 34450092

He X, Caoili EM, Avram AM, Miller BS, Else T. 18F-FDG-PET/CT evaluation of indeterminate adrenal masses in noncancer patients. *J Clin Endocrinol Metab.* 2021;106(5):1448-1459. PMID: 33524123

3 ANSWER: E) Start hydrocortisone, 50 mg oral 3 times a day, and fludrocortisone, 0.1 mg daily

This patient has tuberculosis and is treated with rifampicin. He most likely had compensated adrenal insufficiency at the time of initial diagnosis. Although initial symptoms can be due to the underlying infection, hyperkalemia, hyponatremia, and elevated ACTH are suggestive of impending adrenal insufficiency. Rifampicin induces CYP3A4, which increases cortisol metabolism. While physiologically only a small fraction of cortisol is metabolized through 6β-hydroxylation by CYP3A4, induction of this enzyme can significantly increase (10-fold) this fraction and become a clinically relevant deactivating pathway. Common inducers of CYP3A4 are mitotane, rifampicin, carbamazepine, phenytoin, and St. John's Wort. The patient has symptoms and signs of adrenal insufficiency on the verge of adrenal crisis and should be treated immediately. Higher-than-physiologic doses are necessary, and therapy in this case should include fludrocortisone (Answer E), as there is initial evidence that tuberculosis has caused some primary adrenal insufficiency. Due to the increased metabolism and subacute presentation, replacement with 10 mg and 5 mg hydrocortisone (Answer D) would not be enough.

Rifampicin should be continued to treat tuberculosis. Holding rifampicin (Answer A) would decrease metabolism but not address the underlying cause of adrenal insufficiency and the effect would be delayed and not immediate.

Adrenal insufficiency can be caused by autoimmune adrenalitis (21-hydroxylase antibodies), destruction (eg, infection or hemorrhage), hereditary conditions (eg, adrenoleukodystrophy), surgery (bilateral adrenalectomy), or infiltration (eg, sarcoidosis or lymphoma). Further workup (Answer B) is not indicated.

Adrenal biopsy (Answer C) in adrenal insufficiency should only be considered in patients with bilateral adrenal pathology and if the cause cannot be determined by other diagnostic procedures.

EDUCATIONAL OBJECTIVE
Identify medications that induce CYP3A4 as a cause of increased hydrocortisone metabolism.

REFERENCE(S)

Thijs E, Wierckx K, Vandecasteele, Van den Bruel A. Adrenal insufficiency, be aware of drug interactions! *Endocrinol Diabetes Metab Case Rep.* 2019;2019:19-0062. PMID: 31581123

Bornstein SR, Allolio B, Arlt W, et al. Diagnosis and treatment of primary adrenal insufficiency: an Endocrine Society clinical practice guideline. *J Clin Endocrinol Metab.* 2016;101(2):364-389. PMID: 26760044

4   ANSWER: E) Transthoracic echocardiography

This patient has classic features of Carney complex. Carney complex has a multitude of manifestations, the most common being perioral and mucosal freckling, cutaneous and cardiac myxomas, primary pigmented adrenal nodular disease with cortisol excess, large-cell calcifying Sertoli-Leydig–cell tumors of the testis, and GH-excess/acromegaly.

This patient has a history of adrenal Cushing syndrome, typical clinical findings of perioral freckling, and evidence of large-cell calcifying Sertoli-Leydig cell tumors of the testis, making Carney complex the likely diagnosis. Genetic testing could be ordered to evaluate for pathogenic variants in the *PRKAR1A* gene. However, up to one-third of patients with Carney complex who have typical clinical features do not have an identifiable pathogenic variant in this gene and should still be treated based on a clinical diagnosis. In adults, the greatest morbidity (eg, stroke) and mortality are associated with cardiac myxomas. Therefore, this patient should undergo imaging with transthoracic surface echocardiography of the heart (Answer E) or cardiac MRI.

Physical examination and additionally screening should be done annually, but cardiac evaluation is the first priority. In addition to annual echocardiography, the general screening procedures to consider for adults with Carney complex are testicular ultrasonography (annually), thyroid ultrasonography (Answer D) (baseline examination), transabdominal ultrasonography of the ovaries (baseline examination), evaluation for cortisol and GH excess (including urinary free cortisol levels) (annually), and measurement of serum IGF-1 (Answer A).

Measurement of morning 17-hydroxyprogesterone, androstenedione, and DHEA-S (Answer B) is usually done to evaluate for congenital adrenal hyperplasia. Although testicular tumors (adrenal rests) can be observed in patients with congenital adrenal hyperplasia, the history of Cushing syndrome would not be consistent with congenital adrenal hyperplasia.

While testicular biopsy (Answer C) could confirm the presence of large-cell calcifying Sertoli-Leydig–cell tumors, this procedure is usually not necessary, as the diagnosis can be made by imaging in a patient with Carney complex. Imaging follow-up will be important, but screening for a cardiac myxoma, which bears the highest morbidity and mortality in patients with Carney complex, is more important.

EDUCATIONAL OBJECTIVE

Identify Carney complex by clinical features and strategize surveillance for hereditary syndromes based on morbidity.

REFERENCE(S)

Bouys L, Bertherat J. Management of endocrine disease: Carney complex: clinical and genetic update 20 years after the identification of the CNC1 (PRKAR1A) gene. *Eur J Endocrinol.* 2021;184(3):R99-R109. PMID: 33444222

5 ANSWER: A) Counsel to seek alternatives to facet injections

This scenario is a common referral to an adrenal clinic. The patient has received exogenous steroids over the course of years (facet joint injections), has symptoms and signs of hypercortisolism (weight gain, hypertension, and worsening diabetes), suppressed cortisol, and an incidental adrenal nodule. The correct recommendation is to reduce exogenous steroids and seek alternative strategies for back pain management (Answer A). Exogenous steroids received by injection are often highly potent and can suppress the adrenal axis 4 weeks or longer.

This patient's adrenal nodule is small and has a benign appearance. Any clinically significant cortisol production by the small nodule (cortisol-producing adenomas tend to be 2-4 cm) is unlikely and would result in normal or high cortisol levels. Further evaluation for hypercortisolism is not needed.

The patient has hypertension and an adrenal nodule and is on 2 antihypertensive medications. This warrants screening for primary aldosteronism with aldosterone and renin, but not a confirmatory study with 24-hour urine collection following salt loading (Answer C).

He has a low morning cortisol level, which is explained by suppression of the adrenal axis by exogenous steroids. He does not have any symptoms or signs of adrenal insufficiency and therefore no further workup or therapy is needed (Answers D and E).

Although opioids can lead to adrenal insufficiency, this would not occur in the absence of symptoms. Thus, opioids do not need to be stopped (Answer B).

The adrenal nodule does not need further imaging workup, as it is benign by imaging features. One could consider continued sporadic tests for hypercortisolism after avoiding exogenous glucocorticoids.

EDUCATIONAL OBJECTIVE

Identify causes of exogenous Cushing syndrome.

REFERENCE(S)

Stout A, Friedly J, Standaert CJ. Systemic absorption and side effects of locally injected glucocorticoids. *PM R.* 2019;11(4):409-419. PMID: 30925034

6 ANSWER: B) Recommend no intervention now

This patient has elevated levels of DHEA-S without clinically subjectively significant symptoms, and no therapy is needed at this point (Answer B). The differential diagnosis of elevated DHEA-S levels includes adrenal tumors, with a specific concern for adrenal cancer, congenital adrenal hyperplasia, 3β-hydroxysteroid dehydrogenase deficiency, and polycystic ovary syndrome. This patient had imaging excluding an adrenal tumor. The ovary is not a significant source of DHEA-S, and imaging is not indicated. Classic 3β-hydroxysteroid dehydrogenase deficiency leads to congenital adrenal hyperplasia with virilization and adrenal insufficiency with salt wasting. However, a nonclassic presentation often shows milder expression, mainly with menstrual irregularity. This patient's dynamic testing shows a normal cortisol response and an increase in 17-hydroxypregnenolone, but not to the level that would be expected with 3β-hydroxysteroid dehydrogenase deficiency. Therefore, no treatment for adrenal insufficiency (Answer C) is necessary.

Nonclassic 3β-hydroxysteroid dehydrogenase deficiency is best treated with antiandrogens, such as spironolactone and/or axis suppression with low-dosage nighttime dexamethasone. However, dexamethasone (Answer D) should only be considered for fertility, and spironolactone (Answer E) should be considered if the patient wishes to treat symptoms of hyperandrogenism (but only with adequate contraception).

This patient does not have classic or nonclassic 3β-hydroxysteroid dehydrogenase deficiency. She has elevated DHEA-S, and she has no subjective concerns. Therefore, no therapy is necessary. Of note, her weight loss is significant (BMI reduction from 28 to 22 kg/m^2), which significantly lowers the risk profile in an Asian patient. The presumptive diagnosis is polycystic ovary syndrome with DHEA-S elevation.

Women with polycystic ovary syndrome often have an increased LH-to-FSH ratio, but gonadotropins (Answer A) are not part of the diagnostic criteria. This patient already fulfilled 2 criteria in the past (oligomenorrhea and hyperandrogenemia).

EDUCATIONAL OBJECTIVE
Identify causes of elevated DHEA-S.

REFERENCE(S)

Pang SY, Lerner AJ, Stoner E, et al. Late-onset adrenal steroid 3 beta-hydroxysteroid dehydrogenase deficiency. I. A cause of hirsutism in pubertal and postpubertal women. *J Clin Endocrinol Metab.* 1985;60(3):428-439. PMID: 2982896

Pang S. Congenital adrenal hyperplasia owing to 3 beta-hydroxysteroid dehydrogenase deficiency. *Endocrinol Metab Clin North Am.* 2001;30(1):81-99, vi-vii. PMID: 11344940

Miller WL, Auchus RJ. The molecular biology, biochemistry, and physiology of human steroidogenesis and its disorders. *Endocr Rev.* 2011;32(1):81-151. PMID: 21051590

7 ANSWER: C) Recommend no changes

Treatment of 21-hydroxylase deficiency requires glucocorticoid to replace cortisol deficiency and to limit the rise in ACTH, thus controlling the adrenal-derived androgen excess. Relatively tight control of androgen (and thus estrogen) excess is necessary in childhood to prevent premature development of secondary sexual characteristics and bone maturation. Serum 17-hydroxyprogesterone, which accumulates immediately before the enzymatic block, is used for diagnosis and is also measured to titrate therapy in children. 17-Hydroxyprogesterone is a very

sensitive measure of disease control when small amounts of androgens and estrogens are detrimental. In adults, disease control is relaxed somewhat as tolerated, because small amounts of adrenal-derived sex steroid compared with gonadal synthesis are not damaging. Overtreatment can cause iatrogenic Cushing syndrome with long-term complications. Scenarios requiring intensified therapy in adults include when women are attempting pregnancy and when men have testicular adrenal rest tumors.

This woman, who has no androgen excess symptoms, regular menses, and absence of cushingoid features, has disease control that is clinically at goal. Not surprisingly, her androstenedione and testosterone levels are in the normal female reference range, and her plasma renin activity is normal. 17-Hydroxyprogesterone tends to rise before the next dose of hydrocortisone, but a high 17-hydroxyprogesterone level alone—especially just before a hydrocortisone dose—is not an indication for intensified therapy. Hence, no change in therapy is indicated (Answer C).

Increasing in the hydrocortisone dosage (Answer B) or further dividing her dose (Answer A) is not necessary. In fact, her hydrocortisone dosage could be reduced slightly, but that is not a listed option. Note that DHEA-S is typically low and rarely elevated in the setting of classic 21-hydroxylase deficiency. Dexamethasone given at bedtime is the most effective way to prevent the early-morning ACTH rise and thus control the androgen excess. However, dexamethasone is difficult to titrate and easily causes iatrogenic Cushing syndrome, particularly when given at bedtime (Answer E). A dosage of 1 mg daily is far too high for a small adult such as this patient. Stopping fludrocortisone (Answer D) would cause volume depletion, so it should not be discontinued.

EDUCATIONAL OBJECTIVE
Guide the treatment of congenital adrenal hyperplasia on the basis of clinical and laboratory information.

REFERENCE(S)

Auchus RJ, Arlt W. Approach to the patient: the adult with congenital adrenal hyperplasia. *J Clin Endocrinol Metab.* 2013;98(7):2645-2655. PMID: 23837188

Arlt W, Willis DS, Wild SH, et al; United Kingdom Congenital Adrenal Hyperplasia Adult Study Executive (CaHASE). Health status of adults with congenital adrenal hyperplasia: a cohort study of 203 patients. *J Clin Endocrinol Metab.* 2010;95(11):5110-5121. PMID: 20719839

Casteràs A, De Silva P, Rumsby G, Conway GS. Reassessing fecundity in women with classical congenital adrenal hyperplasia (CAH): normal pregnancy rate but reduced fertility rate. *Clin Endocrinol (Oxf).* 2009;70(6):833-837. PMID: 19250265

8   ANSWER: A) Laparoscopic right adrenalectomy

This patient has significant ACTH-independent hypercortisolism with low ACTH, abnormal cortisol suppression with dexamethasone, and mildly elevated urinary free cortisol. Macronodular adrenocortical hyperplasia is observed on CT imaging. Unlike what is observed with unilateral adenomas, progression to overt hypercortisolism is common in macronodular hyperplasia. Cortisol production in this condition roughly correlates with adrenal size, and when there is significant asymmetry, unilateral adrenalectomy of the larger side (Answer A) often induces remission and clinical improvement. However, recurrence of hypercortisolism from further hyperplasia of the remaining gland might occur in the future.

Observation (Answer C) would not be appropriate for a patient with this degree of hypercortisolism who has a clear etiology and marked symptoms.

Pasireotide (Answer D) is a pan-somatostatin receptor agonist that is approved for the treatment of Cushing disease but not ACTH-independent hypercortisolism.

Spironolactone and metformin (Answer E) would treat the blood pressure and hyperglycemia but not the cushingoid features and the catabolic actions of cortisol.

MRI of the adrenal glands (Answer B) would only confirm the fact that these are lipid-rich cortical adenomas and would not provide additional diagnostic or therapeutic value. A few studies have attempted to define useful parameters for adrenal venous sampling that quantify the amount of cortisol coming from each adrenal. Unlike in the setting of primary aldosteronism, both sides are always producing cortisol, although not always symmetrically, and nearly always proportionate to size.

Alternatively, this patient could consider medical management with mifepristone or levoketoconazole, both of which are FDA-approved for this indication. One could also consider off-label use of ketoconazole (not FDA-approved) or osilodrostat (only approved for pituitary Cushing disease).

EDUCATIONAL OBJECTIVE
Manage macronodular adrenocortical hyperplasia.

REFERENCE(S)

Debillon E, Velayoudom-Cephise FL, Salenave S, et al. Unilateral adrenalectomy as a first-line treatment of Cushing's syndrome in patients with primary bilateral macronodular adrenal hyperplasia. *J Clin Endocrinol Metab.* 2015;100(12):4417-4424. PMID: 26451908

Xu Y, Rui W, Qi Y, et al. The role of unilateral adrenalectomy in corticotropin-independent bilateral adrenocortical hyperplasias. *World J Surg.* 2013;37(7):1626-1632. PMID: 23592061

Acharya R, Dhir M, Bandi R, Yip L, Challinor S. Outcomes of adrenal venous sampling in patients with bilateral adrenal masses and ACTH-independent Cushing's syndrome. *World J Surg.* 2019;43(2):527-533. PMID: 30232569

Ueland GÅ, Methlie P, Jøssang DE, et al. Adrenal venous sampling for assessment of autonomous cortisol secretion. *J Clin Endocrinol Metab.* 2018;103(12):4553-4560. PMID: 30137397

Young WF Jr, du Plessis H, Thompson GB, et al. The clinical conundrum of corticotropin-independent autonomous cortisol secretion in patients with bilateral adrenal masses. *World J Surg.* 2008;32(5):856-862. PMID: 18074172

9 ANSWER: C) Refer for laparoscopic right adrenalectomy

The evaluation of ACTH-independent hypercortisolism prompted by the incidental discovery of an adrenocortical adenoma is slightly different than screening for Cushing disease based on clinical suspicion. For an adrenal adenoma, the dexamethasone-suppression test evaluates autonomous cortisol production when ACTH is completely suppressed, and its sensitivity is the highest among the conventional tests. Additional tests that assess the chronic state of the hypothalamic-pituitary-adrenal axis in these patients use a first-morning plasma ACTH measurement and a random DHEA-S measurement, which is an ACTH-dependent product of the adrenal cortex. Urinary free cortisol excretion is elevated in a minority of patients and is not a very sensitive test for detecting subtle hypercortisolism of any type.

A substantial body of literature now documents the long-term health consequences of mild autonomous cortisol excess, most commonly derived from adrenal adenomas. These tumors are typically larger than 2.4 cm in diameter, as in this patient, and although exact minimal criteria for mild autonomous cortisol excess are debated, the 3 main tests (ACTH, DHEA-S, and dexamethasone-suppressed cortisol) are all consistently abnormal in this patient. She was initially clinically observed because she had only osteoporosis and borderline hypertension as possible manifestations of hypercortisolism. However, hypertension has now worsened and she has developed obesity and diabetes. The DHEA-S concentration has further decreased because of persistent hypercortisolism of adrenal origin (suppression of pituitary ACTH drive). The major morbidity that improves with adrenalectomy is hypertension. However, autonomous cortisol excess from adrenal adenomas is associated with a host of other conditions, such as osteoporosis, glucose intolerance, cardiovascular events, and death, thus justifying the recommendation for surgical right adrenalectomy (Answer C).

Retrospective and prospective studies have shown that patients without elevated urinary free cortisol excretion might benefit from surgery.

Thus, delaying medical or surgical therapy until urinary free cortisol is clearly elevated (Answer A) is incorrect. Also, this degree of cortisol excess can cause morbidities.

The patient does not have ACTH-dependent Cushing syndrome and therefore petrosal sinus sampling (Answer D) is not indicated.

There is also no concern for adrenocortical carcinoma, as there is only insidious worsening of symptoms and the mass appears to be benign with a density of less than −5 Hounsfield units. Therefore, imaging for malignant transformation (Answer B) is incorrect.

Surgery as a final therapy is preferred over any medical treatment, including mifepristone (Answer E), which is indicated for patients with failed surgery or those who are not surgical candidates.

Indeed, this patient needed postsurgical hydrocortisone replacement due to suppression of the contralateral adrenal gland—post hoc evidence for presurgical hypercortisolism.

EDUCATIONAL OBJECTIVE
Guide the management of patients with subclinical Cushing syndrome and mild autonomous cortisol excess.

REFERENCE(S)

Morelli V, Reimondo G, Giordano R, et al. Long-term follow-up in adrenal incidentalomas: an Italian multicenter study. *J Clin Endocrinol Metab.* 2014;99(3):827-834. PMID: 24423350

Chiodini I, Morelli V, Salcuni AS, et al. Beneficial metabolic effects of prompt surgical treatment in patients with an adrenal incidentaloma causing biochemical hypercortisolism. *J Clin Endocrinol Metab.* 2010;95(6):2736-2745. PMID: 20375210

Di Dalmazi G, Vicennati V, Garelli S, et al. Cardiovascular events and mortality in patients with adrenal incidentalomas that are either non-secreting or associated with intermediate phenotype or subclinical Cushing's syndrome: a 15-year retrospective study. *Lancet Diabet Endocrinol.* 2014;2(5):396-405. PMID: 24795253

10 ANSWER: B) Adrenocortical carcinoma

Functional benign adrenal adenomas nearly always produce a single active hormone as their final product. Large cortisol-producing adenomas sometimes co-secrete aldosterone, but usually one hormone excess is dominant, while the second is mild. In contrast, overt, clinically manifested excess of more than one active steroid, such as glucocorticoid and androgen excess, is characteristic of adrenal cancer. Furthermore, the rapid progression of androgen excess alone, with very high testosterone and virilization (voice deepening), is worrisome for an adrenal or ovarian tumor. The mineralocorticoid excess in this patient, which is disproportionate to the cortisol and aldosterone concentrations, suggests elevation of cortisol precursors, primarily corticosterone and 11-deoxycorticosterone. Adrenal carcinomas tend to be relatively deficient in 11β-hydroxylase activity, leading to elevation of 11-deoxycortisol and further upstream intermediates, which can account for the robust androgen and mineralocorticoid excess with normal or modestly elevated cortisol. In particular, the elevation of DHEA-S in parallel to testosterone and the 11-deoxycortisol elevation is almost pathognomonic for adrenocortical carcinoma (Answer B). Hypokalemia in patients with adrenal cancer can arise from severe hypercortisolism overwhelming 11β-hydroxysteroid dehydrogenase type 2 in the kidney, mineralocorticoid production, or compression of the kidney and renal vasculature causing hyperreninemic hyperaldosteronism.

Macronodular adrenocortical hyperplasia (Answer C) typically manifests with pure cortisol excess, and the mineralocorticoid excess is due to cortisol and parallels cortisol production. DHEA-S is typically normal in hypercortisolemic patients with macronodular hyperplasia rather than suppressed as is often the case in hypercortisolemic patients with unilateral adrenal cortical adenomas, but this preservation of DHEA-S does not account for the profound androgen excess in this patient.

While mild or nonclassic 11β-hydroxylase deficiency (Answer D) has been described, affected patients have mild androgen excess and rarely have hypertension; the abrupt onset in this vignette is also inconsistent with a genetic etiology.

Anabolic steroid abuse (Answer A) could account for the androgen excess but not the mineralocorticoid excess.

Ovarian hyperthecosis (Answer E) is another cause of hirsutism and hyperandrogenemia. However, onset is usually more insidious and testosterone levels are not as elevated as they are in this patient. Most importantly, DHEA-S is usually not significantly elevated in the setting of ovarian hyperthecosis.

EDUCATIONAL OBJECTIVE
Suspect adrenocortical carcinoma on the basis of clinical features.

REFERENCE(S)
Arlt W, Biehl M, Taylor AE, et al. Urine steroid metabolomics as a biomarker tool for detecting malignancy in adrenal tumors. *J Clin Endocrinol Metab.* 2011;96(12):3775-3784. PMID: 21917861

Messer CK, Kirschenbaum A, New MI, Unger P, Gabrilove JL, Levine AC. Concomitant secretion of glucocorticoid, androgens, and mineralocorticoid by an adrenocortical carcinoma: case report and review of literature. *Endocr Pract.* 2007;13(4):408-412. PMID: 17669719

Fassnacht M, Dekkers OM, Else T, et al. European Society of Endocrinology clinical practice guidelines on the management of adrenocortical carcinoma in adults, in collaboration with the European Network for the Study of Adrenal Tumors M. *Eur J Endocrinol.* 2018;179(4):G1-G46. PMID: 30299884

11 ANSWER: E) *VHL*

The susceptibility genes for pheochromocytoma and paraganglioma are listed (*see table on the next page*).

Classic von Hippel–Lindau syndrome involves retinal and cerebellar hemangioblastomas, pancreatic islet-cell tumors, and renal cell cancer, but pheochromocytoma can also be part of the syndrome and is sometimes the only manifestation. In contrast to the biochemical profile of pheochromocytomas associated with multiple endocrine neoplasia 2A and 2B,

Syndrome	Gene(s)	Tumor locations	Hormone products	Other features
Familial paraganglioma type 1	SDHD	Head and neck paraganglioma, multiple; mediastinal paraganglioma; rarely adrenal medulla	NE, DA, or none	Clear cell renal cell carcinoma, gastrointestinal stromal tumor, pituitary adenoma, pulmonary chondroma
Familial paraganglioma type 2	SDHAF2	Head and neck paraganglioma, multiple; rarely adrenal medulla	Unknown	Unknown
Familial paraganglioma type 3	SDHC	Head and neck paraganglioma; mediastinal paraganglioma	NE or none	Unknown
Familial paraganglioma type 4	SDHB	Abdominal and pelvic paraganglioma; mediastinal paraganglioma; rarely adrenal medulla	NE, DA, or none	Often malignant paraganglioma; clear cell renal cell carcinoma, gastrointestinal stromal tumor, pituitary adenoma, pulmonary chondroma
Familial paraganglioma	SDHA	Head and neck or other paraganglioma; adrenal medulla	Unknown	Unknown
Multiple endocrine neoplasia type 2A and 2B	RET	Adrenal medulla, bilateral	E>>NE	Medullary thyroid carcinoma, hyperparathyroidism; marfanoid habitus and mucosal ganglioneuromas (2B only)
Neurofibromatosis type 1	NF1	Adrenal medulla	E or E and NE	Café-au-lait spots, neurofibromas, carcinoid tumors, peripheral nerve sheath tumors
von Hippel–Lindau syndrome	VHL	Adrenal medulla, bilateral; rarely paraganglioma	NE>>DA	Retinal and central nervous system hemangioblastomas, clear cell renal cell carcinoma, pancreatic islet-cell tumors, other
Familial pheochromocytoma	TMEM127	Adrenal medulla	NE and E	Renal cell carcinoma
Familial pheochromocytoma	MAX	Adrenal medulla, bilateral	NE and E	Unknown
Fumarate hydratase deficiency	FH	Head and neck paraganglioma; adrenal medulla	NE	Papillary renal cell carcinoma, uterine fibroids, cutaneous leiomyoma

Abbreviations: DA, dopamine; E, epinephrine; NE, norepinephrine.

Courtesy of Rich Auchus.

pheochromocytomas in von Hippel–Lindau syndrome almost invariably produce norepinephrine and normetanephrine. Thus, given this patient's laboratory test results, the gene most likely responsible for pheochromocytoma in her kindred is *VHL* (Answer E).

Establishing a genetic diagnosis is important, as it will inform future surveillance for other associated tumors. In this case, the patient should be monitored for renal cell cancer and pancreatic neuroendocrine tumors. Confirming a genetic diagnosis also serves as the basis for further family cascade screening (first-degree relatives are at 50% risk of carrying the same pathogenic variant). Evaluation would be indicated even in the absence

of a positive family history, as roughly one-third of all patients with von Hippel–Lindau syndrome do not have a positive family history.

Pathogenic variants in the *SDH* genes (Answer D) predispose to the development of paragangliomas, and pathogenic variants in *TMEM127* and *MAX* are rare causes of pheochromocytoma.

RET pathogenic variants (Answer C), which cause multiple endocrine neoplasia type 2A and 2B, are a more common cause of bilateral pheochromocytoma. However, tumors associated with these syndromes almost invariably produce epinephrine and metanephrine.

Pheochromocytoma is not a characteristic tumor of Carney complex, which is caused by pathogenic variants in the *PRKAR1A* gene (Answer B).

Patients with neurofibromatosis type 1 can have bilateral pheochromocytomas. Neurofibromatosis type 1 remains a clinical diagnosis with the presence of other features, such as neurofibromas, Lisch nodules, and axillary freckling.

Germline pathogenic variants in the *KCNJ5* gene (Answer A) can cause familial hyperaldosteronism but do not predispose to pheochromocytoma.

EDUCATIONAL OBJECTIVE
Compare the genetics and hormonal function of different familial pheochromocytoma syndromes.

REFERENCE(S)
Pacak K, Wimalawansa SJ. Pheochromocytoma and paraganglioma. *Endocr Pract.* 2015;21(4):406-412. PMID: 25716634

Fishbein L, Merrill S, Fraker DL, Cohen DL, Nathanson KL. Inherited mutations in pheochromocytoma and paraganglioma: why all patients should be offered genetic testing. *Ann Surg Oncol.* 2013;20(5):1444-1450. PMID: 23512077

12 ANSWER: D) Perform bilateral adrenalectomy

This woman has a metastatic, low-grade foregut neuroendocrine tumor with a pancreatic primary tumor. Originally, this tumor showed only features of gastrinoma, and predictably, she showed slow progression and good hormonal control with lanreotide. With time, clones from this tumor can acquire the capacity to produce other hormones, and this patient has rapidly progressive hypercortisolism typical of ectopic ACTH syndrome. Pancreatic neuroendocrine tumors that produce ACTH often co-secrete gastrin, so the index of suspicion for ectopic ACTH syndrome is quite high, and the history, physical examination findings, and laboratory findings corroborate the diagnosis. The most important point in this patient's management is that the tumor burden is not her most pressing immediate problem; rather, it is her hypercortisolism. She is at high risk for psychosis, opportunistic infections, and venous thrombosis. Prompt control of her Cushing syndrome is indicated with medical and/or surgical management. Bilateral adrenalectomy (Answer D) is the best step now.

Ketoconazole (Answer B) is most likely not potent enough to immediately control hypercortisolism.

One could consider using mifepristone. The patient's potassium would need to be corrected first, as mifepristone could lead to significant hypokalemia due to rising cortisol levels, overwhelming 11β-hydroxysteroid dehydrogenase type 2 in the kidney and leading to activation of the mineralocorticoid receptor. Alternatively, osilodrostat or metyrapone (both off-label) could be used to control hypercortisolism through CYP11B1 inhibition.

Lanreotide and octreotide are likely equivalent in their ability to treat paraneoplastic hormone production. However, control of the high ACTH and cortisol levels with a somatostatin analogue is unlikely. Thus, changing to octreotide (Answer A) is incorrect.

Cytotoxic chemotherapy (Answer E) for neuroendocrine tumors is reserved for low- and intermediate-grade tumors with significant progression or high-grade neuroendocrine tumors, including small cell lung cancer, but will not control paraneoplasting Cushing syndrome in a short time frame.

Gallium 68 DOTATATE can be helpful, as it provides high-resolution PET-CT images and is generally considered more sensitive than ^{111}In-pentetreotide scintigraphy. Lutetium DOTATATE therapy (Answer C) is a valuable tool for therapy but is unlikely to control hypercortisolism.

EDUCATIONAL OBJECTIVE
Manage ectopic ACTH syndrome resulting from a metastatic neuroendocrine tumor.

REFERENCE(S)
Kamp K, Alwani RA, Korpershoek E, Franssen GJ, de Herder WW, Feelders RA. Prevalence and clinical features of the ectopic ACTH syndrome in patients with gastroenteropancreatic and thoracic neuroendocrine tumors. *Eur J Endocrinol.* 2016;174(3):271-280. PMID: 26643855

Ejaz S, Vassilopoulou-Sellin R, Busaidy NL, et al. Cushing syndrome secondary to ectopic adreno-corticotropic hormone secretion: the University of Texas MD Anderson Cancer Center Experience. *Cancer.* 2011;117(19):4381-4389. PMID: 21412758

Isidori AM, Kaltsas GA, Pozza C, et al. The ectopic adrenocorticotropin syndrome: clinical features, diagnosis, management, and long-term follow-up. *J Clin Endocrinol Metab.* 2006;91(2):371-377. PMID: 16303835

Ilias I, Torpy DJ, Pacak K, Mullen N, Wesley RA, Nieman LK. Cushing's syndrome due to ectopic corticotropin secretion: twenty years' experience at the National Institutes of Health. *J Clin Endocrinol Metab.* 2005;90(8):4955-4962. PMID: 15914534

13 ANSWER: C) Measurement of plasma free fractionated metanephrines

The finding of an incidental adrenal nodule in a patient with a known malignancy always raises the possibility of metastatic disease. The primary malignancies most commonly associated with adrenal metastasis include lung cancer, breast cancer, gastrointestinal cancers, and melanoma. The history of breast cancer, the large right adrenal nodule with a high attenuation value, and the positive PET scan should raise the possibility of metastatic disease in this patient. A percutaneous CT-guided aspiration biopsy (Answer D) is certainly warranted in patients in whom metastatic disease may change the prognosis or therapeutic plan. However, biochemical evaluation of an adrenal nodule (Answer C) is *always* required before any attempts to perform a CT-guided biopsy or to remove the nodule surgically (Answer E). Adrenal venous sampling (Answer A) is only indicated to distinguish a steroid-secreting neoplasm (usually aldosterone-secreting) from bilateral adrenal hyperplasia.

Pheochromocytoma must always be excluded in patients with incidental adrenal nodules that have an attenuation value greater than 15 Hounsfield units. An aspiration biopsy may result in a catastrophic outcome in a patient with an unsuspected pheochromocytoma. Fluorodeoxyglucose PET yields positive uptake in 70% to 80% of patients with both benign and malignant pheochromocytomas. Therefore, plasma free fractionated metanephrines (Answer C) or 24-hour urinary catecholamines and metanephrines should be measured before any further intervention in this patient. This woman had marked elevation of plasma free metanephrines and eventually had successful laparoscopic right adrenalectomy for removal of her pheochromocytoma.

In this vignette, the overnight low-dose (1-mg) dexamethasone-suppression test yielded an abnormal cortisol concentration of 2.2 µg/dL (60.7 nmol/L) (normal, <1.8 µg/dL [<49.7 nmol/L]). However, in this patient, the abnormal result is confounded by the use of tamoxifen. Similar to estrogen, tamoxifen raises the level of the binding protein for cortisol—corticosteroid-binding globulin—and makes it impossible to interpret the result of a dexamethasone-suppression test (thus, Answer B is incorrect). If there is concern about a cortisol-secreting adenoma or possibly an adrenal nodule associated with ACTH-dependent Cushing syndrome, other studies, such as measurement of late-night salivary cortisol, urinary cortisol, and basal ACTH, should be considered.

EDUCATIONAL OBJECTIVE
Order appropriate biochemical tests to exclude pheochromocytoma in all patients with adrenal nodules and an indeterminate attenuation value.

REFERENCE(S)
Vikram R, Yeung HDW, Macapinlac HA, Iyer RB. Utility of PET/CT in differentiating benign from malignant adrenal nodules in patients with cancer. *Am J Roentgenol.* 2008;191(5):1545-1551. PMID: 18941099

Shulkin BL, Thompson NW, Shapiro B, Francis IR, Sisson JC. Pheochromocytomas: imaging with 2-[fluorine- 18]fluoro-2-deoxyglucose-D-glucose PET. *Radiology.* 1999;212(1):35-41. PMID: 10405717

Yu R, Nissen NN, Dhall D, Wei M. Pheochromocytoma in patients suspected of harboring adrenal metastasis: management and clinical predictors. *Endocr Pract.* 2008;14(8):967-972. PMID: 19095594

14 ANSWER: D) Plasma ACTH measurement

The biochemical diagnosis of Cushing syndrome currently relies on 3 diagnostic studies: 24-hour urinary free cortisol excretion, late-night salivary cortisol measurement, and the overnight 1-mg dexamethasone-suppression test. None of these studies is perfect, and they all have limitations. The value of any of these tests depends greatly on the pretest probability of Cushing syndrome. This woman has a very high pretest probability of Cushing syndrome on the basis of her history and physical examination findings. Therefore, even a normal study (urinary free cortisol) is not enough to dismiss the diagnosis. Urinary free cortisol is a very poor screening test for Cushing syndrome, with only 70% to 75% sensitivity. In contrast, late-night salivary cortisol measurement has 95% to 100% sensitivity for the diagnosis of ACTH-dependent Cushing syndrome if immunoassay methodology is used. However, late-night salivary cortisol does not provide good sensitivity in patients with adrenal-dependent Cushing syndrome. The overnight 1-mg dexamethasone-suppression test also has very good sensitivity and a very high positive predictive value. Unfortunately, the overnight 1-mg dexamethasone-suppression test is associated with a significant number of false-positive results. Securing dexamethasone levels after the test helps to provide evidence that the study was performed correctly. Because the patient described in this vignette has overt clinical features of Cushing syndrome, as well as marked elevations of late-night salivary cortisol and an abnormal result from the low-dose dexamethasone-suppression test, the diagnosis of endogenous hypercortisolism has been confirmed.

The initial test for the differential diagnosis of Cushing syndrome is measurement of plasma ACTH (Answer D). If ACTH levels are greater than 25 pg/mL (>5.5 pmol/L), the diagnosis of an ACTH-secreting neoplasm is likely and pituitary MRI (Answer E) is warranted. ACTH levels less than 10 pg/mL (<2.2 pmol/L) suggest adrenal-dependent hypercortisolism, for which adrenal CT (Answer A) is indicated. However, many current ACTH assays cannot reliably measure suppressed levels in patients with ACTH-independent hypercortisolism.

Therefore, adrenal imaging should be considered in patients with a plasma ACTH concentration in the range of 10 to 25 pg/mL (2.2 to 5.5 pmol/L). No imaging studies should supersede measurement of plasma ACTH.

The dexamethasone corticotropin-releasing hormone test (Answer B) has been used to distinguish physiologic hypercortisolism from pathologic hypercortisolism; however, results of this test have been reported to be abnormal in many conditions (eg, depression) associated with physiologic activation of the hypothalamic-pituitary-adrenal axis.

The high-dose dexamethasone-suppression test (Answer C) is not reliable in the differential diagnosis of Cushing syndrome.

EDUCATIONAL OBJECTIVE

Recommend measurement of plasma ACTH as the initial differential diagnostic test in the evaluation of Cushing syndrome.

REFERENCE(S)

Findling JW, Raff H. Cushing's syndrome: important issues in diagnosis and treatment. *J Clin Endocrinol Metab.* 2006;91(10):3746-3753. PMID: 16868050

Kidambi S, Raff H, Findling JW. Limitations of nocturnal salivary cortisol and urine free cortisol in the diagnosis of mild Cushing's syndrome. *Eur J Endocrinol.* 2007;157(6):725-731. PMID: 18057379

Alexandraki KI, Grossman AB. Is urinary free cortisol of value in the diagnosis of Cushing syndrome? *Curr Opin Endocrinol Diabetes Obes.* 2011;18(4):259-263. PMID: 21681089

Pecori Giraldi F, Saccani A, Cavagnini F; Study Group on the Hypothalamo-Pituitary-Adrenal Axis of the Italian Society of Endocrinology. Assessment of ACTH assay variability: a multi-center study. *Eur J Endocrinol.* 2011;164(4):505-512. PMID: 21252174

15 ANSWER: A) Measure serum aldosterone and plasma renin activity

The recommended functional evaluation of an incidentally discovered adrenal mass includes:

- Measurement of plasma or urinary metanephrines to exclude pheochromocytoma
- Overnight dexamethasone-suppression test to exclude hypercortisolemia
- Measurement of plasma renin and serum aldosterone (Answer A) to exclude primary aldosteronism (only in hypertensive patients)

This patient had normal results for the first 2 tests. While plasma metanephrine measurement has many false-positive results, the test has high negative predictive value, and further testing for pheochromocytoma (Answer C) is not necessary.

If the dexamethasone-suppression test result were equivocal, serum DHEA-S and plasma ACTH (Answer B) could be used to further assess for autonomous cortisol excess, but these tests are not necessary if the dexamethasone-suppression test result is normal. Furthermore, clinically significant hypercortisolemia is uncommon if an adrenal adenoma is smaller than 2.4 cm in diameter.

Because this patient has hypertension, he should be screened for primary aldosteronism, even with a normal serum potassium level. Of normokalemic hypertensive patients with an incidental adrenal tumor, 5% to 10% have primary aldosteronism. In fact, this patient did have primary aldosteronism, and after evaluation, he underwent left adrenalectomy with subsequent improvement in his blood pressure.

Characterization of adrenal nodules by imaging is the mainstay to diagnose potential malignancy. Hounsfield units (HU) before and after contrast can be very helpful. However, measurement of HU should only be done on homogeneous lesions. As a first step, the density of this mass should be measured before contrast application. If the density on this noncontrast CT is less than 10 HU, then this is a lipid-rich adenoma, and no further imaging follow-up is required. If the density of the mass is indeterminate (>10 HU), there are 3 options: (1) immediate further imaging characterization (eg, MRI [Answer D]); (2) repeated imaging in 6 to 12 months (Answer E); or (3) surgery. However, in the absence of a clear classification as an indeterminate mass, evaluation for primary aldosteronism should be conducted first. In addition, this small

homogeneous mass with a density of 8 HU is clearly identified as a lipid-rich adenoma. Even if not definitively a benign, lipid-rich adenoma, repeated imaging or further imaging evaluation is more reasonable than surgery.

EDUCATIONAL OBJECTIVE
Evaluate an incidentally discovered adrenal tumor for hormone production.

REFERENCE(S)

Zeiger MA, Siegelman SS, Hamrahian AH. Medical and surgical evaluation and treatment of adrenal incidentalomas. *J Clin Endocrinol Metab*. 2011;96(7):2004-2015. PMID: 21632813

Bernini G, Moretti A, Argenio G, Salvetti A. Primary aldosteronism in normokalemic patients with adrenal incidentalomas. *Eur J Endocrinol*. 2002;146(4):523-529. PMID: 11916621

Fassnacht M, Arlt W, Bancos I, et al. Management of adrenal incidentalomas: European Society of Endocrinology Clinical Practice Guideline in collaboration with the European Network for the Study of Adrenal Tumors. *Eur J Endocrinol*. 2016;175(2):G1-G34. PMID: 27390021

16 ANSWER: C) Hypoparathyroidism

The combination of mucocutaneous candidiasis, ectodermal dysplasia, and autoimmune adrenal insufficiency establishes a diagnosis of polyglandular autoimmune syndrome (APS) type 1. APS type 1 is an autosomal recessive disorder due to pathogenic variants in the autoimmune regulatory (*AIRE*) gene, which is necessary for the thymus to eliminate autoreactive T cells. About 60% of patients with APS type 1 develop adrenal insufficiency, usually in adolescence or adulthood after first acquiring mucocutaneous candidiasis, ectodermal dysplasia, and hypoparathyroidism as children. Hypoparathyroidism (Answer C) develops in more than 80% of patients with pathogenic variants in the *AIRE* gene, often as a first or second manifestation, although rarely patients develop adrenal insufficiency before hypoparathyroidism. In patients with apparently isolated adrenal insufficiency, genetic testing for *AIRE* pathogenic variants or testing for autoantibodies against cytokines, including interleukin-22, interferon α2, and interferon-ω, can identify patients with APS type 1. Positive 21-hydroxylase antibodies in a patient with APS type 1 predict current or future adrenal insufficiency in nearly 100% of cases.

The horizontal bands on teeth develop because of enamel hypoplasia, part of the ectodermal dysplasia in this syndrome, which also involves the nails. The syndrome is also called APECED (autoimmune polyendocrinopathy–candidiasis–ectodermal dysplasia).

In contrast to APS type 2, autoimmune thyroid diseases (Answers B and D) and type 1 diabetes (Answer E) occur in only 10% of patients with APS type 1. Gonadal failure (Answer A) occurs in approximately 50% and almost exclusively in females. Other frequent autoimmune manifestations in APS type 1 include hepatitis, alopecia, vitiligo, pernicious anemia, and chronic diarrhea.

EDUCATIONAL OBJECTIVE
List the endocrinopathies associated with polyglandular autoimmune syndrome type 1.

REFERENCE(S)

Eriksson D, Dalin F, Eriksson GN, et al. Cytokine autoantibody screening in the Swedish Addison Registry identifies patients with undiagnosed APS1. *J Clin Endocrinol Metab.* 2018;103(1):179-186. PMID: 29069385

Orlova EM, Sozaeva LS, Kareva MA, et al. Expanding the phenotypic and genotypic landscape of autoimmune polyendocrine syndrome type 1. *J Clin Endocrinol Metab.* 2017;102(9):3546-3556. PMID: 28911151

Bruserud Ø, Oftedal BE, Landegren N, et al. A longitudinal follow-up of autoimmune polyendocrine syndrome type 1. *J Clin Endocrinol Metab.* 2016;101(8):2975-2783. PMID: 27253668

17 ANSWER: B) Decrease in testosterone
This man has ectopic ACTH syndrome, a characteristic paraneoplastic syndrome resulting from small cell lung cancer, which is a type of high-grade neuroendocrine tumor. Ketoconazole inhibits several enzymes in cortisol biosynthesis, primarily P450 17A1 (17-hydroxylase/17,20-lyase), P450 11A1 (cholesterol side-chain cleavage enzyme), and P450 11B1 (11β-hydroxylase). For this reason, ketoconazole is used off-label to treat Cushing syndrome, but it has also been used to treat prostate cancer because inhibition of P450 17A1 and P450 11A1 rapidly and effectively lowers testosterone production at these dosages (Answer B). Consequently, men with hypercortisolemia managed with ketoconazole often require testosterone supplementation.

Metyrapone and osilodrostat primarily inhibit P450 11B1 and thus increase 11-deoxycortisol, but ketoconazole simultaneously inhibits P450 11A1 and P450 17A1, preventing a rise in 11-deoxycortisol (thus, Answer D is incorrect).

Although ACTH can rise with medical therapy in Cushing disease, this rise does not occur in ectopic ACTH syndrome due to neuroendocrine carcinomas (thus, Answer C is incorrect).

An increase in corticosteroid-binding globulin is seen with mitotane, but no change occurs with ketoconazole per se (thus, Answer A is incorrect).

Ketoconazole can cause gynecomastia due to disproportionate reduction in testosterone relative to slight decreases in estradiol, but estradiol does not rise with treatment (thus, Answer E is incorrect).

EDUCATIONAL OBJECTIVE
Anticipate adverse effects of ketoconazole therapy for Cushing syndrome.

REFERENCE(S)

Valassi E, Crespo I, Gich I, Rodriguez J, Webb SM. A reappraisal of the medical therapy with steroidogenesis inhibitors in Cushing's syndrome. *Clin Endocrinol (Oxf).* 2012;77(5):735-742. PMID: 22533782

Castinetti F, Guignat L, Giraud P, et al. Ketoconazole in Cushing's disease: is it worth a try? *J Clin Endocrinol Metab.* 2014;99(5):1623-1630. PMID: 24471573

Fleseriu M. Medical treatment of Cushing disease: new targets, new hope. *Endocrinol Metab Clin North Am.* 2015;44(1):51-70. PMID: 25732642

Ryan CJ, Halabi S, Ou S-S, Vogelzang NJ, Kantoff P, Small EJ. Adrenal androgen levels as predictors of outcome in prostate cancer patients treated with ketoconazole plus antiandrogen withdrawal: results from a cancer and leukemia group B study. *Clin Cancer Res.* 2007;13(7):2030-2037. PMID: 17404083

18 ANSWER: E) No changes

Primary aldosteronism causes more end-organ damage than equivalent degrees of essential hypertension, particularly on the kidney, heart, and vasculature. Proteinuria and renal insufficiency are common complications that improve with targeted treatment, either surgery or mineralocorticoid receptor antagonist therapy. Similar to the early stages of diabetic nephropathy, primary aldosteronism is a state of renal hyperfiltration, and targeted therapy often uncovers occult kidney damage, manifest as a rise in serum creatinine. In an older individual with longstanding hypertension and evidence of kidney damage, a rise in creatinine is expected with surgical cure or medical treatment of primary aldosteronism with a mineralocorticoid receptor antagonist. The goals of medical therapy are to normalize blood pressure and serum potassium and to stabilize deterioration of kidney function. Most authorities also target increasing plasma renin at least to measurable levels, but the increase in renin can take months to years. Consequently, given normal blood pressure and serum potassium on this regimen, the rise in creatinine to a new stable value is expected, and no changes should be made (Answer E).

Reducing the eplerenone dosage to 50 mg daily (Answer D), which did not previously adequately control his blood pressure, is a mistake. Dosage adjustments of a mineralocorticoid receptor antagonist should be made slowly, with gradual up-titration (as was done in this case), because several weeks are required to observe steady-state changes in blood pressure.

Spironolactone is, if anything, more potent than eplerenone on a milligram-for-milligram basis, and the dosage of 100 mg daily (Answer A) might be excessive and cause hyperkalemia. In addition, there is no reason to change.

Given his age and duration of hypertension, he is most likely to have a degree of fixed hypertension even with proper treatment of the primary aldosteronism, and his blood pressure would probably rise if amlodipine were discontinued (Answer B).

Eplerenone should not be discontinued (Answer C). A β-adrenergic blocker such as atenolol, which lowers plasma renin, is often used in high-renin hypertension.

EDUCATIONAL OBJECTIVE
Titrate medical therapy for primary aldosteronism.

REFERENCE(S)
Reincke M, Rump LC, Quinkler M, et al; Participants of German Conn's Registry. Risk factors associated with a low glomerular filtration rate in primary aldosteronism. *J Clin Endocrinol Metab.* 2009;94(3):869-875. PMID: 19116235

Fourkiotis V, Vonend O, Diederich S, et al; Mephisto Study Group. Effectiveness of eplerenone or spironolactone in preserving renal function in primary aldosteronism. *Eur J Endocrinol.* 2012;168(1):75-81. PMID: 23033260

Sechi LA, Colussi G, Di Fabio A, Catena C. Cardiovascular and renal damage in primary aldosteronism: outcomes after treatment. *Am J Hypertens.* 2010;23(12):1253-1260. PMID: 20706195

Byrd JB, Turcu AF, Auchus RJ. Primary aldosteronism. *Circulation.* 2018;138(8):823-835. PMID: 30359120

19 ANSWER: D) No further diagnostic studies

Approximately 15% to 20% of aldosterone-producing adenomas larger than 1.5 cm co-secrete cortisol. The autonomous cortisol secretion is usually mild, and affected patients often lack any overt evidence of hypercortisolism. Aldosterone-producing adenomas rarely consist of only zona glomerulosa–derived cells. As an aldosterone-producing adenoma grows, glucocorticoid oversecretion by the tumor may become apparent or detectable by biochemical testing. After adrenalectomy, the patient may have suppression of the endogenous hypothalamic-pituitary-adrenal axis with hypocortisolism and, as expected, suppression of the renin-angiotensin system with hypoaldosteronism. Accordingly, patients may experience signs and symptoms of adrenal insufficiency and glucocorticoid withdrawal, as well as hyperkalemia. There have been reports of adrenal insufficiency after unilateral adrenalectomy for a "nonsecretory" adrenal nodule. Patients with both primary aldosteronism and autonomous cortisol secretion have a high incidence of cardiovascular events, which mandates an aggressive diagnostic and therapeutic strategy.

Because the degree of ACTH-independent hypercortisolism is mild and subclinical, the hypothalamic-pituitary-adrenal axis often recovers promptly and the patient may do well and not need any diagnostic testing or therapeutic intervention. The recovery of the hypothalamic-pituitary-adrenal axis after suppression by either endogenous or exogenous corticosteroid excess follows a typical pattern: initially, the hypothalamus and pituitary recover until ACTH levels actually exceed the normal range to provoke growth and increased steroidogenesis from the atrophic adrenal cortex. Thus, the elevated ACTH and low cortisol mimic the biochemical findings of primary adrenal insufficiency, but, in fact, provide reassurance that hypothalamic-pituitary-adrenal function is recovering nicely. Basal physiologic hydrocortisone therapy and stress-dose management are usually required until there is full recovery of adrenal function. No further diagnostic studies are needed in this patient (Answer D). The hypoaldosteronism can usually be managed conservatively by encouraging liberal salt intake (increasing distal renal sodium delivery) and a low-potassium diet. Occasionally, patients may need mineralocorticoid replacement with fludrocortisone.

This patient's biochemical findings clearly show postoperative hypocortisolism. Because oral contraceptives increase the major binding protein for cortisol (corticosteroid-binding globulin), the low cortisol level is enough to establish a diagnosis of cortisol deficiency.

21-Hydroxylase antibodies (Answer B) are a hallmark of classic autoimmune adrenalitis, which is unlikely in this patient. Her elevated ACTH and low serum cortisol provide enough evidence for adrenal insufficiency.

Since adrenal androgen production is decreased in both primary and secondary adrenal insufficiency, measuring DHEA-S (Answer A) may be a sensitive indicator of impaired adrenal function; however, hypoadrenalism is already apparent in this patient.

Pituitary imaging (Answer C) would not provide any insight into the recovery of adrenocortical function.

EDUCATIONAL OBJECTIVE
Diagnose adrenal insufficiency after unilateral adrenalectomy for an aldosterone-producing adenoma and recognize the frequency of concomitant and covert autonomous cortisol secretion from some aldosterone- producing adenomas.

REFERENCE(S)

Spath M, Korovkin S, Antke C, Anlauf M, Willenberg HS. Aldosterone- and cortisol-co-secreting adrenal tumors: the lost subtype of primary aldosteronism. *Eur J Endocrinol.* 2011;164(4):447-455. PMID: 21270113

Fisher E, Hanslik G, Pallauf A, et al. Prolonged zona glomerulosa insufficiency causing hyperkalemia in primary aldosteronism after adrenalectomy. *J Clin Endocrinol Metab.* 2012;97(11):3965-3973. PMID: 22893716

Graber AL, Ney RL, Nicholson WE, Island DP, Liddle GW. Natural history of pituitary-adrenal recovery following long-term suppression with corticosteroids. *J Clin Endocrinol Metab.* 1965;25:11-16. PMID: 14252277

Reincke M, Nieke J, Krestin GP, Saeger W, Allolio B, Winkelmann W. Preclinical Cushing's syndrome in adrenal "incidentalomas": comparison with adrenal Cushing's syndrome. *J Clin Endocrinol Metab.* 1992;75(3):826-832. PMID: 1517373

Nakajima Y, Yamada M, Taguchi R, et al. Cardiovascular complications of patients with aldosteronism associated with autonomous cortisol secretion. *J Clin Endocrinol Metab.* 2011;96(8):2512-2518. PMID: 21593113

20

ANSWER: B) Late-night salivary cortisol measurement

Transsphenoidal pituitary microsurgery is the treatment of choice in patients with pituitary ACTH-dependent Cushing syndrome (Cushing disease). In experienced hands, the surgical success rate is 70% to 85%. The presence of immediate postoperative adrenal insufficiency (cortisol <2 µg/dL [<55.2 nmol/L]) usually portends a good outcome, with remission of hypercortisolism. The presence of secondary insufficiency after pituitary surgery for Cushing disease requires glucocorticoid support and is often associated with glucocorticoid withdrawal syndrome. Corticosteroid replacement therapy is provided until the hypothalamic-pituitary-adrenal axis recovers.

Despite the very good initial results published on pituitary surgery for Cushing disease, it has become increasingly apparent that 10% to 20% of patients have a recurrence of hypercortisolism anywhere from 2 to 15 years after their initial successful surgery. Frequently, patients are the first to recognize the recurrence and the signs and symptoms of hypercortisolism are usually much less severe than at their initial presentation. The patient described here had weight gain and blood pressure elevation and was very familiar with the neurocognitive and neuropsychiatric problems associated with hypercortisolism.

There is no consensus regarding the best diagnostic test to establish the diagnosis of recurrent Cushing disease after successful pituitary surgery; however, a preponderance of evidence now suggests that late-night salivary cortisol (Answer B) is the most sensitive diagnostic test to assess for the presence or absence of ACTH-dependent hypercortisolism. The failure of cortisol to reach a nadir around midnight is the earliest detectable biochemical abnormality in patients with Cushing disease who have a normal sleep–wake cycle. It may not be helpful in patients with irregular sleep–wake cycles. Twenty-four–hour urinary cortisol measurement has very poor sensitivity (70%) in the diagnosis of Cushing syndrome and is probably even worse in patients who present with mild recurrence of Cushing disease. Therefore, additional testing is needed, and such patients will not be easily reassured (Answer E).

Although the 2-day low-dose dexamethasone suppression test (Answer A) is of historical interest, it is not a sensitive indicator of early recurrent Cushing disease. It is very clear that many patients with mild ACTH-dependent Cushing syndrome suppress cortisol to relatively low levels after this test.

Pituitary imaging (Answer C) would be indicated only after the presence of recurrent hypercortisolism is established.

Although a frankly elevated basal ACTH level (Answer D) may increase the index of suspicion for recurrence, a normal level would not exclude the presence of hypercortisolism.

This woman had late-night salivary cortisol concentrations of 0.32 µg/dL (8.8 nmol/L) and 0.41 µg/dL (11.4 nmol/L). An overnight 1-mg dexamethasone-suppression test yielded a serum cortisol concentration of 1.4 µg/dL (38.6 nmol/L). Pituitary imaging was equivocal, but transsphenoidal pituitary surgery identified a residual corticotroph adenoma. Its removal resulted in secondary adrenal insufficiency and remission of her hypercortisolism.

EDUCATIONAL OBJECTIVE

Select late-night salivary cortisol measurement as the most sensitive diagnostic test to detect recurrent Cushing disease.

REFERENCE(S)

Bou Khalil R, Baudry C, Guignat L, et al. Sequential hormonal changes in 21 patients with recurrent Cushing's disease after successful pituitary surgery. *Eur J Endocrinol.* 2011;165(5):729-737. PMID: 21885674

Atkinson AB, Kennedy A, Wiggam MI, McCance DR, Sheridan B. Long-term remission rates after pituitary surgery for Cushing's disease: the need for long-term surveillance. *Clin Endocrinol (Oxf).* 2005;63(5):549-559. PMID: 16268808

Patil CG, Prevedello DM, Lad SP, et al. Late recurrences of Cushing's disease after initial successful transsphenoidal surgery. *J Clin Endocrinol Metab.* 2008;93(2):358-362. PMID: 18056770

Findling JW, Raff H, Aron DC. The low-dose dexamethasone suppression test: a reevaluation in patients with Cushing's syndrome. *J Clin Endocrinol Metab.* 2004;89(3):1222-1226. PMID: 15001614

21 ANSWER: A) Discontinue mifepristone and administer dexamethasone, 4 mg every 8 hours

Mifepristone, a derivative of norethindrone, is a progesterone receptor antagonist that has glucocorticoid receptor antagonist activity at higher concentrations. Mifepristone binds to the glucocorticoid receptor with an affinity 4 times higher than that of dexamethasone and about 8 times higher than that of cortisol, but it has little affinity for the mineralocorticoid receptor. It is the only medication currently approved by the US FDA for the treatment of patients with Cushing syndrome. Because it is a potent progesterone receptor antagonist, it is impossible to achieve pregnancy while using this medication. Thus, performing a pregnancy test (Answer D) does not make sense. Mifepristone is orally absorbed, is highly protein-bound, and has a long plasma half-life. It has been shown to improve the clinical manifestations and metabolic derangements associated with endogenous hypercortisolism. Specifically, as seen in this patient, there is a significant reduction in weight, as well as improved insulin sensitivity and glycemic control. However, mifepristone's unique mode of action challenges the endocrinologist monitoring its effectiveness and safety. Glucocorticoid antagonism decreases negative feedback of the hypothalamus and pituitary and leads to increased ACTH and cortisol production in patients with Cushing disease. Because plasma cortisol levels may rise during mifepristone therapy, there is no readily available biomarker to determine the impact of treatment.

The most commonly reported adverse effects in patients receiving mifepristone are nausea, fatigue, headache, arthralgias, vomiting, and decreased appetite. Of course, these symptoms may be manifestations of glucocorticoid withdrawal, but they may also be related to inadequate glucocorticoid activity or adrenal insufficiency. The patient's weight loss with poor appetite and nausea,

as well as the significant reduction in blood pressure with tachycardia, should raise the concern about the possibility of adrenal insufficiency. Because plasma cortisol levels usually increase substantially during mifepristone therapy, the elevated serum cortisol in this woman certainly does not exclude adrenal insufficiency. Ketoconazole (Answer B) is an imidazole derivative that inhibits several adrenal steroidogenic enzymes, thus decreasing cortisol synthesis. Its use in a patient on a glucocorticoid receptor antagonist would be strictly contraindicated. Moreover, mifepristone is metabolized by CYP3A4. Ketoconazole is known to inhibit this enzyme and thereby would further increase mifepristone levels and cause even more pronounced adrenal insufficiency.

Hypokalemia is a well-appreciated adverse effect of mifepristone treatment, occurring in 40% to 50% of patients. Hypokalemia may be associated with alkalosis and edema (as seen in the patient in this vignette) and it usually responds to potassium replacement and a mineralocorticoid receptor antagonist (spironolactone or eplerenone).

Hypokalemia is caused by the marked elevations of cortisol levels with glucocorticoid receptor blockade. Cortisol and aldosterone have the same affinity for the mineralocorticoid receptor. In the kidney, 11β-hydroxysteroid dehydrogenase type 2 converts cortisol to biologically inert cortisone, protecting the mineralocorticoid receptor. The severe hypercortisolemia caused by glucocorticoid receptor antagonism may not be completely inactivated by this enzyme. This impaired intrarenal metabolism of cortisol provides it free access to the mineralocorticoid receptor causing hypokalemic metabolic alkalosis and edema. Therefore, in contrast to patients with primary adrenal insufficiency, hypokalemia rather than hyperkalemia may be seen in patients with mifepristone-induced adrenal insufficiency.

Adrenal insufficiency in patients on mifepristone therapy is diagnosed clinically, and the fatigue, nausea, and decreased blood pressure in this patient should be considered sufficient evidence of this diagnosis. In such patients, mifepristone should be discontinued and dexamethasone should be administered (Answer A). A previous study suggested that 1 mg of dexamethasone daily competes with approximately 400 mg of mifepristone; however, some clinicians suggest administering 2 mg of dexamethasone for every 300 mg of mifepristone to ensure adequate treatment of adrenal insufficiency. Mifepristone can be restarted at a lower dosage and dexamethasone can be withdrawn after the signs and symptoms of adrenal insufficiency have resolved. Because of its long plasma half-life, mifepristone is usually withdrawn for 1 to 2 weeks.

Since mifepristone attenuates glucocorticoid negative feedback, there is some concern about the possibility of pituitary tumor growth. Nonetheless, increases in the size of ACTH-secreting pituitary tumors with administration of glucocorticoid receptor antagonists are rare. Although repeating pituitary MRI (Answer E) in this patient might be a reasonable study after her condition has been stabilized, it certainly does not need to be done immediately and does not take precedent over treating the adrenal insufficiency.

Mifepristone may also cause a reversible TSH increase without any changes in free serum T_4. Presumably, this is related to the attenuation of glucocorticoid-induced negative feedback on TSH secretion. There is no known reason to treat this abnormality (Answer C) unless free serum T_4 decreases. Because mifepristone is a potent antiprogestational agent, the endometrium is exposed to unopposed estrogen and the use of this agent may be associated with endometrial hyperplasia. Occasionally, break-through menstrual bleeding may occur, thus mandating temporary discontinuation of mifepristone.

This woman was actually seen at a local hospital by an endocrinologist who was not familiar with the presentation of mifepristone-induced adrenal insufficiency. Her condition improved with intravenous fluids, and, finally, after further consultation, mifepristone was withdrawn and dexamethasone was administered. Two weeks later, mifepristone was resumed at a lower dosage and the patient did well.

EDUCATIONAL OBJECTIVE
Diagnose and treat mifepristone-induced adrenal insufficiency.

REFERENCE(S)
Fleseriu M, Biller BMK, Findling JW, Molitch ME, Schteingart DE, Gross C; SEISMIC Study Investigators. Mifepristone, a glucocorticoid receptor antagonist, produces clinical and metabolic benefits in patients with Cushing's syndrome. *J Clin Endocrinol Metab.* 2012;97(6):2039-2049. PMID: 22466348

Carroll TB, Findling JW. The use of mifepristone in the treatment of Cushing's Syndrome. *Drugs Today (Barc).* 2012;48(8):509-518. PMID: 22916338

Fleseriu M, Molitch ME, Gross C, Schteingart DE, Vaughan TB 3rd, Biller BMK. A new therapeutic approach in the medical treatment of Cushing's syndrome: glucocorticoid receptor blockade with mifepristone. *Endocr Pract.* 2013;19(2):313-326. PMID: 23337135

22 **ANSWER: C) 24-hour urinary aldosterone and sodium measurement on the third day of a high-salt diet**

For this patient with resistant hypertension, the index of suspicion for primary aldosteronism is high. Nevertheless, the differential diagnosis of resistant hypertension also includes alcohol abuse, medication nonadherence, sleep apnea, and renal insufficiency. Her screening aldosterone-to-renin ratio is at least 23, which is positive; however, this ratio has sensitivity and specificity of only about 80% at a cutoff of 20. For this reason, the guidelines recommend confirmatory testing as the second step in the evaluation.

MR-angiography (Answer D) is appropriate if the renin activity is high, but in this case it is low.

Adrenal CT (Answer A) and adrenal venous sampling (Answer B) are only obtained after the diagnosis is confirmed.

While a 1-mg overnight dexamethasone-suppression test (Answer E) is sometimes part of the workup, it is not used until the diagnosis is confirmed.

The confirmatory tests include:

- Saline infusion (2 L over 4 hours); positive = serum aldosterone >10 ng/dL (>277.4 pmol/L)
- 24-Hour urinary aldosterone measurement on high-salt diet; positive = urinary aldosterone >12-14 µg/24 h (>33.2-38.8 nmol/d) (thus, Answer C is correct)
- Fluxdrocortisone-suppression test; positive = serum aldosterone >6 ng/dL (>166.4 pmol/L)
- Captopril challenge test; positive = no fall in serum aldosterone

The algorithm is shown in the figure.

EDUCATIONAL OBJECTIVE
Follow the steps in the evaluation of primary aldosteronism.

REFERENCE(S)

Funder JW, Carey RM, Mantero F, et al. The management of primary aldosteronism: case detection, diagnosis, and treatment: an Endocrine Society clinical practice guideline. *J Clin Endocrinol Metab.* 2016;101(5):1889-1916. PMID: 26934393

Nishizaka MK, Pratt-Ubunama M, Zaman MA, Cofield S, Calhoun DA. Validity of plasma aldosterone- to-renin activity ratio in African American and white subjects with resistant hypertension. *Am J Hypertens.* 2005;18(6):805-812. PMID: 15925740

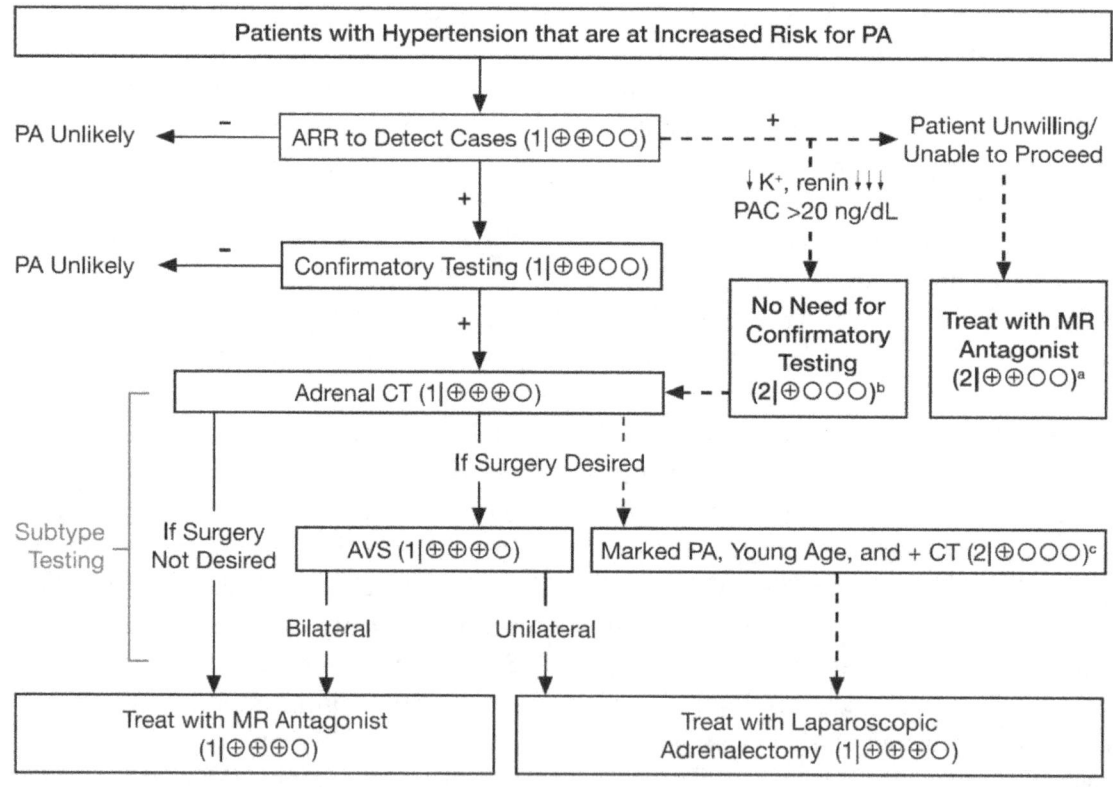

Adapted from Funder JW, et al. *J Clin Endocrinol Metab*, 2016 May;101(5) © Endocrine Society.

Calcium and Bone Board Review

Natalie E. Cusano, MD, MS

1 **ANSWER: A) Calculate her FRAX score**

A "low-trauma" or "fragility" fracture is defined by the World Health Organization as resulting from a trauma equivalent to a fall from standing height or less. While low-trauma rib fractures are considered to be fragility fractures, most experts do not consider rib fractures as osteoporosis-defining. Thus, starting alendronate (Answer C) is incorrect. There is general consensus, including guidelines from the Endocrine Society, that a low-trauma hip fracture is an osteoporosis-defining fracture. Many experts also consider low-trauma vertebral, proximal humerus, pelvis, and distal forearm fractures in the setting of osteopenia as diagnostic of osteoporosis; the American Association of Clinical Endocrinology uses this definition. A fragility fracture outside of these sites in a patient with osteopenia by bone density measurement should prompt use of the FRAX calculator (Answer A) to determine fracture risk and help guide consideration of treatment. Pharmacologic osteoporosis therapy would be recommended for patients with a T-score of −1 to −2.5 and a 10-year probability of 20% or higher for major osteoporotic fractures or 3% or higher for hip fractures based on the US-adapted FRAX tool.

Repeating a bone mineral density test in 2 years (Answer B) without calculation of her FRAX score to determine whether therapy is needed is incorrect.

Hormone therapy (Answer E) can be considered for symptomatic relief of vasomotor symptoms in some women, but it is not indicated as specific therapy for osteoporosis unless bisphosphonates or denosumab therapy is not appropriate.

Increasing her calcium and vitamin D intake (Answer D) is not correct since her calcium intake is sufficient by history and her 25-hydroxyvitamin D level is within the sufficient range.

EDUCATIONAL OBJECTIVE

Diagnose low-trauma fractures and determine a treatment plan.

REFERENCE(S)

Siris ES, Adler R, Bilezikian J, et al. The clinical diagnosis of osteoporosis: a position statement from the National Bone Health Alliance Working Group. *Osteoporos Int.* 2014;25(5):1439-1443. PMID: 24577348

Camacho PM, Petak SM, Binkley N, et al. American Association of Clinical Endocrinologists/American College of Endocrinology clinical practice guidelines for the diagnosis and treatment of postmenopausal osteoporosis-2020 update. *Endocr Pract.* 2020;26(Suppl 1):1-46. PMID: 32427503

Shoback D, Rosen CJ, Black DM, Cheung AM, Murad MH, Eastell R. Pharmacological management of osteoporosis in postmenopausal women: an Endocrine Society guideline update. *J Clin Endocrinol Metab.* 2020;105(3):dgaa048. PMID: 32068863

2 **ANSWER: D) Missed denosumab dose**

A missed dose (Answer D) or abrupt discontinuation of denosumab therapy has been associated with increased risk of multiple vertebral fractures, as early as 7 months from the last dose. Prior vertebral fracture, as in this patient, is a predictor of multiple vertebral fractures after discontinuation of denosumab. Patients on denosumab should be counseled regarding the importance of maintaining treatment every 6 months. Of note, the FDA insert for denosumab recommends considering transition to another antiresorptive agent if denosumab is discontinued. Intravenous bisphosphonate therapy does not appear to maintain bone gains with denosumab as well as oral bisphosphonate therapy does.

Atypical femoral fractures, but not vertebral fractures, are a rare possible complication of prolonged antiresorptive therapy (Answer A).

Her elevated total and bone-specific alkaline phosphatase levels can be explained by her multiple recent fractures and missed denosumab dose. Paget disease (Answer E) is unlikely.

She has a history of stage 1 breast cancer (Answer C), which is unlikely to cause metastasis to her spine.

While aromatase inhibitor therapy has been associated with an increased risk of bone loss and fracture, tamoxifen (Answer B) may be associated with improved bone density and has not been demonstrated to increase fracture risk in postmenopausal woman. Tamoxifen therapy in premenopausal woman, however, may increase risk of bone loss due to competition with circulating estrogen.

EDUCATIONAL OBJECTIVE
Relate the adverse effects of a missed dose or abrupt discontinuation of denosumab therapy.

REFERENCE(S)
Tsourdi E, Langdahl B, Cohen-Solal M, et al. Discontinuation of denosumab therapy for osteo-porosis: a systematic review and position state-ment by ECTS. *Bone.* 2017;105:11-17. PMID: 28789921

Prolia (denosumab). Package insert. Amgen, Inc; 2011.

3 ANSWER: A) Calcium and vitamin D supplementation
A Cochrane review found high-quality evidence that calcium and vitamin D taken together (Answer A) can reduce the likelihood of hip fractures (relative risk, 0.84; 95% CI, 0.74-0.96) and nonvertebral fractures. No effect was noted with calcium or vitamin D supplementation alone (Answers B and D). The optimal intake of calcium and vitamin D is uncertain. Based on the meta-analyses, most experts suggest 1200 mg of calcium (total of diet and supplement) in divided doses, and 800 IU of vitamin D daily for most postmenopausal women with osteoporosis.

Strontium ranelate had been an approved drug for treatment of osteoporosis in Europe and other countries outside the United States, with demonstrated efficacy for vertebral and nonvertebral fractures; however, therapy was associated with possible increased risk of myocardial infarction. Strontium citrate (Answer C), which is used in various supplements, has no clinical trial evidence of fracture prevention efficacy.

A vitamin K_2 preparation (menatetrenone) (Answer E) is approved for use in Japan based on clinical trial data demonstrating reduction in fracture risk in postmenopausal Japanese women. However, the published data are conflicting, and no benefit has been shown in other populations.

EDUCATIONAL OBJECTIVE
Counsel a patient regarding nutritional and supplemental approaches for bone health.

REFERENCE(S)
Avenell A, Mak JCS, O'Connell D. Vitamin D and vitamin D analogues for preventing fractures in post-menopausal women and older men. *Cochrane Database Syst Rev.* 2014;2014(4):CD000227. PMID: 24729336

4 ANSWER: C) Parathyroidectomy in the second trimester
This patient has an elevated serum calcium concentration with concurrently elevated PTH consistent with primary hyperparathyroidism. Her elevated 24-hour urinary calcium excretion excludes familial hypocalciuric hypercalcemia. Primary hyperparathyroidism in pregnancy is associated with a number of maternal complications, including hyperemesis gravidarum, nephrolithiasis, pancreatitis, miscarriage, and preeclampsia. Parathyroidectomy in the second trimester (Answer C) has been associated with favorable outcomes in patients with moderate to severe hypercalcemia during pregnancy in several case reports and case series. Surgery should be avoided in the first trimester (Answer D) if possible.

Cinacalcet (Answer A) is pregnancy category C because it has been shown to cross the placenta, and there are no long-term safety data in pregnancy. However, there have been a few published case reports.

Bisphosphonates and denosumab (Answer B) are pregnancy category D drugs and should be avoided in pregnancy because of adverse fetal skeletal outcomes in animal studies.

Calcitriol levels increase 2- to 5-fold in euparathyroid women in the first trimester of pregnancy to increase intestinal absorption of calcium. The patient's high 1,25-dihydroxyvitamin D level is due to increased production during pregnancy and activation of 1α-hydroxylase activity by PTH. Thus, prednisone (Answer E) is not indicated.

EDUCATIONAL OBJECTIVE
Manage primary hyperparathyroidism in pregnancy.

REFERENCE(S)
Ali DS, Dandurand K, Khan AA. Primary hyperparathyroidism in pregnancy: literature review of the diagnosis and management. *J Clin Med.* 2021;10(13):2956. PMID: 34209340

Bilezikian JP, Khan AA, Silverberg SJ, Fuleihan GEH. Evaluation and management of primary hyperparathyroidism: summary statement and guidelines from the Fifth International Workshop. *J Bone Miner Res.* Forthcoming 2022.

5 ANSWER: C) McCune-Albright syndrome
The radiograph demonstrates irregular, marginated, ground-glass lucencies surrounded by reactive bone. The shaft has an appearance that has been described as a soap bubble. This x-ray is characteristic of fibrous dysplasia, a benign skeletal lesion, most commonly monostotic with a predilection for long bones, ribs, and craniofacial bones. Fibrous dysplasia and McCune-Albright syndrome (OMIM#174800) are skeletal diseases caused by pathogenic postzygotic somatic activating or gain-of-function *GNAS* variants. The fibrous dysplasia/McCune-Albright Syndrome International Consortium defines McCune-Albright syndrome as a combination of fibrous dysplasia and 1 or more extraskeletal feature, or the presence of 2 or more extraskeletal features. Extraskeletal features include:

1. Café-au-lait skin macules with characteristic appearance of jagged, irregular borders (coast of Maine) and a distribution showing the so-called respect of the midline of the body
2. Gonadotropin-independent sex steroid production resulting in precocious puberty, recurrent ovarian cysts in girls and women, or autonomous testosterone production in boys and men
3. Thyroid lesions consistent with fibrous dysplasia/McCune-Albright syndrome with or without nonautoimmune hyperthyroidism
4. GH excess
5. Neonatal hypercortisolism

This patient has evidence of fibrous dysplasia on radiograph, a café-au-lait skin macule with an irregular border on examination, and toxic multinodular goiter, meeting the criteria for McCune-Albright syndrome (Answer C). Given the presence of extraskeletal features, monostotic fibrous dysplasia (Answer D) is incorrect. The remaining answers are not consistent with the patient's radiographic, physical examination, or laboratory findings.

Albright hereditary osteodystrophy (Answer A) is associated with pseudohypoparathyroidism and pseudopseudohypoparathyroidism. It is characterized by brachydactyly (classically described as shortening of the third, fourth, and fifth metacarpals), round facies, short stature, obesity, developmental delay, and subcutaneous calcifications.

Oncogenic osteomalacia (tumor-induced osteomalacia [Answer E]) is caused by small mesenchymal tumors that secrete high levels of FGF-23, producing renal tubular loss of phosphorus.

Fibrodysplasia ossificans progressiva (Answer B) is a disorder in which muscle and connective tissue are gradually replaced by bone (ossified), forming extraskeletal or heterotopic bone that can constrain movement.

EDUCATIONAL OBJECTIVE
Diagnose McCune-Albright syndrome.

REFERENCE(S)

Javaid MK, Boyce A, Appelman-Dijkstra N, et al. Best practice management guidelines for fibrous dysplasia/McCune-Albright syndrome: a consensus statement from the FD/MAS international consortium. *Orphanet J Rare Dis.* 2019;14(1):139. PMID: 31196103

6 ANSWER: C) Increased bone formation; decreased bone resorption

Bone formation and resorption are tightly linked processes. Romosozumab is a monoclonal antibody against sclerostin that has been approved for treatment of postmenopausal women with osteoporosis at high risk for fracture. It results in an uncoupling of the bone remodeling cycle, with an increase in bone formation markers and a decrease in bone resorption markers (Answer C). Of note, romosozumab has been approved by the US FDA with a boxed warning that therapy should not be initiated in patients who have had a myocardial infarction or stroke within the preceding year.

Osteoanabolic therapy with teriparatide and abaloparatide initially results in an increase in bone formation markers with little effect on bone resorption (Answer A); however, because bone formation and resorption are tightly linked, bone resorption markers also rise during therapy (Answer B). The period when bone formation exceeds resorption is termed the "anabolic window." Antiresorptive medications, including bisphosphonates and denosumab, decrease both markers of bone resorption and formation (Answer E). There is no current osteoporosis drug therapy with antiresorptive properties that has no effect on bone formation (Answer D).

EDUCATIONAL OBJECTIVE

Describe the mechanism of action of romosozumab in the management of osteoporosis.

REFERENCE(S)

Cosman F, Crittenden DB, Adachi JD, et al. Romosozumab treatment in postmenopausal women with osteoporosis. *N Engl J Med.* 2016;375(16):1532-1543. PMID: 27641143

7 ANSWER: D) 8 to 12 months

Vitamin D toxicity is not a common cause of hypercalcemia. The liver converts almost all vitamin D to 25-hydroxyvitamin D through the action of several loosely regulated substrate-dependent cytochrome P450-linked oxidases. High concentrations of 25-hydroxyvitamin D may saturate the vitamin D–binding protein, resulting in the greater availability of 1,25-dihydroxyvitamin D at tissue sites. In addition, high concentrations of 25-hydroxyvitamin D may compete to bind at vitamin D receptor sites, producing similar effects as 1,25-dihydroxyvitamin D by initiating translation of vitamin D receptor–responsive genes. The kidney 1α-hydroxylase enzyme is under strict control and limits the production of 1,25-dihydroxyvitamin D, even if large amounts of 25-hydroxyvitamin D are available. In addition to the kidney, however, several other tissues express 1α-hydroxylase, and local paracrine conversion of 25-hydroxyvitamin D to 1,25-dihydroxyvitamin D may also have contributed to this patient's hypercalcemia. In a series of 9 patients with vitamin D intoxication due to an over-the-counter vitamin supplement called Soladek, including the patient in this vignette, there were often other reasons for hypercalcemia (such as lymphoma, granulomatous disease, etc), so that the homeostatic and detoxifying mechanisms were overwhelmed.

The biological half-life of 1,25-dihydroxyvitamin D is only approximately 15 hours, and toxicity due to calcitriol or other active vitamin D concentrations is short-lived. In contrast, vitamin D is highly lipophilic and the half-life of vitamin D ranges from 20 days to months. In this patient with an initial 25-hydroxyvitamin D concentration of 525 ng/mL (1310 nmol/L), it took 12 months (Answer D) for it to drop to 32 ng/mL (79.9 nmol/L) (*see figure on the next page*).

Treatment of vitamin D intoxication includes vigorous intravenous hydration, bisphosphonates, and glucocorticoids, with the caveat that resolution of the high 25-hydroxyvitamin D levels may take weeks or months.

Figure. Change in 25-Hydroxyvitamin D Over Time

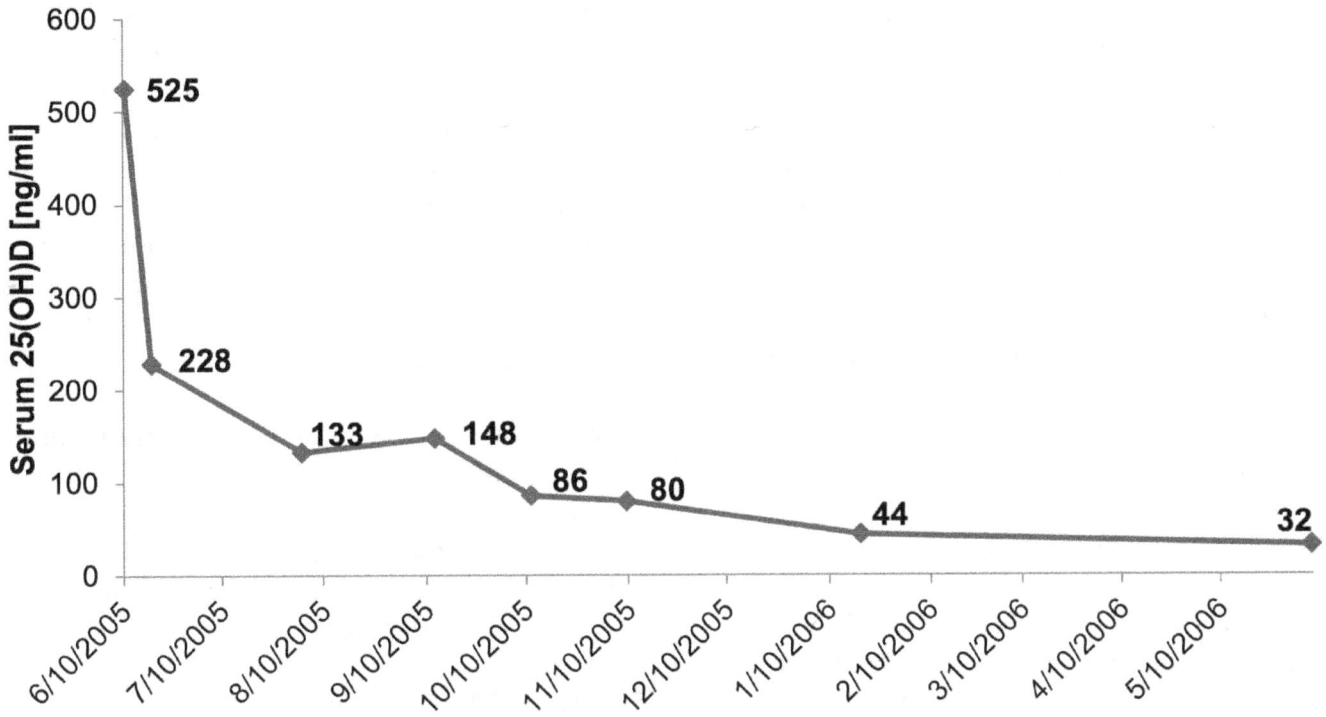

From Lowe H et al. *J Clin Endocrinol Metab*, 2011;96(2) © Endocrine Society.

EDUCATIONAL OBJECTIVE
Identify the timeframe for resolution of vitamin D toxicity.

REFERENCE(S)
Lowe H, Cusano NE, Binkley N, Blaner WS, Bilezikian JP. Vitamin D toxicity due to a commonly available "over the counter" remedy from the Dominican Republic. *J Clin Endocrinol Metab*. 2011;96(2):291-295. PMID: 21123442

Cusano NE, Thys-Jacobs S, and Bilezikian, JP. Hypercalcemia due to vitamin D toxicity. In: Feldman D, Pike JW, Glorieux FH, eds. *Vitamin D*. 3rd ed. Academic Press; 2011: 1381-1402.

8 **ANSWER: D) Severe hypocalcemia**
Chronic kidney disease–mineral and bone disorder (CKD-MBD) describes the systemic changes in mineral, metabolic, hormonal, and bone homeostasis that can increase the risk of fractures, vascular calcification, cardiovascular morbidity, and mortality in patients with stage 3 to 5 chronic kidney disease. Patients with chronic kidney disease have a 2- to 17-fold greater risk of fracture than the general population. Renal osteodystrophy is a broad term describing the various effects of CKD-MBD on bone formation and resorption.

Bone morphology in CKD-MBD is mainly affected by the rate of bone turnover, with a PTH-induced increase in bone resorption (coupled with increased bone formation) generally leading to higher rates of bone turnover. The type and degree of renal osteodystrophy depends on the combination of these factors and the impact of guideline-derived medical interventions. In early chronic kidney disease, bone turnover rates tend to be high, driven by secondary hyperparathyroidism. As chronic kidney disease progresses to end-stage kidney disease, low bone turnover is more prevalent, which may be in large part iatrogenic, due to oversuppression of PTH by medications such as calcium-based phosphate binders, activated vitamin D, and calcimimetics.

It is suggested that patients with chronic kidney disease with evidence of renal osteodystrophy and fracture be diagnosed with osteoporosis, as their bone quality and strength are similarly impaired. Treating low bone density in patients with chronic kidney disease first involves assessing bone turnover. While a bone biopsy is the gold standard, it is an invasive test with limited availability. Serum and plasma bone turnover markers are often used to assess bone turnover. Significantly elevated PTH and bone-specific alkaline phosphatase levels correlate with high bone turnover, and significantly low levels correlate with low bone turnover states. A bone biopsy should be considered in the case of intermediate levels of bone turnover markers.

Treatment of osteoporosis in patients with chronic kidney disease can be challenging. Nephrotoxicity has been reported with bisphosphonates, particularly with intravenous therapy. Pamidronate is associated with focal glomerular sclerosis (especially with multiple high doses) and zoledronic acid has been reported to cause acute tubular injury, even at the 4-mg dose. However, recent data suggest that with careful attention to dosing, infusion rates, and treatment frequency, nephrotoxicity may be rare. Denosumab is not cleared by the kidney and has been used in patients with chronic kidney disease and fractures. While antiresorptive therapies should be avoided in low bone turnover disease, osteoanabolic agents are likely useful. Teriparatide has been studied in small numbers of patients with end-stage kidney disease and low bone turnover.

Denosumab is a human monoclonal antibody against RANK ligand approved for treatment of osteoporosis. It is a very potent inhibitor of osteoclastic bone resorption. Unlike bisphosphonates, denosumab is not cleared via the kidneys and has no effect on kidney function (thus, Answer E is incorrect). The major adverse effect to be expected in this setting is profound, symptomatic hypocalcemia (Answer D) within 7 to 10 days following denosumab administration. Patients at greatest risk for this complication are those with significantly impaired kidney function and high bone turnover with elevated alkaline phosphatase, as demonstrated in this patient. The potent inhibition of osteoclastic bone resorption by denosumab stops the efflux of calcium from bone and can lower serum calcium dramatically. The usual physiologic responses to hypocalcemia, such as a rise in PTH and calcitriol production, that would normally lead to increased renal tubular reabsorption of calcium and increased gut absorption of calcium, will not work in the setting of kidney failure. This woman also has a low vitamin D level and is also at risk for an inadequate homeostatic response due to low vitamin D substrate.

Although cases of osteonecrosis of the jaw (Answer B) have been reported with both bisphosphonates and denosumab, this is very unlikely after a single dose.

Severe flulike syndromes (Answer C) (also known as "acute-phase reactions") are much more common with intravenous bisphosphonates than with denosumab.

Potent antiresorptive agents such as denosumab have not been shown to impair fracture healing (Answer A).

EDUCATIONAL OBJECTIVE
Anticipate the risk of symptomatic hypocalcemia following denosumab in the setting of kidney failure.

REFERENCE(S)
Dave V, Chiang CY, Booth J, Mount PF. Hypocalcemia post denosumab in patients with chronic kidney disease stage 4-5. *Am J Nephrol.* 2015;41(2):129-137. PMID: 25790847

Barta VS, DeVita MV, Rosenstock JL. Chronic kidney disease-mineral and bone disorder (CKD-MBD). *Osteoporosis: A Clinical Casebook.* Cusano NE, ed. Springer; 2021: 109-121.

9 **ANSWER: C) Decreased serum calcium, decreased PTH, no change in bone density**
Cinacalcet is a calcimimetic, working to increase the sensitivity of the calcium-sensing receptor on the parathyroid gland. Cinacalcet is approved by the US FDA for treatment of hypercalcemia in adults with primary hyperparathyroidism for whom parathyroidectomy is indicated on the basis of serum calcium levels, but who are unable to undergo surgery. Cinacalcet has been demonstrated to significantly decrease serum calcium levels; therapy can also decrease PTH concentrations to a lesser extent in patients with primary hyperparathyroidism.

Cinacalcet has no demonstrated effect on bone density. Answer C correctly lists the expected effects on biochemical and bone density parameters in patients with primary hyperparathyroidism treated with cinacalcet. Alendronate significantly improves bone density in patients with primary hyperparathyroidism, similar to its effects in euparathyroid patients, and is routinely used in patients with primary hyperparathyroidism who have low bone density. There are now clinical trial data showing that denosumab also improves bone density in patients with primary hyperparathyroidism. It is important to note there are no fracture data in patients with primary hyperparathyroidism treated with antiresorptive therapy.

EDUCATIONAL OBJECTIVE

Recognize the mechanism of action of cinacalcet in primary hyperparathyroidism.

REFERENCE(S)

Peacock M, Bolognese MA, Borofsky M, et al. Cinacalcet treatment of primary hyperparathyroidism: biochemical and bone densitometric outcomes in a five-year study. *J Clin Endocrinol Metab.* 2009;94(12):4860-4867. PMID: 19837909

Marcocci C, Bollerslev J, Khan AA, Shoback DM. Medical management of primary hyperparathyroidism: proceedings of the fourth International Workshop on the Management of Asymptomatic Primary Hyperparathyroidism. *J Clin Endocrinol Metab.* 2014;99(10):3607-3618. PMID: 25162668

Leere JS, Karmisholt J, Robaczyk M, et al. Denosumab and cinacalcet for primary hyperparathyroidism (DENOCINA): a randomised, double-blind, placebo-controlled, phase 3 trial. *Lancet Diabetes Endocrinol.* 2020;8(5):407-417. PMID: 32333877

10 ANSWER: D) Kidney ultrasonography

Preservation of kidney function is critically important in patients with hypoparathyroidism. In a large Danish study of postoperative patients, risk of kidney calcification was increased 4.8-fold and risk of renal insufficiency was increased 5-fold compared with observations in healthy control participants. International and European guidelines recommend routine monitoring of 24-hour urinary calcium excretion, at least annually or every 2 years. International guidelines recommend kidney imaging at baseline and every 5 years if the patient is asymptomatic or more frequently if clinical symptoms arise. The European guidelines recommend kidney imaging if the patient develops kidney stones or if serum creatinine levels increase. In a direct comparison of ultrasonography and CT in 22 patients with hypoparathyroidism, ultrasonography was found to be superior to CT for detecting nephrocalcinosis. This patient has elevated creatinine, and kidney ultrasonography (Answer D) is recommended by both guidelines.

Patients with hypoparathyroidism have an increased risk of other complications, including cataracts and basal ganglia calcification. Slit-lamp examination for cataracts (but not measurement of intraocular pressure [Answer E]) may be indicated.

Head imaging (Answer C) is indicated for patients with neurologic symptoms.

Bone density assessment (Answer A) is recommended in the international guidelines if a patient otherwise meets criteria for measurement; the European guidelines recommend against routine monitoring of bone density.

While altered tooth morphology may be seen in very young patients with hypoparathyroidism, there are no apparent dental manifestations in adult patients. Routine dental examination (Answer B) can be recommended, but it is not as important as kidney imaging in this patient.

EDUCATIONAL OBJECTIVE

Manage a patient with chronic hypoparathyroidism who is at risk for kidney complications.

REFERENCE(S)

Bilezikian JP, Brandi ML, Cusano NE, et al. Management of hypoparathyroidism: present and future. *J Clin Endocrinol Metab.* 2016;101(6):2313-2324. PMID: 26938200

Bollerslev J, Rejnmark L, Marcocci C, et al; European Society of Endocrinology. European Society of Endocrinology clinical guideline: treatment of chronic hypoparathyroidism in adults. *Eur J Endocrinol*. 2015;173(2):G1-G20. PMID: 26160136

Underbjerg L, Sikjaer T, Mosekilde L, Rejnmark L. Cardiovascular and renal complications to postsurgical hypoparathyroidism: a Danish nationwide controlled historic follow-up study. *J Bone Miner Res*. 2013;28(11):2277-2285. PMID: 23661265

11 ANSWER: D) Genetic testing for pathogenic variants in the multiple endocrine neoplasia type 1 gene (*MEN1*)

It is critical to think about and screen for *MEN1* pathogenic variants (Answer D) in all young patients (<30 years) who present with primary hyperparathyroidism. Up to 10% of patients with primary hyperparathyroidism have a familial (germline) pathogenic variant. Hereditary syndromes should be suspected in anyone with a personal history of other endocrine tumors (especially pancreatic or pituitary) or a family history of parathyroid disease, kidney stones, or pancreatic/pituitary tumors in first-degree relatives. These syndromes should also be suspected and screened for in patients presenting with atypical or multigland parathyroid adenomas at any age. Only 2% to 4% of all patients with primary hyperparathyroidism present with multigland adenomas.

In addition to multiple endocrine neoplasia type 1, other more rare causes of multiorgan syndromic primary hyperparathyroidism include multiple endocrine neoplasia type 2, multiple endocrine neoplasia type 4, and hyperparathyroidism–jaw tumor syndrome. Familial idiopathic primary hyperparathyroidism may be a subtype of hyperparathyroidism–jaw tumor syndrome.

The presence of kidney stones and high urinary calcium excretion excludes familial hypocalciuric hypercalcemia caused by an inactivating variant in the gene encoding the calcium-sensing receptor (*CASR*) (Answer C).

Although a 4D CT of the neck (Answer A) would be reasonable in an older patient with persistent primary hyperparathyroidism, in this young woman it is mandatory to screen for multiple endocrine neoplasia first because that diagnosis would alter the surgical management and medical follow-up.

Another sestamibi scan (Answer E) looking for a second adenoma would not be indicated when all 4 glands may be involved.

Calcium supplementation would not be responsible for these laboratory findings, so cessation of this treatment (Answer B) is not necessary.

EDUCATIONAL OBJECTIVE

Pursue the diagnosis of multiple endocrine neoplasia type 1 in young patients presenting with primary hyperparathyroidism.

REFERENCE(S)

Thakker RV, Newey PJ, Walls GV, et al; Endocrine Society. Clinical practice guidelines for multiple endocrine neoplasia 1 (MEN1). *J Clin Endocrinol Metab*. 2012;97(9):2990-3011. PMID: 22723327

Eastell R, Brandi ML, Costa AG, D'Amour P, Shoback DM, Thakker RV. Diagnosis of asymptomatic primary hyperparathyroidism: proceedings of the Fourth International Workshop. *J Clin Endocrinol Metab*. 2014;99(10):3570-3579. PMID: 25162666

Lassen T, Friis-Hansen L, Rasmussen AK, Knigge U, Feldt-Rasmussen U. Primary hyperparathyroidism in young people. When should we perform genetic testing for multiple endocrine neoplasia 1 (MEN-1)? *J Clin Endocrinol Metab*. 2014;99(11):3983-3987. PMID: 24731012

12 ANSWER: C) Serum cortisol and ACTH

This patient has autoimmune polyendocrine syndrome type 1 (APS type 1) due to a pathogenic variant in the autoimmune regulator gene (*AIRE*) and presents with symptoms and signs of Addison disease. APS type 1 is also known by the acronym APECED (autoimmune polyendocrinopathy-candidiasis-ectodermal dystrophy). The classic presentation includes at least 2 of the following 3 major clinical components: chronic mucocutaneous candidiasis, primary hypoparathyroidism, and autoimmune adrenal insufficiency. The physical examination notes ectodermal dystrophy of the fingernails. Hyperpigmentation from adrenal insufficiency would also be expected on exam. Primary adrenal insufficiency may be diagnosed before clinical symptoms by checking for 21-hydroxylase antibodies, but in this case, serum cortisol and ACTH (Answer C) must be measured immediately. Given the physical examination findings, one would expect to find hyponatremia, hyperkalemia, and elevated ACTH, along with a low or "normal" serum cortisol (which is being maximally stimulated). Pending the results, a formal cosyntropin-stimulation test should be done.

Islet-cell and glutamic acid decarboxylase antibodies (Answer B) can be used for diagnosis of type 1 diabetes mellitus, which can occur in patients with APECED; however, it is much more rare than adrenal insufficiency and prompt diagnosis of adrenal insufficiency is critical.

Hypothyroidism can occur with APECED, although not typically hyperthyroidism (Answer D).

Transglutaminase antibodies (Answer E) can be used to diagnose celiac disease. While up to 80% of patients with APECED have malabsorption or other gastrointestinal illness, celiac disease is not typical.

Carcinoid syndrome can be diagnosed through measurement of 24-hour urinary excretion of 5-hydroxyindoleacetic acid (5-HIAA) (Answer A); however, it is not a feature of APECED and her diarrhea and other symptoms are more concerning for adrenal insufficiency.

EDUCATIONAL OBJECTIVE
Diagnose Addison disease as part of autoimmune polyendocrine syndrome type 1.

REFERENCE(S)

Weiler FG, Dias-da-Silva MR, Lazaretti-Castro M. Autoimmune polyendocrine syndrome type 1: case report and review of literature. *Arq Bras Endocrinol Metabol.* 2012;56(1):54-66. PMID: 22460196

Akirav EM, Ruddle NH, Herold KC. The role of AIRE in human autoimmune disease. *Nat Rev Endocrinol.* 2011;7(1):25-33. PMID: 21102544

Eisenbarth GS, Gottlieb PA. Autoimmune polyendocrine syndromes. *N Engl J Med.* 2004;350(20):2068-2079. PMID: 15141045

Ferre EMN, Rose SR, Rosenzweig SD, et al. Redefined clinical features and diagnostic criteria in autoimmune polyendocrinopathy-candidiasis-ectodermal dystrophy. *JCI Insight.* 2016;1(13):e88782. PMID: 27588307

13   **ANSWER: A) Begin alendronate**
This man has an acute, symptomatic vertebral compression fracture at L1. This warrants intervention with antiresorptive therapy regardless of the DXA results because vertebral fractures are strong independent predictors of both future vertebral and nonvertebral fractures. The correct answer is to begin alendronate (Answer A) because it is an approved and effective therapy in this setting. Repeating DXA now, before therapy initiation, could be considered, although it is unlikely to be helpful given his degenerative arthritis at the spine, and the results would not change the recommendation for therapy.

Teriparatide (Answer B) is contraindicated in a man who has received pelvic irradiation.

A nuclear medicine bone scan (Answer E) is not indicated given the absence of clinical or biochemical evidence (ie, his alkaline phosphatase level is normal) of recurrent bladder cancer or other malignancy.

Patients with acute vertebral fractures from osteoporosis should generally not be referred for vertebral augmentation (kyphoplasty or vertebroplasty [Answer D]) unless severe pain has not responded to medical therapies. Of note, kyphoplasty may be associated with a higher rate of subsequent fracture at adjacent vertebrae.

Because there are no large randomized controlled trials showing antifracture efficacy for testosterone in men with osteoporosis, testosterone therapy (Answer C) should be considered only for hypogonadal men who are symptomatic, have an organic cause of the hypogonadism, have testosterone levels less than 200 ng/dL (<6.9 nmol/L), and/or are not candidates for other therapies. Due to reports of cardiovascular complications, testosterone is not an ideal therapy for a 72-year-old man. In hypogonadal men with benign prostatic hypertrophy, testosterone therapy, along with a 5α-reductase inhibitor such as finasteride, has been given without exacerbating benign prostatic hypertrophy. However, even men with marked hypogonadism have good skeletal responses to bisphosphonate therapy without correction of hypogonadism.

EDUCATIONAL OBJECTIVE

Manage an acute vertebral fracture in an elderly man.

REFERENCE(S)

Watts NB, Adler RA, Bilezikian JP, et al; Endocrine Society. Osteoporosis in men: an Endocrine Society clinical practice guideline. *J Clin Endocrinol Metab.* 2012;97(6):1802-1822. PMID: 22675062

Cosman F, de Beur SJ, LeBoff MS, et al; National Osteoporosis Foundation. Clinician's guide to prevention and treatment of osteoporosis. *Osteoporos Int.* 2014;25(10):2359-2381. PMID: 25182228

McConnell CT Jr, Wippold FJ 2nd, Ray CE Jr, et al. ACR appropriateness criteria for management of vertebral compression fractures. *J Am Coll Radiol.* 2014;11(8):757-763. PMID: 24935074

14 ANSWER: E) Worsening arthritis in the hip

Zoledronic acid should improve the component of pain arising from the pagetic involvement of the patient's left hip, but it is not expected to help the pain due to degenerative arthritis and may not prevent arthritis progression (thus, Answer E is correct and Answer D is incorrect).

Paget disease does not extend across joint spaces and has never been reported to develop in new bones not involved at diagnosis (thus, Answer C is incorrect).

Since she does not have Paget disease in her skull, it will not cause hearing loss (Answer A).

Osteonecrosis of the femoral neck (Answer B) is not more likely after treatment with zoledronic acid in patients with Paget disease of the hip.

Whether all patients with Paget disease should be treated is controversial. Indications for treatment in asymptomatic patients include the following:

- Involvement of a weight-bearing bone (eg, spine or leg)
- Involvement near a joint
- Involvement of the skull
- Serum alkaline phosphatase level greater than 3 times the upper normal limit

Zoledronic acid is clearly the most effective treatment. It normalizes bone turnover markers and maintains normal values for the longest duration of any medication. Normal turnover markers are associated with the normalization of pagetic woven bone to lamellar bone and can eliminate pain arising from pagetic bone. A single dose of zoledronic acid results in many years of disease inactivity in most patients.

EDUCATIONAL OBJECTIVE

Counsel patients that treating Paget disease should effectively eliminate pain attributable to the pagetic bone, but it is not expected to resolve pain due to degenerative arthritis.

REFERENCE(S)

Reid IR, Lyles K, Su G, et al. A single infusion of zoledronic acid produces sustained remissions in Paget disease: data to 6.5 years. *J Bone Miner Res.* 2011;26(9):2261-2270. PMID: 21638319

Langston AL, Campbell MK, Fraser WD, et al; PRISM Trial Group. Randomized trial of intensive bisphosphonate treatment versus symptomatic management in Paget's disease of bone. *J Bone Miner Res.* 2010;25(1):20-31. PMID: 19580457

Ralston SH. Clinical practice. Paget's disease of bone. *N Engl J Med.* 2013;368(7):644-650. PMID: 23406029

15 ANSWER: B) 25-Hydroxyvitamin D

Shown on the radiograph is a Looser zone, characteristic of osteomalacia. Mechanical stress of blood vessels overlying the uncalcified cortical bone affected by osteomalacia is thought to cause "pseudofractures" that appear as transverse zones of rarefaction, sometimes as wide as 1 cm, often multiple, and generally symmetric. Typical locations are the ischium, ilium, pubis, femur, tibia, radius, fibula, lower ribs, and scapula.

This patient was found to have celiac disease, which is causing malabsorption of calcium and vitamin D. Her serum 25-hydroxyvitamin D level (Answer B) was undetectable (<7 ng/mL [<17.5 nmol/L]). Chemical clues to osteomalacia include hypocalcemia, hypophosphatemia, and elevated alkaline phosphatase. Measuring FGF-23 (Answer C), 1,25-dihydroxyvitamin D (Answer A), intact PTH (Answer D), or serum protein electrophoresis (Answer E) would not clarify the diagnosis.

EDUCATIONAL OBJECTIVE
Identify clinical and radiographic findings in osteomalacia (severe vitamin D deficiency).

REFERENCE(S)
Reginato AJ, Falasca GF, Pappu R, McKnight B, Agha A. Musculoskeletal manifestations of osteomalacia: report of 26 cases and literature review. *Semin Arthritis Rheum.* 1999;28(5):287-304. PMID: 10342386

Thacher TD, Clarke BL. Vitamin D insufficiency. *Mayo Clin Proc.* 2011;86(1):50-60. PMID: 21193656

Bhan A, Rao AD, Rao DS. Osteomalacia as a result of vitamin D deficiency. *Endocrinol Metab Clin North Am.* 2010;39(2):321-331. PMID: 20511054

16 **ANSWER: D) Zoledronic acid**
The 2017 guidelines from the American College of Rheumatology recommend pharmacologic treatment for adults 40 years and older with a moderate fracture risk, defined as a glucocorticoid-adjusted FRAX risk of 10% to 19% for major osteoporotic fracture or 1.1% to 2.9% for hip fracture.

Alendronate, risedronate, zoledronic acid (Answer D), teriparatide (Answer C), and denosumab (Answer A) (but not ibandronate [Answer B]) are all FDA approved for management of glucocorticoid-induced osteoporosis. Because there is still controversy about the link between esophageal cancer and oral bisphosphonate use, it may be preferable to start with intravenous zoledronic acid (Answer D) rather than an oral bisphosphonate in a patient with Barrett esophagus.

Teriparatide (Answer C) is usually reserved for patients with prevalent vertebral fractures or much lower vertebral T-scores—in the frankly osteoporotic range.

Given limited safety data, denosumab (Answer A) is generally not recommended as first-line therapy in patients taking multiple immunosuppressive drugs or biologic drugs.

Finally, the low FRAX scores underestimate the fracture risk in patients on long-term glucocorticoid therapy. FRAX does not account for the disproportionate negative effects of glucocorticoids on spinal trabecular bone and does not include spinal bone mineral density in the calculation. Therefore, recommending no therapeutic intervention (Answer E) is incorrect despite the patient's low FRAX scores. Of note, it has been recommended to adjust FRAX scores for patients taking a prednisone dosage greater than 7.5 mg daily or equivalent by multiplying the major osteoporotic fracture risk by 1.15 and hip fracture risk by 1.2.

EDUCATIONAL OBJECTIVE
Determine whether pharmacologic treatment to reduce fracture risk is necessary in a patient taking glucocorticoids.

REFERENCE(S)
Buckley L, Guyatt G, Fink HA, et al. 2017 American College of Rheumatology guideline for the prevention and treatment of glucocorticoid-induced osteoporosis. *Arthritis Rheumatol.* 2017;69(8):1521-1537. PMID: 28585373

Venuturupalli SR, Sacks W. Review of new guidelines for the management of glucocorticoid induced osteoporosis. *Curr Osteoporos Rep.* 2013;11(4):357-364. PMID: 24114241

Leib ES, Saag KG, Adachi JD, et al; FRAX(®) Position Development Conference Members. Official Positions for FRAX(®) clinical regarding glucocorticoids: the impact of the use of glucocorticoids on the estimate by FRAX(®) of the 10 year risk of fracture from Joint Official Positions Development Conference of the International Society for Clinical Densitometry and International Osteoporosis Foundation on FRAX(®). *J Clin Densitom.* 2011;14(3):212-219. PMID: 21810527

17

ANSWER: C) Genetic testing for *GNA11* and *AP2S1* pathogenic variants

Familial hypocalciuric hypercalcemia (FHH) is a rare disease resulting in a rightward shift of a patient's calcium-sensing curve. Patients with FHH do not shut off production of PTH in response to a serum calcium value that for the general population would be considered hypercalcemic. There are 3 variants of the disease: type 1 due to pathogenic variants in the calcium-sensing receptor gene (*CASR*), type 2 caused by pathogenic variants in the guanine nucleotide–binding protein (G-protein) subunit α_{11} gene (*GNA11*), and type 3 due to pathogenic variants in the adaptor-related protein complex 2, sigma 1 subunit gene (*AP2S1*). Patients with FHH have low urinary calcium excretion, calculated with the following formula:

[urine calcium (mg/24 h) × serum creatinine (mg/dL)] / [urine creatinine (mg/24 h) × serum calcium (mg/dL)]

A urinary calcium-to-creatinine ratio less than 0.01 is consistent with a diagnosis of FHH, although patients must be vitamin D replete (>20 ng/mL [>49.9 mmol/L]) with good kidney function for the collection to be interpretable. A patient with no identifiable *CASR* pathogenic variants and clinical concern for FHH should have *GNA11* and *AP2S1* genetic testing (Answer C). This patient was documented to have a pathogenic variant in *AP2S1*. Of note, genetic testing panels are available for evaluating multiple genes associated with hyperparathyroidism, including pathogenic variants in *AP2S1*, *CASR*, *CDC73*, *CDKN1B*, *GNA11*, *MEN1*, and *RET*.

While FHH is a benign disease that does not carry an increased risk of nephrolithiasis or osteoporosis as does primary hyperparathyroidism, patients with FHH type 3 may have significant hypercalcemia and clinical symptoms related to high serum calcium. A case series demonstrated successful cinacalcet therapy for 3 patients with FHH type 3.

Distinguishing between FHH and primary hyperparathyroidism is important, as surgical treatment is not indicated in patients with FHH.

Thus, preoperative localization studies (Answers A and B) or referral to a parathyroid surgeon (Answer E) is incorrect.

Pathogenic variants in the *PHEX* gene (Answer D) result in X-linked hypophosphatasia, a genetic disorder causing rickets and phosphate wasting.

EDUCATIONAL OBJECTIVE
Distinguish familial hypocalciuric hypercalcemia from primary hyperparathyroidism.

REFERENCE(S)
Eastell R, Brandi ML, Costa AG, D'Amour P, Shoback DM, Thakker RV. Diagnosis of asymptomatic primary hyperparathyroidism: proceedings of the Fourth International Workshop. *J Clin Endocrinol Metab.* 2014;99(10):3570-3579. PMID: 25162666

Howles SA, Hannan FM, Babinsky VN, et al. Cinacalcet for symptomatic hypercalcemia caused by AP2S1 mutations. *N Engl J Med.* 2016;374(14):1396-1398. PMID: 27050234

18

ANSWER: B) Increased fluid intake

According to a comprehensive meta-analysis in patients who had a single kidney stone, increased fluid intake (Answer B) was the one intervention shown to reduce recurrent stone disease. Professional guidelines recommended sufficient water intake to achieve a urine volume at or above 2.0 to 2.5 L daily.

Of interest, reducing phosphate-containing soft drink consumption (not offered as an answer option) was moderately helpful. In patients with *multiple* stone episodes—most of whom had already increased their fluid intake—thiazide diuretics (Answer A) and citrate supplements (Answer C) were similarly effective in patients with hypercalciuria, as well as in unselected patients. Hydrochlorothiazide acts to enhance renal calcium reabsorption to reduce urinary calcium excretion and might be an additional measure to consider if he develops more stones.

Hypercalciuria may be caused by increased sodium intake, which leads to increased sodium excretion and an obligatory loss of calcium in the urine; however, this patient's normal urinary sodium excretion indicates that is not the case here. Thus, reducing dietary sodium (Answer E) is incorrect.

His urinary oxalate level is not elevated, so there would be no benefit in reducing his dietary intake of oxalate (Answer D).

EDUCATIONAL OBJECTIVE
Recommend increased fluid intake as a means to reduce the risk of a second kidney stone.

REFERENCE(S)
Fink HA, Wilt TJ, Eldman KE, et al. Medical management to prevent recurrent nephrolithiasis in adults: a systematic review for an American College of Physicians Clinical Guideline [published correction appears in *Ann Intern Med.* 2013;159(3):230-232]. *Ann Intern Med.* 2013;158(7):535-543. PMID: 23546565

Vigen R, Weideman RA, Reilly RF. Thiazides diuretics in the treatment of nephrolithiasis: are we using them in an evidence-based fashion? *Int Urol Nephrol.* 2011;43(3):813-819. PMID: 20737209

Borghi L, Schianchi T, Meschi T, et al. Comparison of two diets for the prevention of recurrent stones in idiopathic hypercalciuria. *N Engl J Med.* 2002;346(2):77-84. PMID: 11784873

19 **ANSWER: B) Risedronate**
This patient has no symptoms of testosterone deficiency and no indication that his mildly low testosterone is "organic." Because there are no large randomized controlled trials showing antifracture effectiveness for testosterone in men with osteoporosis, testosterone therapy (Answers D and E) should only be considered for hypogonadal men who are symptomatic, have an organic cause of hypogonadism, have testosterone levels less than 200 ng/dL (<6.9 nmol/L), and/or are not candidates for other therapies. If he were symptomatic or had lower testosterone levels, testosterone therapy with a 5α-reductase inhibitor such as finasteride could be given without exacerbating his benign prostatic hypertrophy. However, even men with marked hypogonadism respond well to antiresorptive therapy without correction of the hypogonadism.

He should be offered treatment with an agent approved to treat osteoporosis in men and one that reduces fracture risk, such as risedronate (Answer B).

Teriparatide (Answer C) is generally not a first-line agent for osteoporosis and is best reserved for those with vertebral fractures or very low bone mineral density.

Hydrochlorothiazide (Answer A) can be used for management of hypercalciuria, but this patient has a urinary calcium excretion within the reference range for men.

EDUCATIONAL OBJECTIVE
Recommend appropriate management of male osteoporosis in the setting of borderline-low testosterone.

REFERENCE(S)
Watts NB, Adler RA, Bilezikian JP, et al; Endocrine Society. Osteoporosis in men: an Endocrine Society clinical practice guideline. *J Clin Endocrinol Metab.* 2012;97(6):1802-1822. PMID: 22675062

Boonen S, Lorenc RS, Wenderoth D, Stoner KJ, Eusebio R, Orwoll ES. Evidence for safety and efficacy of risedronate in men with osteoporosis over 4 years of treatment: results from the 2-year, open-label, extension study of a 2-year, randomized, double-blind, placebo-controlled study. *Bone.* 2012;51(3):383-388. PMID: 22750403

20 **ANSWER: C) Intravenous bolus of 150 mg calcium gluconate followed by a continuous calcium gluconate infusion of 1 mg/kg per h**
Intravenous calcium should be considered for patients presenting with clinical features of hypocalcemia, including symptoms of paresthesias, carpopedal spasm, bronchospasm or laryngospasm, tetany, seizures, mental status changes, positive Chvostek or Trousseau signs, bradycardia, impaired cardiac contractility, and prolonged QT interval. While some patients with marked hypocalcemia (ie, corrected calcium <7.0 mg/dL [<1.8 mmol/L]) may not be symptomatic, intravenous therapy may be indicated because at those levels, life-threatening features such as laryngeal spasm and seizures can appear acutely.

This patient needs rapid correction of hypocalcemia. Calcium gluconate is preferred over calcium chloride because the latter is more likely to cause vein sclerosis and tissue necrosis if extravasated (thus, Answers A and B are incorrect). Dosing at 1 mg/kg per h would be a total dose of 1680 mg daily for a 70-kg patient (thus, Answer C is correct); a higher rate might be required for patients with a profound calcium deficiency. The dose of intravenous calcium is dangerously high in Answer E. There are case reports using teriparatide (PTH [1-34]) in acute hypocalcemia (Answer D) as an off-label therapy; however, teriparatide typically requires multiple daily dosing to maintain serum calcium in patients with hypoparathyroidism.

Ordering intravenous calcium can be potentially confusing. For intravenous use, a 10-mL ampule of calcium gluconate contains 93 mg of calcium; a 10-mL ampule of 10% calcium chloride contains 272 mg of calcium. In some situations, adding a calcium salt to an intravenous liter bag of 0.9% saline or 5% dextrose requires removing some of the fluid to allow space for the added calcium salt.

EDUCATIONAL OBJECTIVE
Manage acute, severe hypocalcemia.

REFERENCE(S)
Zalonga GP, Chernow B. Hypocalcemia in critical illness. *JAMA*. 1986;256(14):1924-1929. PMID: 3531557

Vetter T, Lohse MJ. Magnesium and the parathyroid. *Curr Opin Nephrol Hypertens*. 2002;11(4):403-410. PMID: 12105390

al-Ghamdi SM, Cameron EC, Sutton RA. Magnesium deficiency: pathophysiologic and clinical overview. *Am J Kidney Dis*. 1994;24(5):737-752. PMID: 7977315

21 ANSWER: C) FGF-23 measurement
This patient has tumor-induced osteomalacia caused by a benign mesenchymal tumor that is secreting FGF-23 (Answer C). This causes renal tubular loss of phosphate and inhibits 1α-hydroxylase, resulting in low 1,25-dihydroxyvitamin D levels. These tumors are typically located in the skin, bones, or connective tissue (eg, sinuses) and may be difficult to localize. Imaging to localize the tumor includes nuclear medicine techniques such as bone scan, octreotide scan, or PET. In difficult cases, serum FGF-23 measurement in selective venous sampling may be used to localize the extremity from which FGF-23 is being secreted. Tumor removal (if it can be located and removed) normalizes renal phosphate handling within hours to days.

Hypophosphatemia induced by tenofovir (and adefovir) is part of a more generalized syndrome known as Fanconi syndrome in which multiple substances such as bicarbonate, glucose, uric acid, potassium, and phosphate are "wasted" in the urine (Answer B). This patient has no evidence of this syndrome.

Low levels of 24,25-dihydroxyvitamin D (Answer A) can be useful to diagnose patients with pathogenic variants in the *CYP24A1* gene who have hypercalcemia and kidney stones.

While the severity of X-linked hypophosphatasia caused by pathogenic variants in *PHEX* (Answer D) varies widely, even among members of the same family, the disease is completely penetrant and not expected to first cause symptoms later in life.

A sestamibi scan (Answer E) is not helpful in diagnosing tumor-induced osteomalacia.

EDUCATIONAL OBJECTIVE
Diagnose tumor-induced osteomalacia by measuring FGF-23.

REFERENCE(S)
Ruppe MD, Jan de Beur SM. Disorders of phosphate homeostasis. In: Rosen CJ, Compston JE, Lian JB, eds. *Primer on the Metabolic Bone Diseases and Disorders of Mineral Metabolism*. Washington, DC: The American Society for Bone and Mineral Research; 2008:601-612.

Jan de Beur SM. Tumor-induced osteomalacia. *JAMA*. 2005;294(10):1260-1267. PMID: 16160135

Andreopoulou P, Dumitrescu CE, Kelly MH, et al. Selective venous catheterization for the localization of phosphaturic mesenchymal tumors. *J Bone Miner Res*. 2011;26(6):1295-1302. PMID: 21611969

22 ANSWER: E) Decrease calcium supplementation

Patients with hypoparathyroidism cannot stimulate renal tubular reabsorption of filtered calcium due to lack of PTH effect on the kidneys. Therefore, calcium and calcitriol supplementation in the management of chronic hypoparathyroidism can lead to hypercalciuria, nephrolithiasis, nephrocalcinosis, and renal insufficiency. Epidemiologic studies have shown markedly increased relative risks (3- to 6-fold) of kidney dysfunction among those with both surgical and nonsurgical hypoparathyroidism. Because of this, it is important to encourage patients to minimize excessive calcium intake, to take the lowest possible calcitriol dosage, and to try to maintain serum calcium in the low-normal or even slightly low range, typically between 8 and 9 mg/dL (2.0-2.3 mmol/L). It is also important to monitor urinary calcium excretion and avoid hypercalciuria. Because this patient has hypercalciuria, continuing the current regimen (Answer D) is not optimal.

The best option is to recommend that she gradually decrease her excessive intake of calcium supplements (Answer E). Patients with hypoparathyroidism can experience unpleasant symptoms of muscle cramps, spasms, and paresthesias, particularly during or after exercise. Therefore, it is important to gradually try to achieve a lower calcium intake that is both safe and tolerable.

The approval of recombinant human PTH (1-84) (Answer B) for management of permanent hypoparathyroidism offers another option, but it is expensive and therapy is reserved for patients who cannot be managed well on conventional therapy. Recombinant human PTH (1-84) is currently not available in the United States due to a voluntary recall of the cartridge device and not due to an issue with the medication itself.

Thiazide diuretics (Answer A) may be useful adjunctive therapy for some patients with persistent hypercalciuria who are unable to decrease calcium intake due to hypocalcemic symptoms. It is reasonable to try a thiazide diuretic in these patients, particularly if serum calcium is on the lower end of normal with persistent hypercalciuria. Often, high dosages (such as 50 mg daily of hydrochlorothiazide or more) are needed to normalize urinary calcium excretion, but some patients respond well to lower dosages. Concomitant potassium-sparing diuretics such as amiloride and low-salt diets may be useful adjunctive therapies. When starting thiazides, serum calcium may rise, allowing reduction in the calcitriol dosage.

Sevelamer (Answer C), a phosphate binder, is not indicated for this mild hyperphosphatemia and would not address the patient's hypercalciuria. Her calcium x phosphate product is less than 55 mg^2/dL^2, so there is no urgency for a phosphate binder.

Other risks for patients with permanent surgical hypoparathyroidism include neuropsychiatric disease, infections, and seizures. Among those with nonsurgical hypoparathyroidism, there is a higher occurrence of ischemic cardiovascular disease, cataracts, and fractures.

EDUCATIONAL OBJECTIVE
Manage chronic surgical hypoparathyroidism.

REFERENCE(S)
Bilezikian JP, Khan A, Potts JT Jr, et al. Hypoparathyroidism in the adult: epidemiology, diagnosis, pathophysiology, target-organ involvement, treatment, and challenges for future research. *J Bone Miner Res.* 2011;26(10):2317-2337. PMID: 21812031

Clarke BL, Brown EM, Collins MT, et al. Epidemiology and diagnosis of hypoparathyroidism. *J Clin Endocrinol Metab.* 2016;101(6):2284-2299. PMID: 26943720

Bilezikian JP, Brandi ML, Cusano NE, et al. Management of hypoparathyroidism: present and future. *J Clin Endocrinol Metab.* 2016;101(6):2313-2324. PMID: 26938200

23 ANSWER: D) Zoledronic acid

A number of clinical trials have demonstrated that women with breast cancer treated with aromatase inhibitors experience higher rates of bone loss and fragility fractures, particularly in the first 1 to 2 years of therapy, compared with rates in women treated with tamoxifen. Thus, recommending no intervention (Answer E) is incorrect. Current recommendations are to optimize calcium and vitamin D supplementation and perform DXA screening. International guidelines recommend antiresorptive treatment for patients initiating aromatase inhibitor therapy with a T-score of −2.0 or less regardless of additional risk factors, for the duration of aromatase inhibitor treatment. In addition, patients with any 2 of the following risk factors should receive antiresorptive therapy: T-score of −1.5 or less, age older than 65 years, low BMI (<20 kg/m^2), family history of hip fracture, personal history of fragility fracture after age 50 years, oral corticosteroid use longer than 6 months, and current cigarette smoking (or history of).

Several large clinical trials in postmenopausal women with early-stage breast cancer have shown that aromatase inhibitor–induced bone loss can be prevented by treatment with antiresorptive agents at the onset of aromatase inhibitor therapy. The drug regimen that has been studied most extensively is intravenous zoledronic acid (Answer D) 4 mg every 6 months, although some experts treat with 5 mg annually despite a lack of clinical trial data. Oral bisphosphonates can also be used in this setting, although clinical trial data are not nearly as extensive. Denosumab, 60 mg subcutaneously every 6 months, has also been shown to reduce both fractures and cancer recurrence in postmenopausal women with early-stage breast cancer.

Calcitonin (Answer A) is a weak antiresorptive agent that would not be appropriate in this patient.

Teriparatide (Answer C) is contraindicated in patients with a history of radiation therapy due to increased risk of osteosarcoma.

Raloxifene (Answer B), a selective estrogen receptor modulator, significantly reduces estrogen receptor–positive breast cancer in women with osteoporosis, but it is not approved for use in women with a diagnosis of breast cancer.

EDUCATIONAL OBJECTIVE
Manage low bone mass in the setting of breast cancer and aromatase inhibitor therapy.

REFERENCE(S)
Hadji P, Aapro MS, Body JJ, et al. Management of aromatase inhibitor-associated bone loss (AIBL) in postmenopausal women with hormone sensitive breast cancer: joint position statement of the IOF, CABS, ECTS, IEG, ESCEO IMS, and SIOG. *J Bone Oncol.* 2017;7:1-12. PMID: 28413771

Wagner-Johnston ND, Sloan JA, Liu H, et al. 5-year follow-up of a randomized controlled trial of immediate versus delayed zoledronic acid for the prevention of bone loss in postmenopausal women with breast cancer starting letrozole after tamoxifen: N03CC (Alliance) trial. *Cancer.* 2015;121(15):2537-2543. PMID: 25930719

Brufsky AM, Harker WG, Beck JT, et al. Final 5-year results of Z-FAST trial: adjuvant zoledronic acid maintains bone mass in postmenopausal breast cancer patients receiving letrozole. *Cancer.* 2012;118(5):1192-1201. PMID: 21987386

Gnant M, Pfeiler G, Steger GG, et al; Austrian Breast and Colorectal Cancer Study Group. Adjuvant denosumab in postmenopausal patients with hormone receptor-positive breast cancer (ABCSG-18): disease-free survival results from a randomised, double-blind, placebo-controlled, phase 3 trial. *Lancet Oncol.* 2019;20(3):339-351. PMID: 30795951

24 ANSWER: B) Measure PTH again in 5 months (before her next denosumab injection)

Denosumab is a known cause of hyperparathyroidism. PTH concentrations can rise within the first 1 to 3 months after an injection, typically decreasing towards normal before the next injection. Measurement of PTH in 5 months (before her next injection) (Answer B) is thus the correct answer. This transient PTH elevation in healthy individuals following inhibition of bone resorption with bisphosphonates or denosumab may be a compensatory mechanism in order to maintain normal serum calcium.

There is no indication to stop denosumab therapy (Answer E) if PTH levels are elevated.

The patient's 25-hydroxyvitamin D level is sufficient, and there is no benefit to further increase vitamin D supplementation (Answer A).

The diagnosis of normocalcemic primary hyperparathyroidism requires elevated PTH concentrations in the absence of secondary causes for hyperparathyroidism. The expert panel from the Fourth International Workshop on the Management of Asymptomatic Primary Hyperparathyroidism recommended that the PTH level remain above the normal range on at least 2 subsequent measurements during a 3- to 6-month period to confirm hyperparathyroidism. Ordering parathyroid imaging (Answer C) or referring to a parathyroid surgeon (Answer D) is incorrect since she has had only a single elevated PTH measurement that may be ascribed to a medication causing hyperparathyroidism.

EDUCATIONAL OBJECTIVE
Identify medications that cause hyperparathyroidism.

REFERENCE(S)

Eastell R, Brandi ML, Costa AG, D'Amour P, Shoback DM, Thakker RV. Diagnosis of asymptomatic primary hyperparathyroidism: proceedings of the Fourth International Workshop. *J Clin Endocrinol Metab.* 2014;99(10):3570-3579. PMID: 25162666

Pawlowska M, Cusano NE. An overview of normocalcemic primary hyperparathyroidism. *Curr Opin Endocrinol Diabetes Obes.* 2015;22(6):413-421. PMID: 26512768

25 ANSWER: E) Working with a dietician to resolve energy deficiency

Relative energy deficiency in sport (RED-S) is a syndrome consisting of disordered eating (or low energy availability), oligomenorrhea/amenorrhea, and decreased bone mineral density. RED-S is a more inclusive and comprehensive term for what was formally referred to as the "female athletic triad."

While this patient's BMI is normal, she has evidence of functional amenorrhea and relative energy deficiency. The Endocrine Society guidelines for functional hypothalamic amenorrhea recommend correcting the energy imbalance (Answer E) to improve function of her hypothalamic-pituitary-ovarian axis, which should also improve bone mineral density.

The guidelines recommend against use of oral contraceptive pills (Answer B) for the sole purpose of regaining menses or improving bone mineral density. There has been lack of clear benefit in studies evaluating bone density effects of oral contraceptive pills vs placebo in women with functional amenorrhea. There are some data that transdermal estrogen with progesterone may be of benefit in women who have not had return of menses after a trial of nutritional, psychological, and/or modified exercise intervention. Transdermal estrogen may improve bone density more than oral contraceptive pills because it does not affect IGF-1 secretion, a bone-trophic hormone that oral contraceptive pills down-regulate.

The guidelines recommend against using bisphosphonates (Answer A), denosumab (Answer C), testosterone, or leptin to improve bone mineral density in women with functional amenorrhea. Short-term teriparatide therapy (Answer D) can be considered in rare cases of women with functional amenorrhea in the setting of delayed fracture healing and very low bone mineral density. This patient has had good fracture healing, and treatment with teriparatide is not indicated.

EDUCATIONAL OBJECTIVE
Treat low bone density in a patient with functional hypothalamic amenorrhea/relative energy deficiency in sport.

REFERENCE(S)

Ackerman KE, Singhal V, Slattery M, et al. Effects of estrogen replacement on bone geometry and microarchitecture in adolescent and young adult oligoamenorrheic athletes: a randomized trial. *J Bone Miner Res.* 2020;35(2):248-260. PMID: 31603998

Gordon CM, Ackerman KE, Berga SL, et al. Functional hypothalamic amenorrhea: an Endocrine Society clinical practice guideline. *J Clin Endocrinol Metab.* 2017;102(5):1413-1439. PMID: 28368518

26 ANSWER: D) Decrease the cinacalcet dosage

This patient's PTH level is lower than the goal in patients undergoing dialysis and may indicate underlying adynamic bone disease. Because of the low PTH and hypocalcemia, the cinacalcet dosage should be decreased (Answer D). Adynamic bone disease, a type of renal osteodystrophy (part of chronic kidney disease–mineral bone disorder [CKD-MBD]), is present in at least one-third of patients receiving dialysis. Adynamic bone disease is characterized by markedly low bone turnover, no accumulation of osteoid, and high fracture risk. Serum PTH levels in adynamic bone disease are relatively low (usually <100 pg/mL [<100 ng/L]) compared with levels in patients undergoing dialysis who have other forms of CKD-MBD.

In patients with end-stage kidney disease, there is resistance to PTH due at least in part to increased N-terminal truncated PTH (7-84), which counteracts the effect of the 1-84 whole molecule on bone. This can be exacerbated by the use of cinacalcet, as well as overly aggressive treatment with calcitriol, both of which reduce PTH secretion. This patient's low alkaline phosphatase level is also consistent with a low bone turnover state.

Increasing the calcitriol dosage (Answer E) would further suppress PTH, which is not a desired outcome. Decreasing the calcitriol dosage (Answer C) may worsen the hypocalcemia.

Teriparatide (Answer B) has been used anecdotally in some patients with end-stage kidney disease, low bone turnover, and fractures, but it is not an approved therapy in this context.

Although denosumab (Answer A) can be used in patients receiving dialysis, it would be inappropriate to administer it now in the face of hypocalcemia, vitamin D deficiency, and probable adynamic bone disease. A potent antiresorptive agent would theoretically worsen the adynamic bone disease and increase fracture risk.

Impaired mineralization, osteitis fibrosa cystica, and mixed renal osteodystrophy are other forms of CKD-MBD, but these diagnoses are unlikely given the laboratory findings. Osteitis fibrosa cystica and high bone turnover are associated with elevated PTH, osteomalacia is associated with very low 25-hydroxyvitamin D, and mixed renal osteodystrophy is associated with both findings.

EDUCATIONAL OBJECTIVE
Diagnose and manage adynamic bone disease in a patient undergoing dialysis.

REFERENCE(S)

Cannata-Andía JB, Rodriguez García M, Gómez Alonso C. Osteoporosis and adynamic bone in chronic kidney disease. *J Nephrol.* 2013;26(1):73-80. PMID: 23023723

Hruska KA, Mathew S. Chronic kidney disease mineral bone disorder (CKD-MBD). In: Rosen CJ, Compston JE, Lian JB, eds. *Primer on the Metabolic Bone Diseases and Disorders of Mineral Metabolism.* The American Society for Bone and Mineral Research; 2008:343-349.

Brandenburg VM, Floege J. Adynamic bone disease: bone and beyond. *NDT Plus.* 2008;1(3):135-147. PMID: 25983860

Kidney Disease: Improving Global Outcomes (KDIGO) CKD-MBD Work Group. KDIGO clinical practice guideline for the diagnosis, evaluation, prevention, and treatment of chronic kidney disease-mineral and bone disorder (CKD-MBD). *Kidney Int Suppl.* 2009;(Suppl 113):S1-S130. PMID: 19644521

27 ANSWER: C) Calcium citrate, 600 mg 4 times daily

Absorption of calcium carbonate is pH-dependent. In one experiment, only 1% of 500 mg of calcium carbonate was dissolved in 500 mL of water after 1 hour at 98.6°F (37°C) at a neutral pH, with 100% dissolving at a pH of 2.5, similar to that observed in the stomach. Proton-pump inhibitors inhibit the parietal cell H+ K+ATPase pump, leading to suppressed acid secretion and increased stomach pH. There have been multiple case reports of acute hypocalcemia in patients with hypoparathyroidism on calcium carbonate subsequently treated with a proton-pump inhibitor. Absorption of calcium citrate is not pH-dependent, and patients with hypoparathyroidism who will be starting a proton-pump inhibitor should be transitioned to a regimen of calcium citrate (Answer C) since calcium carbonate (Answers A and B) is not well absorbed in this setting.

While there are case reports of teriparatide (PTH[1-34]) use (Answers D and E) in acute hypocalcemia, it is off-label and not standard treatment. In addition, teriparatide typically requires multiple daily dosing to maintain serum calcium in patients with hypoparathyroidism.

Hydrochlorothiazide (Answer B) can be used to treat hypercalciuria, but it is not used for acute hypocalcemia.

Of note, there are also multiple cases of euparathyroid individuals developing functional hypoparathyroidism caused by hypomagnesemia related to proton-pump inhibitor use, since the secretion of PTH is magnesium-dependent.

EDUCATIONAL OBJECTIVE
Recognize problems with calcium absorption in the setting of proton-pump inhibitor use.

REFERENCE(S)

Bilezikian JP, Brandi ML, Cusano NE, et al. Management of hypoparathyroidism: present and future. *J Clin Endocrinol Metab.* 2016;101(6):2313-2324. PMID: 26938200

Epstein M, McGrath S, Law F. Proton-pump inhibitors and hypomagnesemic hypoparathyroidism. *N Engl J Med.* 2006;355(17):1834-1836. PMID: 17065651

Milman S, Epstein EJ. Proton pump inhibitor-induced hypocalcemic seizure in a patient with hypoparathyroidism. *Endocr Pract.* 2011;17(1):104-107. PMID: 21041166

Vallejo F, Sum M. Acute hypocalcemia from proton pump inhibitor use. In: *Hypoparathyroidism: A Clinical Casebook.* Cusano NE, ed. Switzerland: Springer; 2020:9-15.

28 ANSWER: B) 25-Hydroxyvitamin D measurement

Although this patient may have Paget disease, other causes of elevated alkaline phosphatase must be considered before proceeding to bone scan, including vitamin D deficiency and/or secondary hyperparathyroidism, particularly given his age and chronic kidney disease. This patient was indeed found to have vitamin D deficiency with secondary hyperparathyroidism. Thus, measurement of 25-hydroxyvitamin D (Answer B) is the correct next step. Although he has been taking 2000 IU of vitamin D daily, this is not enough to maintain a normal 25-hydroxyitamin D level in some patients after bariatric surgery.

Serum levels of 1,25-dihyroxyvitamin D are regulated primarily by PTH levels, which in turn are regulated by calcium and/or vitamin D. 1,25-Dihydroxyvitamin D levels do not reflect vitamin D stores, and in vitamin D deficiency, 1,25-dihydroxyvitamin D levels are normal or even elevated due to secondary hyperparathyroidism. Thus, measuring 1,25-dihydroxyvitamin D (Answer A) is incorrect.

In this patient, a whole-body bone scan (Answer E) may be spuriously abnormal, showing multiple areas of uptake due to increased bone turnover.

Serum C-telopeptide (Answer C) may be elevated, but its measurement would not help determine the cause of his elevated alkaline phosphatase.

A skeletal survey (Answer D) would be helpful if multiple myeloma were the suspected diagnosis, which is not the case.

EDUCATIONAL OBJECTIVE
Rule out vitamin D deficiency and secondary hyperparathyroidism before evaluating for Paget disease.

REFERENCE(S)

Karefylakis C, Näslund I, Edholm D, Sundbom M, Karlsson FA, Rask E. Vitamin D status 10 years after primary gastric bypass: gravely high prevalence of hypovitaminosis D and raised PTH levels. *Obes Surg.* 2014;24(3):343-348. PMID: 24163201

29 ANSWER: D) Type 1 collagen α 1 and 2 genes (*COL1A1/COL1A2*)

This patient has the mildest form of osteogenesis imperfecta, known as type 1. Inheritance is autosomal dominant, but many pathogenic variants can occur de novo, so the family history may be negative. Patients with osteogenesis imperfecta type 1 have normal stature and little or no skeletal deformity. Fractures occur in childhood or adolescence and decrease markedly after puberty.

As is the case in this vignette, affected patients may then present in middle age with "osteoporosis." In 50% of patients, there is early-onset hearing loss before age 40 years. On physical examination, there may be blue sclerae and easy bruising. Joint laxity may be present, but dentinogenesis imperfecta is usually absent. Diagnosis is made by sequencing the genes that encode type 1 collagen (α1 and α2) (*COL1A1*/*COL1A2*) (Answer D). Pathogenic variants in *COL1A1* or *COL1A2* that cause decreased amounts of normal collagen lead to the mild phenotype seen in patients with osteogenesis imperfecta type 1. Pathogenic variants that disrupt the formation of the normal type I collagen triple helix cause the lethal phenotype seen in type IIA. Posttranslational defects in the interferon-induced transmembrane protein 5 gene (*IFITM5*), FK506-binding protein 10 gene (*FKBP10* [*FKBP65*]), and cartilage-associated protein gene (*CRTAP*) are among the causes of osteogenesis imperfecta in the 10% patients without pathogenic variants in *COL1A1* or *COL1A2*.

The main therapy for osteogenesis imperfecta remains bisphosphonates (intravenous pamidronate and zoledronic acid and oral bisphosphonates). Denosumab has been used in rare case reports. Teriparatide does not dramatically change clinical outcomes. It is hoped that the sclerostin inhibitor romosozumab may have some effectiveness in decreasing fractures in osteogenesis imperfecta, but this awaits clinical trials.

Osteoprotegerin (Answer B) is a cytokine and decoy receptor for the receptor activator of nuclear factor kappa B ligand (RANKL). By binding to RANKL, it reduces differentiation of precursors to osteoclasts and blocks osteoclast production and proliferation, thus reducing bone resorption. Pathogenic variants in this gene have been associated with osteoarthritis but not with the phenotype illustrated in this vignette.

Pathogenic variants in the gene encoding the LDL receptor-related protein 5 (Answer A) are involved with the canonical Wnt pathway. Loss-of-function variants can cause osteoporosis-pseudoglioma syndrome, while gain-of-function variants result in a high bone mass phenotype.

Pathogenic variants in the vitamin D receptor gene (Answer E) can be found in vitamin D–resistant rickets, but this would be accompanied by a high 1,25-dihydroxyvitamin D level, as well as hypophosphatemia, hypocalcemia, and osteomalacia.

Sclerostin, produced by the *SOST* gene (Answer C), is produced by osteocytes and has antianabolic effects on bone formation by suppressing Wnt signaling. Inactivating variants in the *SOST* gene cause syndromes of high bone mass (sclerosteosis and van Buchem disease).

EDUCATIONAL OBJECTIVE
Diagnose osteogenesis imperfecta type 1 (the mildest form).

REFERENCE(S)

Van Dijk FS, Sillence DO. Osteogenesis imperfecta: clinical diagnosis, nomenclature and severity assessment [published correction appears in *Am J Med Genet A*. 2015;167A(5):1178]. *Am J Med Genet A*. 2014;164A(6):1470-1481. PMID: 24715559

Thomas IH, DiMeglio LA. Advances in the classification and treatment of osteogenesis imperfecta. *Curr Osteoporos Rep*. 2016;14(1):1-9. PMID: 26861807

Shapiro JR, Thompson CB, Wu Y, Nunes M, Gillen C. Bone mineral density and fracture rate in response to intravenous and oral bisphosphonates in adult osteogenesis imperfecta. *Calcif Tissue Int*. 2010;87(2):120-129. PMID: 20544187

30 ANSWER: E) Primary hyperparathyroidism

Primary hyperparathyroidism (Answer E) is one of the most common endocrine disorders and is diagnosed in the setting of hypercalcemia with an elevated or inappropriately normal PTH. This patient's PTH concentration, although technically within normal limits, is inappropriate in the setting of hypercalcemia. In primary hyperparathyroidism, PTH facilitates the conversion of 25-hydroxyvitamin D to 1,25-dihydroxyvitamin D, and up to 25% of patients have frankly elevated 1,25-dihydroxyvitamin D levels.

Familial hypocalciuric hypercalcemia (FHH) (Answer B) is a rare, benign disorder caused by loss-of-function pathogenic variants in the gene encoding the calcium-sensing receptor. Patients with FHH usually have a positive family history, although a given patient could represent an index case. The extremely high penetrance of FHH ensures that virtually all patients develop hypercalcemia by their third decade. In FHH, 24-hour urinary calcium excretion is typically less than 100 mg with a calcium-to-creatinine clearance ratio less than 0.01, while typically the ratio is greater than 0.02 in patients with primary hyperparathyroidism. It can be difficult to distinguish between FHH and primary hyperparathyroidism when the ratio is between 0.01 and 0.02; however, patients must be vitamin D replete (>20 ng/mL [>49.9 mmol/L]) with good kidney function for the collection to be interpretable. In younger patients, genetic testing may assist with making the diagnosis.

In granulomatous disease (Answer C), while 1,25-dihydroxyvitamin D is typically elevated because macrophages in the granulomas synthesize the active metabolite of vitamin D, PTH levels are also suppressed. PTH levels would also be suppressed in the case of calcitriol toxicity (Answer A).

In humoral hypercalcemia of malignancy (Answer D), PTH levels are classically undetectable because endogenous PTH is suppressed and PTHrP, a major cause of humoral hypercalcemia of malignancy, is not detected by immunoassays for PTH.

EDUCATIONAL OBJECTIVE
Diagnose primary hyperparathyroidism.

REFERENCE(S)

Cusano NE, Bilezikian JP. Parathyroid hormone in the evaluation of hypercalcemia. *JAMA.* 2014;312(24):2680-2681. PMID: 25536261

Eastell R, Brandi ML, Costa AG, D'Amour P, Shoback DM, Thakker RV. Diagnosis of asymptomatic primary hyperparathyroidism: proceedings of the Fourth International Workshop. *J Clin Endocrinol Metab.* 2014;99(10):3570-3579. PMID: 25162666

Diabetes Mellitus, Section 1 Board Review

Vivian A. Fonseca, MD

1 **ANSWER: B) Improvement in glucose tolerance**

Somatostatin receptor ligand therapy (octreotide) decreases insulin secretion. Because octreotide is being discontinued, insulin secretion will no longer be decreased (Answer A). Pegvisomant blocks the GH receptor and therefore improves insulin sensitivity without affecting secretion. Glucose tolerance is expected to improve (Answer B) after this patient has taken pegvisomant for 3 months. Therefore, the risk of new-onset diabetes is reduced, so type 2 diabetes mellitus (Answer C) would not be an expected outcome. Insulin resistance is expected to improve, not worsen (Answer E). GH concentrations actually rise with pegvisomant, not decrease (Answer D).

EDUCATIONAL OBJECTIVE

Predict the effect of pegvisomant on glucose tolerance in a patient with acromegaly.

REFERENCE(S)

Barkan AL, Burman P, Clemmons DR, et al. Glucose homeostasis and safety in patients with acromegaly converted from long-acting octreotide to pegvisomant. *J Clin Endocrinol Metab.* 2005;90(10):5684-5691. PMID: 16076947

2 **ANSWER: C) Liver enzymes**

Nonalcoholic fatty liver disease (NAFLD) is a serious risk factor for insulin resistance and the progression to type 2 diabetes mellitus, as well as for overall mortality once diabetes develops. Thus, of the listed options, liver enzymes (Answer C) are the best predictor of the risk for developing diabetes.

LDL cholesterol (Answer B) is not a good predictor of progression to type 2 diabetes, whereas high triglycerides and low HDL cholesterol may be better.

Low testosterone (Answer E) is common in men with obesity, as well as in men with diabetes, but it does not predict progression to diabetes.

The presence of glutamic acid decarboxylase antibodies (Answer A) suggests autoimmunity and type 1 diabetes rather than type 2 diabetes.

Microalbuminuria (Answer D) can occur in individuals with obesity who do not have diabetes in whom it is a marker of endothelial dysfunction and is associated with cardiovascular disease. However, it is not a good predictor of progression to diabetes.

EDUCATIONAL OBJECTIVE

Identify abnormal liver enzymes as a predictor of the risk for developing type 2 diabetes mellitus.

REFERENCE(S)

Haffner SM. Relationship of metabolic risk factors and development of cardiovascular disease and diabetes. *Obesity.* 2006;14(Suppl 3):121S-127S. PMID: 16931493

Yki-Järvinen H. Non-alcoholic fatty liver disease as a cause and a consequence of metabolic syndrome. *Lancet Diabetes Endocrinol.* 2014;2(11):901-910. PMID: 24731669

3 **ANSWER: D) Repeat hemoglobin A_{1c} measurement**

The American Diabetes Association guidelines suggest that in asymptomatic individuals, a test result diagnostic of diabetes should be repeated to rule out laboratory error unless the diagnosis is clear on clinical grounds (thus, Answer A is incorrect). It is preferable that the same test be repeated for confirmation because there is a greater likelihood of concurrence. If results from 2 different tests are available for a given patient, and the results are discordant, the test that has a result above the diagnostic cut point should be repeated, and the diagnosis should be made based on the confirmed test. Therefore, the best next step to determine whether this patient has diabetes is to repeat the hemoglobin A_{1c} measurement (thus, Answer D is correct and Answer E is incorrect).

While some consider oral glucose tolerance testing (Answer C) to be the gold standard, a borderline result may lead to additional confusion.

There is no history in this vignette to suggest the presence of abnormal hemoglobin, so hemoglobin electrophoresis (Answer B) is incorrect.

EDUCATIONAL OBJECTIVE
Summarize conflicts in diagnostic testing for diabetes mellitus.

REFERENCE(S)
American Diabetes Association. 2. Classification and diagnosis of diabetes: standards of medical care in diabetes. *Diabetes Care.* 2021;44(Suppl 1):S15-S33. PMID: 33298413

4 ANSWER: E) Raise the low-alarm threshold level
Continuous glucose monitoring sensors measure glucose in interstitial fluid, which creates a physiologic lag when values are compared with capillary blood glucose readings. As a result, a patient may have hypoglycemia without it being recognized by the continuous glucose monitoring sensor, unless the threshold is increased (thus, Answer E is correct and Answers, A, B, C, and D are incorrect). The use of trend arrows also helps recognize glucose trends.

EDUCATIONAL OBJECTIVE
Explain the difference between blood and interstitial fluid glucose and resulting discrepancies in glucose measurement.

REFERENCE(S)
Shang T, Zhang JY, Thomas A, et al. Products for monitoring glucose levels in the human body with noninvasive optical, noninvasive fluid sampling, or minimally invasive technologies. *J Diabetes Sci Technol.* 2022;16(1):168-214. PMID: 34120487

5 ANSWER: A) Add midodrine hydrochloride
Midodrine (Answer A) is approved for the treatment of postural hypotension related to autonomic neuropathy. Fludrocortisone is also commonly used, but it may increase edema.

Lisinopril is needed for nephropathy, and discontinuation (Answer D) is not the best next step.

Salt intake may need to be increased (not decreased [Answer C]), and indeed sodium bicarbonate could be prescribed for patients with postural hypotension.

While phentermine (Answer B) can raise blood pressure, it also increases heart rate and is not used for postural hypotension related to autonomic neuropathy.

EDUCATIONAL OBJECTIVE
Manage severe postural hypotension due to diabetic autonomic neuropathy.

REFERENCE(S)
Gibbons CH, Schmidt P, Biaggioni I, et al. The recommendations of a consensus panel for the screening, diagnosis, and treatment of neurogenic orthostatic hypotension and associated supine hypertension. *J Neurol.* 2017;264(8):1567-1582. PMID: 28050656

Arora RR, Bulgarelli RJ, Ghosh-Dastidar S, Colombo J. Autonomic mechanisms and therapeutic implications of postural diabetic cardiovascular abnormalities. *J Diabetes Sci Technol.* 2008;2(4):645-657. PMID: 19885241

6 ANSWER: D) *KCNJ11*
This patient has neonatal diabetes, which is rarely an autoimmune condition that presents in the first year of life. The lack of a strong family history makes it unlikely that she has another form of monogenic diabetes. The most common abnormality leading to neonatal diabetes is a pathogenic variant in the *KCNJ11* gene (Answer D), which is known to encode the "sulfonylurea receptor." Affected patients respond well to sulfonylureas and do not need insulin. Autoimmune disease (such as classic type 1 diabetes) is rare in the first year of life. Pathogenic

variants in the *GCK* (Answer A), *HNF1A* (Answer B), *HNF4A* (Answer C), and *SLC2A2* (Answer E) genes are associated with other forms of monogenic diabetes that often resemble type 2 diabetes.

EDUCATIONAL OBJECTIVE

Suspect monogenic diabetes and differentiate among genetic etiologies.

REFERENCE(S)

Fajans SS, Bell GI, Polonsky KS. Molecular mechanisms and clinical pathophysiology of maturity-onset diabetes of the young. *N Engl J Med.* 2001;345(13):971-980. PMID: 11575290

Hattersley A, Bruining J, Shield J, Njolstad P, Donaghue KC. The diagnosis and management of monogenic diabetes in children and adolescents. *Pediatr Diabetes.* 2009;10(Suppl 12):33-42. PMID: 19754616

Murphy R, Ellard S, Hattersley AT. Clinical implications of a molecular genetic classification of monogenic beta-cell diabetes. *Nat Clin Pract Endocrinol Metab.* 2008;4(4):200-213. PMID: 18301398

Kavvoura FK, Owen KR. Maturity onset diabetes of the young: clinical characteristics, diagnosis and management. *Pediatr Endocrinol Rev.* 2012;10(2):234-242. PMID: 23539835

7 ANSWER: D) Recommend no additional therapy

Studies have shown that in normotensive, normoalbuminuric individuals with type 1 diabetes, there is no renal protective benefit from ACE inhibitors (Answer A), angiotensin-receptor blockers (Answer B), or SGLT-2 inhibitors (Answer C). Many physicians prescribe these agents in the hopes that they will help if used early, but this is not the case. Early use may limit the effectiveness of these medications later. None of these agents should be started to prevent the development of nephropathy, as there is no evidence of benefit (thus, Answer D is correct).

EDUCATIONAL OBJECTIVE

Explain that there are no data on prophylactic treatment of nephropathy in normotensive individuals with type 1 diabetes mellitus.

REFERENCE(S)

Mauer M, Zinman B, Gardiner R, et al. Renal and retinal effects of enalapril and losartan in type 1 diabetes. *N Engl J Med.* 2009;361(1):40-51. PMID: 19571282

8 ANSWER: D) MRI

Distinguishing between osteomyelitis and neuropathic osteoarthropathy of the foot frequently presents a clinical and radiological challenge in patients with diabetes. Studies have shown that MRI (Answer D) may help distinguish between the 2 diagnoses. In patients with osteomyelitis, increased signal intensity and other abnormalities are usually seen within the bone marrow. However, decreased signal intensity is seen in the setting of Charcot foot.

Although both bone scan (Answer B) and CT (Answer C) are likely to show an abnormality, there are no features to resolve the differential diagnosis as with MRI.

Biopsy (Answer A) would provide a definitive diagnosis, but it is invasive and is therefore not the first step in diagnosis.

EDUCATIONAL OBJECTIVE

Select MRI as the appropriate diagnostic imaging to distinguish between osteomyelitis and Charcot foot.

REFERENCE(S)

Marmolejo VS, Arnold JF, Ponticello M, Anderson CA. Charcot foot: clinical clues, diagnostic strategies, and treatment principles. *Am Fam Physician.* 2018;97(9):594-599. PMID: 29763252

9 ANSWER: D) Pramlintide

Pramlintide (Answer D), an analogue of the naturally occurring hormone amylin, increases satiety, decreases body weight, slows gastric emptying, and suppresses glucagon secretion in conjunction with insulin in both type 1 and type 2 diabetes. It is associated with a modest degree of weight loss in most individuals. None of the other listed drugs are US FDA approved for type 1 diabetes, although they are frequently used off label.

Metformin (Answer B) is generally considered weight neutral or associated with a mild degree of weight loss. It has been shown in some studies to reduce the amount of insulin required, but it has no significant effect on hemoglobin A_{1c} levels or cardiovascular outcomes. Metformin is also not approved by the US FDA for use in type 1 diabetes because of a relative concern regarding risk of lactic acidosis.

α-Glucosidase inhibitors (Answer C) have been tested in type 1 diabetes and have some effect on postprandial glucose levels and body weight, but they do not significantly reduce hemoglobin A_{1c} values in individuals with type 1 diabetes.

There is some evidence that GLP-1 receptor agonists (Answer E) have beneficial effects on β-cell function, but this evidence is largely in animals. However, research is ongoing to investigate this potential beneficial effect in humans, particularly in the settings of recent-onset type 1 diabetes and islet-cell transplant.

Although SGLT-2 inhibitors (Answer A) may improve glycemic control and cause weight loss, they have not been adequately studied in persons with type 1 diabetes, nor are they recommended or approved for use in this setting. Also, SGLT-2 inhibitors may increase the risk of diabetic ketoacidosis. Some GLP-1 receptor agonists and SGLT-2 inhibitors may be selected based on their cardio-renal benefits if the patient has chronic kidney disease or congestive heart failure, etc. However, none of these situations is present in this vignette.

EDUCATIONAL OBJECTIVE

Recommend adjunctive treatments for management of type 1 diabetes mellitus.

REFERENCE(S)

Lebovitz HE. Adjunct therapy for type 1 diabetes mellitus. *Nat Rev Endocrinol.* 2010;6(6):326-334. PMID: 20404854

George P, McCrimmon RJ. Potential role of non-insulin adjunct therapy in type 1 diabetes. *Diabet Med.* 2013;30(2):179-188. PMID: 22804102

Taylor SI, Blau JE, Rother KI, Beitelshees AL. SGLT2 inhibitors as adjunctive therapy for type 1 diabetes: balancing benefits and risks. *Lancet Diabetes Endocrinol.* 2019;7(12):949-958. PMID: 31585821

10 ANSWER: E) Not sufficiently decrease blood glucose levels

SGLT-2 inhibitors are the newest class of drugs for the treatment of type 2 diabetes. They act by reducing the renal threshold for glucose excretion, thereby lowering blood glucose by increasing renal glucose clearance. These drugs do cause weight loss, as monotherapy and in combination, although the mechanism is not fully understood. In clinical trials, weight loss persists for at least 6 to 12 months and often longer (thus, Answer A is incorrect).

Although SGLT-2 inhibitors can transiently worsen the estimated glomerular filtration rate, in the longer term they provide renal protection (thus, Answer C is incorrect). Likewise, no adverse effects on blood pressure or hepatic function have been described (thus, Answers B and D are incorrect).

The glucose-lowering effects of SGLT-2 inhibitors are dependent on the estimated glomerular filtration rate, and hemoglobin A_{1c} lowering decreases to approximately 0.4% at rates below 60 mL/min per 1.73 m². In this woman with an estimated glomerular filtration rate of 38 mL/min per 1.73 m², the addition of empagliflozin is unlikely to help achieve her hemoglobin A_{1c} goal.

EDUCATIONAL OBJECTIVE

Determine when an SGLT-2 inhibitor is appropriate in the treatment of type 2 diabetes mellitus.

REFERENCE(S)

Abdul-Ghani MA, Norton L, Defronzo RA. Role of sodium-glucose cotransporter 2 (SGLT 2) inhibitors in the treatment of type 2 diabetes. *Endocr Rev.* 2011;32(4):515-531. PMID: 21606218

Neuen BL, Young T, Heerspink HJL, et al. SGLT2 inhibitors for the prevention of kidney failure in patients with type 2 diabetes: a systematic review and meta-analysis. *Lancet Diabetes Endocrinol.* 2019;7(11):845-854. PMID: 31495651

11

ANSWER: E) Use professional diagnostic continuous glucose monitoring to guide treatment

In this case, the hemoglobin A_{1c} value of 8.2% (66 mmol/mol) correlates with an estimated average glucose concentration of 189 mg/dL (10.5 mmol/L), a number that is very different from the downloaded value from the patient's meter (128 mg/dL [7.1 mmol/L]). This could mean that the patient is not monitoring at the times of highest blood glucose levels or that the meter is not accurate (which was checked). It could also reflect that some factor is interfering with the reliability of the hemoglobin A_{1c} assay. β-Thalassemia is associated with falsely elevated hemoglobin A_{1c} values. Measuring fructosamine is a good option to confirm this suspicion, but this choice was not offered. Relying on self-monitored blood glucose levels to guide treatment used to be the best management strategy. Continuous glucose monitoring is probably the best option in such patients, but professional diagnostic continuous glucose monitoring (Answer E) for 2 to 4 weeks may be a more affordable option. Glycated albumin measurement is also now available; it is more stable than fructosamine and is not affected by anemia.

A problem in carbohydrate counting would not cause the discrepancy between the hemoglobin A_{1c} level and the average glucose concentration, and adjustment of the ratio (Answer D) would not help.

Titrating the insulin glargine dosage (Answer B) would not address or correct the discrepancy between the hemoglobin A_{1c} level and the average glucose concentration. Also, increasing the insulin glargine dosage may worsen daytime hypoglycemia.

There is no evidence to support the use of a GLP-1 receptor agonist (Answer A) in patients with type 1 diabetes, and the combination may worsen daytime hypoglycemia.

Although insulin pump therapy (Answer C) might be a good treatment option for many reasons, it also does not address or correct the discrepancy between the hemoglobin A_{1c} and the average glucose concentration.

EDUCATIONAL OBJECTIVE

Explain the relationship between hemoglobin A_{1c} and estimated average glucose values and identify factors that can interfere with hemoglobin A_{1c} measurement.

REFERENCE(S)

Kahn R, Fonseca V. Translating the A1C assay. *Diabetes Care.* 2008;31(8):1704-1707. PMID: 18540045

Nathan DM, Kuenen J, Borg R, Zheng H, Schoenfeld D, Heine RJ; A1c-Derived Average Glucose Study Group. Translating the A1C assay into estimated average glucose values [published correction appears in *Diabetes Care.* 2009;32(1):207]. *Diabetes Care.* 2008;31(8):1473-1478. PMID: 18540046

Wiwanitkit V. Problem of using hemoglobin A1C measurement in endemic area of hemoglobinopathy. *Prim Care Diabetes.* 2007;1(3):173-175. PMID: 18632040

Battelino T, Danne T, Bergenstal RM, et al. Clinical targets for continuous glucose monitoring data interpretation: recommendations from the International Consensus on Time in Range. *Diabetes Care.* 2019;42(8):1593-1603.

Desouza CV, Holcomb RG, Rosenstock J, et al. Results of a study comparing glycated albumin to other glycemic indices. *J Clin Endocrinol Metab.* 2020;105(3):677-687. PMID: 31650161

12

ANSWER: B) Exenatide

Exenatide (Answer B) is relatively contraindicated in such patients because of reports of acute kidney injury. In clinical trials in patients with advanced chronic kidney disease, GLP-1 receptor agonists such as dulaglutide and semaglutide have been found to be safe.

SGLT-2 inhibitors (Answer D), including dapagliflozin, canagliflozin, and empagliflozin, inhibit glucose absorption in the proximal tubule, causing glucosuria, weight loss, and improved glycemic control. A reduced dosage is recommended in patients with a glomerular filtration rate in the range of 45 to 60 mL/min per 1.73 m². However, these agents have been used at lower estimated glomerular filtration rates, such as that observed in this patient, in clinical trials of patients with chronic kidney disease (eg, CREDENCE, DAPA CKD) and have been found to be safe.

Although glyburide would have to be discontinued in this patient, glimepiride could be used cautiously in a patient with an estimated glomerular filtration rate less than 60 mL/min per 1.73 m^2, so not all sulfonylureas (Answer E) must be discontinued. Additionally, glipizide, another sulfonylurea, can be continued in patients with a reduced glomerular filtration rate without dosage adjustment.

Neither insulin (Answer A) nor pioglitazone (Answer C) is contraindicated in patients with chronic kidney disease.

EDUCATIONAL OBJECTIVE
Identify effects of diabetes medications on kidney impairment.

REFERENCE(S)
American Diabetes Association Professional Practice Committee; Boris Draznin, Aroda AR, Bakris G, et al. 9. Pharmacologic approaches to glycemic treatment: standards of medical care in diabetes-2022. *Diabetes Care.* 2022;45(Suppl 1):S125-S143. PMID: 34964831

Inzucchi SE, Lipska KJ, Mayo H, Bailey CJ, McGuire DK. Metformin in patients with type 2 diabetes and kidney disease: a systematic review. *JAMA.* 2014;312(24):2668-2675. PMID: 25536258

Kalra S. Sodium glucose co-transporter-2 (SGLT2) inhibitors: a review of their basic and clinical pharmacology. *Diabetes Ther.* 2014;5(2):355-366. PMID: 25424969

Arjona Ferreira JC, Corry D, Mogensen CE, et al. Efficacy and safety of sitagliptin in patients with type 2 diabetes and ESRD receiving dialysis: a 54-week randomized trial [published correction appears in *Am J Kidney Dis.* 2013;62(4):847]. *Am J Kidney Dis.* 2013;61(4):579-587. PMID: 23352379

McGill JB, Sloan L, Newman J, et al. Long-term efficacy and safety of linagliptin in patients with type 2 diabetes and severe renal impairment: a 1-year, randomized, double-blind, placebo-controlled study. *Diabetes Care.* 2013;36(2):237-244. PMID: 23033241

Sampanis CH. Management of hyperglycemia in patients with diabetes mellitus and chronic renal failure. *Hippokratia.* 2008;12(1):22-27. PMID: 18923754

13 ANSWER: B) Basal insulin daily plus rapid-acting insulin analogue (eg, insulin aspart) every 6 hours when his blood glucose is >180 mg/dL (>10.0 mmol/L) to achieve most blood glucose values between 140 and 180 mg/dL (7.8-10.0 mmol/L)

It is now widely accepted that proper attention to glycemic management both in the intensive care unit and in the general medical-surgical wards is an important aspect of high-quality, safe inpatient care. A 2009 American Association of Clinical Endocrinologists–American Diabetes Association consensus statement endorsed the use of intravenous insulin in the intensive care unit setting, targeting blood glucose values between 140 and 180 mg/dL (7.8-10.0 mmol/L). In this vignette, the patient's postoperative blood glucose is clearly uncontrolled, placing him at increased risk of infection, among other potential complications.

Scheduled basal insulin given once daily combined with rapid-acting insulin analogue given every 6 hours when blood glucose is above the upper limit of his target range (Answer B) is an appropriate regimen for this man while he remains on nothing-by-mouth status. The dose of basal insulin could also be appropriately split into a twice-daily regimen.

A regular insulin sliding-scale regimen (Answer D) would reduce glucose levels to some degree, but it has been associated with increased rates of both hyperglycemia and hypoglycemia when compared with regimens that include some basal insulin.

Aspart premixed insulin such as 70/30 (Answer A) has little role in the hospital setting because it is an inflexible product and does not allow for adjustments in the dose of the intermediate insulin separate from the dose of the rapid-acting insulin analogue (and vice versa).

GLP-1 receptor agonists such as liraglutide (Answer E) should be used only in outpatients and they have no current role in the hospital setting.

Intravenous insulin infusion (Answer C) could be used, but many hospitals are not equipped to manage insulin infusions outside of the intensive care unit, and the titration target should be 140 to 180 mg/dL, not 80 to 110 mg/dL.

EDUCATIONAL OBJECTIVE
Manage preexisting diabetes mellitus in hospitalized patients.

REFERENCE(S)
Moghissi ES, Korytkowski MT, DiNardo M, et al; American Association of Clinical Endocrinologists; American Diabetes Association. American Association of Clinical Endocrinologists and American Diabetes Association consensus statement on inpatient glycemic control. *Diabetes Care.* 2009;32(6):1119-1131. PMID: 19429873

Lleva RR, Inzucchi SE. Hospital management of hyperglycemia. *Curr Opin Endocrinol Diabetes Obes.* 2011;18(2):110-118. PMID: 21358407

14 ANSWER: C) Measure serum vitamin B_{12}

This patient has new neuropathic symptoms superimposed on a history and examination findings consistent with peripheral polyneuropathy. The symptoms and physical findings suggest posterior column and upper motor neuron disease, and in this setting, a positive Romberg sign and Babinski response would likely be present. Although this may represent progression of diabetic neuropathy, the latter findings are not typical for this alone. He has anemia, and the combination of neurologic and hematologic disturbance is compatible with vitamin B_{12} deficiency. Use of metformin has been associated with decreased plasma vitamin B_{12} levels in up to 30% of patients, and this medication doubles the risk of clinically significant B_{12} deficiency. While the mechanism is not entirely clear, most evidence points to interference with food-derived B_{12} absorption, primarily in the ileum. Replacement with oral or parenteral vitamin B_{12} is usually successful and precludes discontinuation of metformin.

Numerous laboratory testing options are available to assess for the presence of B_{12} deficiency. Serum vitamin B_{12} measurement (Answer C) is most commonly used for initial assessment, while others, such as measurement of holotranscobalamin, methylmalonic acid, or homocysteine, are reserved for confirmatory testing.

Findings on electromyography and nerve conduction studies (Answer E) would most likely be abnormal in this man, but they are not specific for subacute combined degeneration (neuropathy due to vitamin B_{12} deficiency).

Vitamin B_6, pyridoxine, has a role in serotonin and norepinephrine metabolism and in the formation of myelin. Clinical symptoms of B_6 deficiency are bilateral, distal limb numbness (appears early) and distal limb burning paresthesia (replaces numbness later in the course). Distal limb weakness is rare. Thus, measuring vitamin B_6 (Answer B) is not the best next step.

This patient's presentation is not consistent with spinal or nerve root irritation from C-spine disease, which can manifest as pain in the neck and pain and numbness or weakness radiating down to the shoulder, arm, and hand. Thus, MRI of the cervical spine (Answer D) is incorrect.

γ-Glutamyltransferase (Answer A) would be elevated if he had alcohol-related neuropathy, but that is not suggested by his history.

EDUCATIONAL OBJECTIVE
Diagnose adverse effects of metformin.

REFERENCE(S)
Pierce SA, Chung AH, Black KK. Evaluation of vitamin B_{12} monitoring in a veteran population on long-term, high-dose metformin therapy. *Ann Pharmacother.* 2012;46(11):1470-1476. PMID: 23115224

Pflipsen MC, Oh RC, Saguil A, Seehusen DA, Seaquist D, Topolski R. The prevalence of vitamin B(12) deficiency in patients with type 2 diabetes: a cross-sectional study. *J Am Board Fam Med.* 2009;22(5):528-534. PMID: 19734399

Ting RZ-W, Szeto CC, Chan MH, Ma KK, Chow KM. Risk factors of vitamin B(12) deficiency in patients receiving metformin. *Arch Intern Med.* 2006;166(18):1975-1979. PMID: 17030830

Ward PCJ. Modern approaches to the investigation of vitamin B12 deficiency. *Clin Lab Med.* 2002;22(2):435-445. PMID: 12134470

15 ANSWER: A) Add sulfonylurea therapy

New-onset diabetes after transplant (NODAT) occurs in approximately one-third of all patients who receive a kidney transplant. Risk factors include increased age, obesity, African American or Hispanic ethnicity, family history of diabetes, and certain antirejection medications, including glucocorticoids. NODAT can be defined as the presence of diabetes symptoms (including polyuria, polydipsia, and unexplained weight loss) and a random plasma glucose value of 200 mg/dL or greater ($\geq$11.1 mmol/L), a fasting plasma glucose value of 126 mg/dL or greater ($\geq$7.0 mmol/L), or a 2-hour plasma glucose value of 200 mg/dL or greater ($\geq$11.1 mmol/L) any time after transplant.

A stepwise approach is recommended for managing NODAT, beginning with lifestyle management and oral treatment with a sulfonylurea (Answer A). Of note, metformin is often used as first-line pharmacotherapy in the treatment of kidney transplant recipients with NODAT. The benefits potentially counter some of the weight gain associated with immunosuppressant regimens. In addition, the safety concern regarding the risk of lactic acidosis risk is not considered to be a factor in well-functioning allografts. No oral agents have been studied in the prevention of NODAT.

Thiazolidinediones (Answer B) are not recommended because of their adverse effect on fluid retention.

Because glucocorticoid use is associated with hyperglycemia, a decreased dosage (not increased [Answer C]) is recommended, if possible, in the context of transplant protection.

Insulin therapy is only recommended after oral therapy and should be used to maintain hemoglobin A_{1c} levels below 7.0% (<53 mmol/mol), not 8.0% (64 mmol/mol) (Answer D).

EDUCATIONAL OBJECTIVE
Identify new-onset diabetes after transplant and recommend appropriate treatment.

REFERENCE(S)
Sharif A. Should metformin be our antiglycemic agent of choice post-transplantation? *Am J Transplant.* 2011;11(7):1376-1381. PMID: 21564529

16 ANSWER: D) Discontinue insulins glargine and lispro and switch to regular U500 insulin 3 times daily

Insulin is the preferred therapeutic option for patients with persistent hyperglycemia that fails to respond to other agents. However, in patients requiring more than 200 units of insulin daily, the volume of insulin becomes a problem, both in terms of patient comfort and pharmacokinetics. Large-volume insulin injections are poorly absorbed. In these cases, U500 insulin should be considered (Answers B or D). There is increasing evidence of more reliable delivery of insulin and successful outcomes with the use of U500 insulin in patients such as the one presented. Although the formulation of U500 is similar to that of regular insulin, the duration of action is up to 13 to 24 hours, permitting adequate delivery with 2 or 3 injections per day. Long-acting insulin is therefore no longer needed; insulin glargine can be discontinued (Answer D). Fortunately, U500 pens are now available.

Given the severity of this patient's hyperglycemia, switching to insulin degludec (Answer E), even at a higher dosage, or adding linagliptin (Answer A) is unlikely to achieve a target hemoglobin A_{1c} level less than 7.0% (<53 mmol/mol).

Switching to insulin pump therapy (Answer C) is not desirable because large volumes of insulin, either by injection or pump, are poorly absorbed and are unlikely to achieve the target hemoglobin A_{1c} level.

EDUCATIONAL OBJECTIVE
Treat extreme insulin resistance with U500 insulin.

REFERENCE(S)

Hood RC, Arakaki RF, Wysham C, Li YG, Settles JA, Jackson JA. Two treatment approaches for human regular U-500 insulin in patients with type 2 diabetes not achieving adequate glycemic control on high-dose U-100 insulin therapy with or without oral agents: a randomized, titration-to-target clinical trial. *Endocr Pract.* 2015;21(7):782-793. PMID: 25813411

Quinn SL, Lansang MC, Mina D. Safety and effectiveness of U-500 insulin therapy in patients with insulin-resistant type 2 diabetes mellitus. *Pharmacotherapy.* 2011;31(7):695-702. PMID: 21923457

Lane WS, Cochran EK, Jackson JA, et al. High-dose insulin therapy: is it time for U-500 insulin? *Endocr Pract.* 2009;15(1):71-79. PMID: 19211405

Garg R, Johnston V, McNally PG, Davies MJ, Lawrence IG. U-500 insulin: why, when and how to use in clinical practice. *Diabetes Metab Res Rev.* 2007;23(4):265-268. PMID: 17109474

17 ANSWER: B) Once-daily basal insulin, plus correction insulin dose regimen every 4 to 6 hours

Subcutaneous insulin is the recommended treatment for glycemic management in postoperative patients with type 2 diabetes who are in a noncritical care unit. If the patient were in the critical care setting, continuous intravenous insulin infusion (Answer A) would be the recommended method of glycemic management. However, if the patient is in a noncritical care setting, as in this case, a regimen of scheduled subcutaneous insulin injections is the best method for achieving glycemic targets.

This patient's glycemic status warrants basal insulin in addition to correction dose insulin. As she is not eating, meal insulin will not be provided. The dosing frequency of correction insulin depends on the type of insulin used. If a rapid-acting analogue is used, it may be given every 4 hours, and if regular insulin is used, it will be given every 6 hours (Answer B). These time intervals correspond to the known duration of action of each insulin and will help avoid stacking of insulin and resulting hypoglycemia. Injections should align with meals and bedtime or every 4 to 6 hours if the patient is not consuming meals (thus, Answer C is incorrect).

Evidence clearly shows that sliding-scale insulin used alone (Answer E) is associated with increased rates of both hypoglycemia and hyperglycemia and its use is therefore not recommended. In addition, evidence from randomized controlled trials has demonstrated that a scheduled basal plus bolus treatment regimen results in better glycemic control and reduced hospital complications when compared with outcomes with sliding-scale insulin alone in general surgery patients with type 2 diabetes, further making the case for a basal plus bolus regimen. When this patient begins to eat, scheduled meal insulin will be added to her regimen.

Restarting home medications without insulin (Answer D) is incorrect, as the patient has nausea and also may be at risk of lactic acidosis.

EDUCATIONAL OBJECTIVE
Manage inpatient insulin treatment in the noncritical care setting.

REFERENCE(S)

American Diabetes Association Professional Practice Committee; Draznin B, Aroda VR, Bakris G, et al. 16. Diabetes care in the hospital: standards of medical care in diabetes-2022. *Diabetes Care.* 2022;45(Suppl 1):S99-S104. PMID: 34964884

Umpierrez GE, Smiley D, Jacobs S, et al. Randomized study of basal-bolus insulin therapy in the inpatient management of patients with type 2 diabetes undergoing general surgery (RABBIT 2 surgery). *Diabetes Care.* 2011;34(2):256-261. PMID: 21228246

18 ANSWER: B) C-peptide, glutamic acid decarboxylase antibodies, and insulinoma-associated protein 2 antibodies

Ketosis-prone diabetes, previously referred to as Flatbush diabetes or type 1b diabetes, has been increasingly recognized since the mid-1990s. In the United States, 20% to 50% of newly diagnosed patients are Black or Hispanic. Although these patients present with diabetic ketoacidosis, predicting the duration of insulin therapy has been a therapeutic challenge. To facilitate the understanding of the diagnosis and insulin management subsequent to the acute diabetic ketoacidosis episode, 4 classification systems have been developed focusing on β-cell autoimmunity measured by glutamic acid decarboxylase and insulinoma-associated protein 2 antibodies and β-cell function assessed by the C-peptide concentration (thus, Answer B is correct). The system of classification that most accurately (99% sensitivity and 96% specificity) predicts the need for insulin treatment 12 months after presentation with diabetic ketoacidosis is known as the Aβ system.

EDUCATIONAL OBJECTIVE
Choose the appropriate classification system for predicting duration of insulin therapy in ketosis-prone diabetes.

REFERENCE(S)
Banerji MA, Dham S. A comparison of classification schemes for ketosis-prone diabetes. *Nat Clin Pract Endocrinol Metab.* 2007;3(7):506-507. PMID: 17489086

Balasubramanyam A, Garza G, Rodriguez L, et al. Accuracy and predictive value of classification schemes for ketosis-prone diabetes. *Diabetes Care.* 2006;29(12):2575-2579. PMID: 17130187

Mauvais-Jarvis F, Sobngwi E, Porcher R, et al. Ketosis-prone type 2 diabetes in patients of sub-Saharan African origin: clinical pathophysiology and natural history of beta-cell dysfunction and insulin resistance. *Diabetes.* 2004;53(3):645-653. PMID: 14988248

19 ANSWER: D) Progressively initiate more vigorous regular exercise

This relatively healthy woman with type 2 diabetes who has no symptoms to suggest coronary heart disease should be able to initiate regular exercise with slow progression as tolerated (Answer D). Although type 2 diabetes is associated with a 2-fold increased risk of coronary heart disease, national guidelines from the American Diabetes Association currently do not recommend routine screening of asymptomatic patients with high cardiovascular disease risk because cardiac outcomes are not improved as long as cardiac risk factors are being treated. Randomized controlled trials have also found no clinical benefit of screening asymptomatic patients with type 2 diabetes and normal results from electrocardiography.

An exercise tolerance test (Answer B) and stress echocardiography (Answer C) have some value in determining risk for cardiac events; however, screening asymptomatic patients with diabetes is not currently recommended. Exercise stress tests have comparable sensitivity and specificity in patients with and without diabetes (approximately 50% and 80%, respectively), and stress echocardiography is even more accurate in predicting events. Cardiac rehabilitation (Answer A) is generally recommended for patients with recent interventions or other comorbidities.

EDUCATIONAL OBJECTIVE
Provide patients with diabetes mellitus exercise recommendations in the setting of managing cardiovascular disease risk.

REFERENCE(S)
American Diabetes Association Professional Practice Committee. 10. Cardiovascular disease and risk management: standards of medical care in diabetes-2022. *Diabetes Care.* 2022;45(Suppl 1):S144-S174. PMID: 34964815

Patel NB, Balady GJ. Diagnostic and prognostic testing to evaluate coronary artery disease in patients with diabetes mellitus. *Rev Endocr Metab Disord.* 2010;11(1):11-20. PMID: 20225090

20 ANSWER: A) Alirocumab, 75 mg every 2 weeks

Recommendations for lipid-lowering treatment have been revised such that treatment initiation and the initial statin dosage are personalized on the basis of risk profile. For persons with diabetes, a high-potency statin (ie, atorvastatin, 80 mg daily, or rosuvastatin, 40 mg daily) is recommended, although some patients may not tolerate these dosages. Atorvastatin, 60 mg daily, (Answer B) is unlikely to reduce his LDL-cholesterol concentration lower than his current medication already has.

Additional benefit may be obtained by adding high-potency fish oil such as icosapent ethyl for those with high triglycerides or a PCSK9 inhibitor such as alirocumab or evolocumab if LDL cholesterol remains high as in this case. Subgroup analysis of the alirocumab trials demonstrated greatest benefit in secondary benefit for those with an LDL-cholesterol concentration greater than 100 mg/dL (>2.59 mmol/L). Because this patient's LDL-cholesterol concentration is greater than 100 mg/dL (>2.59 mmol/L) but his triglyceride concentration is normal, alirocumab (Answer A) would be the best addition, rather than icosapent ethyl (Answer D). Clinical trials have shown that individuals at high risk for cardiovascular disease have a significant reduction in further cardiovascular events with an aggressive regimen of high-intensity lipid-lowering therapy.

Pravastatin (Answer E) is a less potent statin, and lowering the statin dosage/intensity in a patient at high risk is not appropriate.

Ezetimibe (Answer C) in combination with statin therapy has been shown to reduce cardiovascular events, but in the IMPROVE IT trial, the achieved LDL-cholesterol concentration was 55 mg/dL (1.42 mmol/L), which may not be possible in this case.

EDUCATIONAL OBJECTIVE
Recommend appropriate intensive lipid-lowering therapy in patients with type 2 diabetes mellitus and coronary artery disease.

REFERENCE(S)
Stone NJ, Robinson JG, Lichtenstein AH, Bairey Merz CN, Blum CB, et al. 2013 ACC/AHA guideline on the treatment of blood cholesterol to reduce atherosclerotic cardiovascular risk in adults: a report of the American College of Cardiology/American Heart Association Task Force on Practice Guidelines [published correction appears in *J Am Coll Cardiol.* 2014;63(25 Pt B):3024-3025]. *J Am Coll Cardiol.* 2014;63(25 Pt B):2889-2934. PMID: 24239923

American Diabetes Association Professional Practice Committee. 10. Cardiovascular disease and risk management: standards of medical care in diabetes-2022. *Diabetes Care.* 2022;45(Suppl 1):S144-S174. PMID: 34964815

Schwartz GG, Steg PG, Szarek M, et al; ODYSSEY OUTCOMES Committees and Investigators. Alirocumab and cardiovascular outcomes after acute coronary syndrome. *N Engl J Med.* 2018;379(22):2097-2107. PMID: 30403574

Jellinger PS, Handelsman Y, Rosenblit PD, et al. American Association of Clinical Endocrinologists and American College of Endocrinology guidelines for management of dyslipidemia and prevention of cardiovascular disease. *Endocr Pract.* 2017;23(Suppl 2):1-87. PMID: 28437620

21 ANSWER: D) Oral glucose tolerance test

CFRD is the result of a primary defect of insulin secretion due in part to nonautoimmune destruction of β cells (mainly) and α cells in the pancreas, so both insulin and glucagon secretion are defective. However, histologic studies have reported variability in the degree of islet-cell destruction. This indicates there are other factors contributing to insulin deficiency in CFRD, perhaps "collateral damage" from fibrosis and fatty infiltration or islet amyloid. The presence of CFRD strongly correlates with poorer clinical status, reflected by reduced pulmonary function and nutritional status, increased frequency of acute pulmonary exacerbations, and significant sputum pathogens. Annual screening for CFRD in all patients with cystic fibrosis is recommended beginning by 10 years of age, consistent with guidelines from the American Diabetes Association, Cystic Fibrosis Foundation, Pediatric Endocrine Society, and International Society for Pediatric and Adolescent Diabetes. The best method to screen for and diagnose CFRD is the oral glucose tolerance test (Answer D).

Hemoglobin A_{1c} (Answer C) and fasting plasma glucose measurement (Answer A) should not be used for screening because they have low sensitivity for detecting CFRD. This has been confirmed in several studies. In these patients, hemoglobin A_{1c} is often normal, regardless of the degree of hyperglycemia. In 1 study, only 16% of patients with cystic fibrosis had elevated hemoglobin A_{1c} values at the time of CFRD diagnosis. Also, waiting for symptoms to prompt screening for CFRD (Answer E) is not a good strategy. In a population of pediatric patients with cystic fibrosis in Toronto, only 2.7% were clinically recognized as having CFRD, but with oral glucose tolerance testing of asymptomatic adolescents (aged 10 to 18 years), 17% were found to have impaired glucose tolerance and 13% had CFRD without fasting hyperglycemia. The recommended treatment for CFRD is insulin, albeit this is based on few clinical trials.

Fructosamine (Answer B) is not used for diabetes screening.

EDUCATIONAL OBJECTIVE
Recommend the best screening method for cystic fibrosis–related diabetes mellitus.

REFERENCE(S)
Moran A, Pillay K, Becker DJ, Acerini CL; International Society for Pediatric and Adolescent Diabetes. ISPAD Clinical Practice Consensus Guidelines 2014. Management of cystic fibrosis-related diabetes in children and adolescents. *Pediatr Diabetes*. 2014;15(Suppl 20):65-76. PMID: 25182308

O'Shea D, O'Connell J. Cystic fibrosis related diabetes. *Curr Diab Rep*. 2014;14(8):511. PMID: 24915888

Kelly A, Moran A. Update on cystic fibrosis-related diabetes [published correction appears in *J Cyst Fibros*. 2014;13(1):119]. *J Cyst Fibros*. 2013;12(4):318-331. PMID: 23562217

22 **ANSWER: D) Start insulin**
This patient presents with a form of type 1 diabetes that may be seen in adults—latent autoimmune diabetes in adults (LADA). Persons with LADA can progress to the need for insulin very slowly, over years, or more rapidly, as in this patient. LADA may be present in up to 30% of patients with a clinical diagnosis of type 2 diabetes. Compared with type 2 diabetes, LADA is generally associated with lower BMI, lower triglycerides,

higher HDL cholesterol, and lower prevalence of hypertension. The Immunology of Diabetes Society has proposed the following criteria for LADA: age at onset of at least 30 years, positive for at least 1 autoantibody associated with type 1 diabetes, and not requiring insulin within the first 6 months after diagnosis. Many experts think the latter criterion is too subjective. This patient's continued symptomatic hyperglycemia and lack of response to metformin are clues to the correct diagnosis. The family history of autoimmune disease also points to the correct diagnosis. Failure to recognize it can delay appropriate treatment. The diagnosis is confirmed by the seropositivity of the antibodies (glutamic acid decarboxylase antibodies being the most sensitive immune parameter), especially if the titer is high.

This patient requires insulin (Answer D) to control his hyperglycemia; no other intervention has been well studied or shown to be effective in treating LADA. Thus, adding a sulfonylurea (Answer C), an SGLT-2 (Answer A), or a GLP-1 receptor agonist (Answer B) is incorrect.

EDUCATIONAL OBJECTIVE
Diagnose latent autoimmune diabetes in adults (LADA) in a patient misdiagnosed as having type 2 diabetes and review treatment implications.

REFERENCE(S)
O'Neil KS, Johnson JL, Panak RL. Recognizing and appropriately treating latent autoimmune diabetes in adults. *Diabetes Spectr*. 2016;29(4):249-252. PMID: 27899877

Laugesen E, Ostergaard JA, Leslie RD; Danish Diabetes Academy Workshop and Workshop Speakers. Latent autoimmune diabetes of the adult: current knowledge and uncertainty. *Diabet Med*. 2015;32(7):843-852. PMID: 25601320

Liao Y, Xiang Y, Zhou Z. Diagnostic criteria of latent autoimmune diabetes in adults (LADA): a review and reflection. *Front Med*. 2012;6(3):243-247. PMID: 22843304

Naik RG, Brooks-Worrell BM, Palmer JP. Latent autoimmune diabetes in adults. *J Clin Endocrinol Metab*. 2009;94(12):4635-4644. PMID: 19837918

23 ANSWER: C) Gastric-emptying study

In insulin-treated patients with diabetes, gastroparesis (delayed gastric emptying) may lead to unexplained hypoglycemia, particularly early in the postprandial period. Gastroparesis often occurs in patients with longstanding diabetes and concomitant microvascular complications. Most patients with gastroparesis present with upper gastrointestinal symptoms, although the correlation of symptoms with delayed gastric emptying is weak, and some patients are asymptomatic. The rate of gastric emptying regulates the delivery of carbohydrates to the small intestine, and it has a major effect on postprandial blood glucose. Variations in the rate of gastric emptying account for 35% of the variance in the initial rise of blood glucose after a 75-g glucose load in healthy persons and those with diabetes. Nuclear medicine scintigraphy, or a gastric-emptying study (Answer C), remains the criterion standard for assessing gastric emptying, although inconsistency in its use may affect its diagnostic accuracy.

Although adrenal insufficiency can be a cause of unexplained hypoglycemia in a patient with type 1 diabetes, it is a less likely diagnosis in a patient with normal blood pressure and electrolytes and without symptoms of orthostasis. Thus, a cosyntropin-stimulation test (Answer B) is incorrect.

This patient is frustrated and stressed about her situation, and while psychiatric evaluation (Answer D) and counseling may be helpful in coping with any chronic condition, this approach is unlikely to uncover the cause of her hypoglycemia.

Similarly, because she has had ongoing and recent nutrition counseling, suboptimal carbohydrate counting skills (Answer E) are unlikely to be the reason for her frequent unexplained hypoglycemia.

Abdominal CT (Answer A) is incorrect, as CT will not diagnose gastroparesis. Other CT findings are irrelevant in this case.

EDUCATIONAL OBJECTIVE

Diagnose the etiology of unexplained recurrent hypoglycemia and glycemic variability.

REFERENCE(S)

Phillips LK, Deane AM, Jones KL, Rayner CK, Horowitz M. Gastric emptying and glycaemia in health and diabetes mellitus. *Nat Rev Endocrinol.* 2015;11(2):112-128. PMID: 25421372

Chang J, Rayner CK, Jones KL, Horowitz M. Diabetic gastroparesis and its impact on glycemia. *Endocrinol Metab Clin North Am.* 2010;39(4):745-762. PMID: 21095542

Samsom M, Bharucha A, Gerich JE, Hermann K, Limmer J, Linke R, et al. Diabetes mellitus and gastric emptying: questions and issues in clinical practice. *Diabetes Metab Res Rev.* 2009;25(6):502-514. PMID: 19610128

Ma J, Rayner CK, Jones KL, Horowitz M. Diabetic gastroparesis: diagnosis and management. *Drugs.* 2009;69(8):971-986. PMID: 19496627

24 ANSWER: E) Tissue transglutaminase IgA antibodies

About 5% of persons with type 1 diabetes develop celiac disease. Only a minority of children and adolescents with type 1 diabetes and celiac disease present with gastrointestinal symptoms. More common initial findings include unpredictable blood glucose measurements and recurrent episodes of hypoglycemia because of erratic intestinal absorption of nutrients. Thus, elevated tissue transglutaminase IgA antibodies (Answer E) would most likely explain her hypoglycemia.

Less than 1% of children with type 1 diabetes have autoimmune adrenalitis (Addison disease) (Answer A). In one report, about 2% of children with type 1 disease had circulating antibodies to steroid 21-hydroxylase (Answer D). Although less common than celiac disease, this condition is associated with decreased insulin requirement and increased frequency of hypoglycemia, hyperpigmentation, hypotension, hyponatremia, and hyperkalemia (none of which is present in this patient).

Hyperthyroidism (Answer B) is rare in patients with type 1 diabetes (1%-2%) and can lead to higher blood glucose values due to insulin resistance, not hypoglycemia. In addition, except for weight loss, this patient has no symptoms or physical findings to suggest Graves disease.

Antibodies to glutamic acid decarboxylase (a 65-kD protein) (Answer C) are found in about 70% of patients with type 1 diabetes at the time of diagnosis. They could very well be high in this patient, but this would not explain her hypoglycemia.

EDUCATIONAL OBJECTIVE
Recognize hypoglycemia resulting from celiac disease in type 1 diabetes mellitus and describe its presentation.

REFERENCE(S)
Khoury N, Semenkovich K, Arbeláez AM. Coeliac disease presenting as severe hypoglycaemia in youth with type 1 diabetes. *Diabet Med.* 2014;31(12):e33-e36. PMID: 24805141

Abid N, McGlone O, Cardwell C, McCallion W, Carson D. Clinical and metabolic effects of gluten free diet in children with type 1 diabetes and coeliac disease. *Pediatr Diabetes.* 2011;12(4 Pt 1):322-325. PMID: 21615651

Warncke K, Fröhlich-Reiterer EE, Thon A, Hofer SE, Wiemann D, Holl RW; DPV Initiative of the German Working Group for Pediatric Diabetology; German BMBF Competence Network for Diabetes Mellitus. Polyendocrinopathy in children, adolescents, and young adults with type 1 diabetes: a multicenter analysis of 28,671 patients from the German/Austrian DPV-Wiss database. *Diabetes Care.* 2010;33(9):2010-2012. PMID: 20551013

25 ANSWER: C) Metformin

Despite this man's modestly increased risk for cardiovascular disease, metformin (Answer C) remains the first-line agent of choice in international guidelines for diabetes management, including the 2018 American Diabetes Association and European Association for the Study of Diabetes Consensus Report on management of hyperglycemia in type 2 diabetes and subsequent guidelines. He does not have established atherosclerotic cardiovascular disease, chronic kidney disease, or congestive heart failure. Metformin should be combined with comprehensive lifestyle changes (including weight management and physical activity) if hemoglobin A_{1c} is above target, as is the case in this patient.

The major change in the new guidelines is based on accumulating evidence that specific SGLT-2 inhibitors and GLP-1 receptor agonists improve cardiovascular outcomes, as well as secondary outcomes such as heart failure and progression of kidney disease, in patients with established cardiovascular disease or chronic kidney disease. Therefore, subsequent guidance in this overall approach when another drug is required is based on the presence or absence of established atherosclerotic cardiovascular disease or chronic kidney disease. Because this patient has newly diagnosed diabetes, a modestly elevated hemoglobin A_{1c}, and no evidence of established cardiovascular disease or nephropathy, incorporation of an SGLT-2 inhibitor (Answer A) or a GLP-1 receptor agonist (Answer B) into his antihyperglycemic medication regimen is not indicated. Importantly, patients with newly diagnosed diabetes were not included in the diabetes cardiovascular outcomes trials (except for those evaluating drugs for chronic kidney disease and congestive heart failure), and therefore the effectiveness and cost-effectiveness of newer and more expensive drugs cannot be evaluated.

DPP-4 inhibitors (Answer D) do not confer advantages in terms of cardiovascular disease or kidney outcomes.

This man's calculated 10-year risk of heart disease or stroke is 14.1%. In patients with diabetes mellitus at higher risk, especially those with multiple risk factors or those 50 to 75 years of age, it is reasonable to recommend a high-intensity statin to reduce LDL cholesterol by 50% or more. The American College of Cardiology/American Heart Association guidelines therefore suggest treatment with a high-intensity statin. This patient is taking atorvastatin, 40 mg daily. High-intensity dosing for atorvastatin is 80 mg daily, unless down-titration is required if the patient is unable to tolerate this dosage. He should be advised to increase his atorvastatin dosage to 80 mg daily. In addition, based on his age and calculated cardiovascular disease risk greater than 10%, he should be advised to start taking aspirin, 81 mg daily, as long as he is not at increased risk for bleeding and is willing to take it daily for at least 10 years.

EDUCATIONAL OBJECTIVE
Explain how atherosclerotic cardiovascular disease risk is incorporated into selection of medications used to treat type 2 diabetes mellitus.

REFERENCE(S)
CV Risk Calculator. Ahead Research, Inc. November 11, 2021. Available at: http://www.cvriskcalculator.com/

Davies MJ, D'Alessio DA, Fradkin J, et al. Management of hyperglycemia in type 2 diabetes, 2018. A consensus report by the American Diabetes Association (ADA) and the European Association for the Study of Diabetes (EASD). *Diabetes Care*. 2018;41(12):2669-2701. PMID: 30291106

Grundy SM, Stone NJ, Bailey AL, et al. 2018 AHA/ ACC/AACVPR/AAPA/ABC/ACPM/ADA/AGS/ AphA/ASPC/NLA/PCNA guideline on the management of blood cholesterol: a report of the American College of Cardiology/American Heart Association Task Force on Clinical Practice Guidelines. *J Am Coll Cardiol*. 2019;73(24):e285-e350. PMID: 20423393

26 ANSWER: B) Begin sildenafil
This patient has longstanding diabetes, macrovascular disease, retinopathy, and peripheral and autonomic neuropathy. It is not surprising that he has erectile dysfunction given the key role that endothelial function and autonomic innervation have in penile tumescence.

Use of phosphodiesterase 5 inhibitors such as sildenafil (Answer B) is the mainstay of therapy for erectile dysfunction. Although patients with diabetes do not respond as well as those without diabetes, response rates are still approximately 50%. This patient may have a reduced chance of responding because of his longstanding erectile dysfunction and other comorbidities; nonetheless, neither the presence of endothelial dysfunction nor autonomic neuropathy predicts response to sildenafil. The simplicity and safety of phosphodiesterase 5 inhibitor treatment make it the best first step in this patient's management. Although use of nitrates is a contraindication for use of drugs such as sildenafil, the presence of cardiovascular disease is not.

Improvement of glycemic control (Answer C) has not been demonstrated to improve sexual function in cases of erectile dysfunction.

Intracavernosal alprostadil (Answer A) and penile implants (Answer D) are effective treatments, but they are more invasive than sildenafil and are thus relegated to second- or third-line therapy.

It should also be noted that many medications, including antihypertensive agents (ie, metoprolol, which this patient is taking), antidepressants, antianxiety and anticonvulsant drugs, antihistamines, and some nonsteroidal antiinflammatory agents (eg, naproxen and indomethacin) may also cause erectile dysfunction. If his neuropathy and/or cardiac disease were not so advanced, it would be worth asking his cardiologist to consider substituting another class of antihypertensive drug for the β-adrenergic blocker.

EDUCATIONAL OBJECTIVE
Manage erectile dysfunction in the setting of diabetes mellitus.

REFERENCE(S)
Price D, Hackett G. Management of erectile dysfunction in diabetes: an update for 2008. *Curr Diab Rep*. 2008;8(6):437-443. PMID: 18990299

Pegge NC, Twomey AM, Vaughton K, Gravenor MB, Ramsey MW, Price DE. The role of endothelial dysfunction in the pathophysiology of erectile dysfunction in diabetes and in determining response to treatment. *Diabet Med*. 2006;23(8):873-878. PMID: 16911625

Diabetes Mellitus, Section 2 Board Review

Marie E. McDonnell, MD

27 **ANSWER: C) One or more insulin-to-carbohydrate ratios must be adjusted**

Automated insulin delivery systems that adjust insulin delivery rates in response to interstitial glucose levels transmitted by continuous glucose monitoring systems (hybrid closed loop) are more globally accessible to insulin-requiring people with diabetes. While each hybrid closed-loop system has unique characteristics, they all depend on accurate and well-timed dosing of insulin for food intake to achieve glycemic goals. The insulin-to-carbohydrate ratio requires regular adjustment (Answer C) until goal time in range is achieved. The sensitivity factor programmed for correction boluses (Answer A) is not relevant in automated insulin delivery systems, as correction boluses are administered according to the electronic algorithms, which include machine-learning approaches to determine correction insulin doses.

Most systems have achieved similar glycemic targets in populations studied; for example, approximately 70% time in range using the 70 to 180 mg/dL (3.9-10.0 mmol/L) glucose range as recommended by a recent international consensus panel. In most patients, achieving this time in range leads to a mean blood glucose value between 145 and 155 mg/dL (8.0-8.6 mmol/L). Based on published studies, this can be achieved when the algorithm is used more than 90% of the time, making this patient's use adequate (thus, Answer D is incorrect).

Her total daily insulin dose is relatively high, which, if programmed lower into the pump, could result in the automated insulin delivery algorithm delivering insufficient correction boluses. A too-high programmed total daily insulin requirement (Answer B) could result in overly aggressive insulinization, which would not explain a higher-than-expected mean blood glucose value.

EDUCATIONAL OBJECTIVE

Optimize hybrid closed-loop automated insulin delivery systems for individual patients.

REFERENCE(S)

Battelino T, Danne T, Bergenstal RM, et al. Clinical targets for continuous glucose monitoring data interpretation: recommendations from the International Consensus on Time in Range. *Diabetes Care.* 2019;42(8):1593-1603. PMID: 31177185

Breton MD, Kovatchev BP. One year real-world use of the Control-IQ advanced hybrid closed-loop technology. *Diabetes Technol Ther.* 2021;23(9): 601-608. PMID: 33784196

28 **ANSWER: C) Continue with the new meter (the glucose discrepancy is within the US FDA acceptable range)**

People with diabetes are increasingly exposed to new devices on a regular basis, either due to helpful technological advances or coverage changes dictated by their health insurance companies based on variables that may change intermittently, including cost and supply. Many patients report not being aware of accuracy limitations of glucose monitoring devices. As a result, people with diabetes often compare devices and seek input from their care team on differences they identify. Per the US FDA, when comparing measurements from 2 glucose monitoring devices, and when comparing results from a single device with glucose concentrations measured in a certified laboratory, 95% of all readings must be within 15% of each other and 99% must be within 20% of each other. Based on the results of this patient's tests performed within a few minutes and from the same fingerstick, the discrepancy she identified (approximately 18%) is within these parameters. She should continue with the new meter (thus, Answer C is correct and Answer B is incorrect).

In addition, accuracy does not change with reduced battery life, so replacing the battery (Answer D) is not the best advice.

Standard point-of-care glucose meters intended for personal use are internally- or factory-calibrated and do not allow for additional calibration (Answer A). The patient should be counseled to continue use of a single glucose meter.

EDUCATIONAL OBJECTIVE
Counsel patients on the acceptable accuracy limitations of point-of-care glucose monitoring systems according to the US FDA.

REFERENCE(S)
Stedman M, Rea R, Duff CJ, et al. The experience of blood glucose monitoring in people with type 2 diabetes mellitus (T2DM). *Endocrinol Diabetes Metab.* 2022;5(2):e00302. PMID: 34921531

U.S. Department of Health and Human Services, Food and Drug Administration, Center for Devices and Radiological Health. Self-Monitoring Blood Glucose Test Systems for Over-the-Counter Use. Guidance for Industry and Food and Drug Administration Staff. Available at: https://www.fda.gov/media/87721/download. Accessed June 2022.

29 ANSWER: A) Anti-CD3 monoclonal antibody

Type 1 diabetes mellitus is an autoimmune disease that in recent years has been characterized as progressing in 3 stages in the setting of having 2 or more detectable type 1 diabetes autoantibodies. Stage 1 is asymptomatic with normoglycemia, stage 2 is asymptomatic with any degree of glucose intolerance (as in this case), and stage 3 is overt diabetes with marked hyperglycemia and symptoms. Tepilizumab, an anti-CD3 monoclonal antibody (Answer A), was recently shown to delay the onset of type 1 diabetes from this stage in those with at least 1 family member with type 1 diabetes.

Comprehensive lifestyle modification (Answer B) and liraglutide (Answer D) have been found to delay the onset of type 2 diabetes, but not type 1 diabetes.

In a randomized controlled trial, verapamil (Answer E) prolonged β-cell function in combination with standard insulin therapy in patients with recently diagnosed type 1 diabetes. As this patient does not yet have diabetes based on hemoglobin A_{1c} and glucose values, verapamil is incorrect.

Basal insulin (Answer C) has not been documented to delay the onset of type 1 diabetes.

EDUCATIONAL OBJECTIVE
Identify stage 2 type 1 diabetes mellitus in a young person with prediabetes.

REFERENCE(S)
Type 1 Diabetes TrialNet. Understanding the stages of type 1 diabetes. Available at: https://www.trialnet.org/. Accessed June 2022.

Herold KC, Bundy BN, Long SA, et al. An anti-CD3 antibody, teplizumab, in relatives at risk for type 1 diabetes [published correction appears in *N Engl J Med.* 2020;382(6):586]. *N Engl J Med.* 2019;381(7):603-613. PMID: 31180194

Ovalle F, Grimes T, Xu G, et al. Verapamil and beta cell function in adults with recent-onset type 1 diabetes. *Nat Med.* 2018;24(8):1108-1112. PMID: 29988125

30 ANSWER: D) Start insulin infusion and potassium repletion

This patient has diabetic ketoacidosis (DKA) in the setting of severe COVID-19, with classic biochemical characteristics of pregnancy. Her blood glucose concentration is below 250 mg/dL (<13.9 mmol/L) (often referred to as "euglycemic DKA"), and her anion gap appears to be normal but is elevated for pregnancy (normal anion gap in pregnancy is approximately 8.5 mEq/L). DKA is defined by a detectable elevation in plasma ketones, as seen with this patient's elevated β-hydroxybutyrate, and also by a bicarbonate concentration of 18 mEq/L or lower. In pregnancy, serum bicarbonate is normally lower (18-26 mEq/L) than in the nonpregnant state due to compensation for chronic respiratory alkalosis, so one can often overestimate the severity of DKA in pregnancy by assuming a greater bicarbonate deficit than is actually present. While relatively mild, her condition warrants standard treatment for DKA. Thus, observation (Answer B) is incorrect. Intravenous fluids should be administered, followed by potassium repletion and insulin infusion (Answer D). In contrast, bicarbonate infusion (Answer C) in the setting of DKA in both pregnant and nonpregnant adults should only be considered if the blood pH is very low (≤6.9).

Although lactated Ringer's solution (Answer A) may reduce the risk of hyperchloremic metabolic acidosis when compared with normal saline, saline is a sufficient and potentially preferred fluid for intravascular volume repletion. Switching to lactated Ringer's would be reasonable to consider at some point, but it should not be prioritized over insulin therapy.

EDUCATIONAL OBJECTIVE
Diagnose diabetic ketoacidosis and normal alterations in acid–base physiology during pregnancy.

REFERENCE(S)

Palermo NE, Sadhu AR, McDonnell ME. Diabetic ketoacidosis in COVID-19: unique concerns and considerations. *J Clin Endocrinol Metab.* 2020;105(8):dgaa360. PMID: 32556147

Sibai BM, Viteri OA. Diabetic ketoacidosis in pregnancy. *Obstet Gynecol.* 2014;123(1):167-178. PMID: 24463678

Abbassi-Ghanavati M, Greer LG, Cunningham FG. Pregnancy and laboratory studies: a reference table for clinicians. *Obstet Gynecol.* 2009;114(6):1326-1331. PMID: 19935037

31 ANSWER: E) Reduce all basal rates by 10% to 15% and deactivate the hybrid closed-loop algorithm in her pump

This patient is in the first trimester of pregnancy and is appropriately worried that her glucose control is suboptimal during the important weeks of fetal development. While her patterns are common in the first trimester, they must be addressed. Thus, simply providing reassurance (Answer D) is incorrect.

Automated insulin delivery systems used in hybrid closed-loop subcutaneous insulin pumps have not been widely tested in pregnancy and can be most problematic when insulin needs are changing rapidly. Such systems should be used with caution since the goal of achieving good control without hypoglycemia can "backfire" by adding to the glycemic instability most characteristic of the first trimester. This is due to several factors, including lower insulin sensitivity before 16 weeks, unique glucose excursions in pregnancy and other less well-established concerns such as accuracy of continuous glucose monitoring in pregnancy. The automated insulin delivery algorithms are designed to "suspend on low" or "suspend before low," where basal rates are intentionally interrupted until the glucose concentration is higher than the low threshold, usually 70 mg/dL (3.9 mmol/L). During the first trimester of pregnancy, there is a steeper rapid rise and fall of glucose around meals, particularly when women are dosing insulin to achieve a 1-hour target concentration less than 140 mg/dL (<7.8 mmol/L). If the overall insulin delivery is too high, as is more common in the first trimester, the automated algorithm can lead to frequent suspensions of basal insulin and a frustrating pattern of both low and high blood glucose despite careful attention overall to insulin management in highly engaged patients, as in this vignette.

Given both her stage of pregnancy and her high percentage of time spent with a glucose concentration less than 70 mg/dL (<3.9 mmol/L), she clearly requires a reduction in her basal insulin rates. A reduction of 10% to 15% reduction (Answer E) targeting the overnight period when she is at highest risk of hypoglycemia is reasonable. In addition, given her diligence and hypoglycemia awareness, the automated insulin delivery algorithm should be turned off at this time to allow her to appropriately correct mild hypoglycemia and avoid rebound hyperglycemia. Continuing the automated insulin delivery algorithm later in pregnancy could be considered, but this would have to be assessed depending on whether the target blood glucose achievable by the algorithm is consistent with targets recommended during pregnancy.

Discontinuation of insulin pump therapy (Answer A) is generally not recommended in pregnancy.

Continuous glucose monitoring, when used in addition to blood glucose monitoring, can reduce macrosomia and neonatal hypoglycemia in pregnancy complicated by type 1 diabetes. Thus, it should not be discontinued (Answer B).

Even though her percentage of time spent with a glucose concentration above 180 mg/dL (>10.0 mmol/L) is elevated, her report and download indicate that this is mostly rebound hyperglycemia following low blood glucose; thus, increasing her basal rates (Answer C) would exacerbate the problem.

EDUCATIONAL OBJECTIVE
Identify common glycemic patterns in pregnant patients with type 1 diabetes mellitus and recommend the best treatment approaches.

REFERENCE(S)
García-Patterson A, Gich I, Amini SB, Catalano PM, de Leiva A, Corcoy R. Insulin requirements throughout pregnancy in women with type 1 diabetes mellitus: three changes of direction. *Diabetologia.* 2010;53(3):446-451. PMID: 20013109

Feig DS, Donovan LE, Corcoy R, et al; CONCEPTT Collaborative Group. Continuous glucose monitoring in pregnant women with type 1 diabetes (CONCEPTT): a multicentre international randomised controlled trial. *Lancet.* 2017;390(10110):2347-2359. PMID: 28923465

American Diabetes Association Professional Practice Committee; Draznin B, Aroda VR, et al. 15. Management of diabetes in pregnancy: *standards of medical care in diabetes-2022. Diabetes Care.* 2022;45(Suppl 1):S232-S243. PMID: 34964864

32 ANSWER: E) Refer to a program for behavioral lifestyle change

This patient has been referred for a mildly low testosterone concentration but is more worried about his increased risk of diabetes and expresses concern mostly about microvascular complications resulting from chronic hyperglycemia. During the Diabetes Prevention Program (DPP) trial (1996-2001), adults at high risk of developing diabetes were randomly assigned to a behavioral lifestyle program plus placebo (n = 1082) or to metformin, 850 mg twice daily (n = 1073). Participants originally assigned to metformin continued to receive metformin in a follow-up outcomes study (2002-present). Behavioral lifestyle intervention was found to be more effective, with a relative risk reduction of approximately 60%, as has been shown in other trials such as the Finish Diabetes Prevention Study. In the DPP, metformin (Answer C) was less effective than lifestyle intervention with a relative risk reduction of approximately 30%, but it appeared to be even less potent in adults older than 60 years. Thus, this patient should be referred to a program for behavioral lifestyle change (Answer E).

Acarbose (Answer A) modestly reduced progression to type 2 diabetes in the STOP-NIDDM trial, but it is contraindicated in persons with inflammatory bowel disease, which this patient has.

While testosterone (Answer D) has been preliminarily studied as a potential player in diabetes prevention, there are no prospective randomized controlled trials published that directly test this hypothesis. In the T4DM trial, there appeared to be a preventive effect with a relative risk reduction of 0.49 in addition to general lifestyle advice. The ongoing TRAVERSE study will most likely help answer this question. In addition, testosterone concentrations may improve with weight loss because of a subsequent rise in SHBG levels (value not provided in this case). Moreover, this patient's testosterone concentration is only modestly reduced and given his mildly elevated PSA, it is best to defer testosterone treatment.

Lastly, this patient's LDL-cholesterol concentration is elevated and should be addressed to reduce overall cardiometabolic risk. However, given that he does not have established diabetes or heart disease, a reasonable first step is dietary intervention rather than statin therapy (Answer B). Additionally, starting a statin in the setting of prediabetes increases the likelihood of developing overt diabetes and would not be consistent with the patient's stated personal health goals at this time.

EDUCATIONAL OBJECTIVE

Describe interventions that have been shown to delay the onset of diabetes mellitus in older adults.

REFERENCE(S)

Yassin A, Haider A, Haider KS, et al. Testosterone therapy in men with hypogonadism prevents progression from prediabetes to type 2 diabetes: eight-year data from a registry study. *Diabetes Care.* 2019;42(6):1104-1111. PMID: 30862651

Diabetes Prevention Program Research Group. Long-term effects of metformin on diabetes prevention: identification of subgroups that benefited most in the diabetes prevention program and diabetes prevention program outcomes study. *Diabetes Care.* 2019;42(4):601-608. PMID: 30877090

33 ANSWER: B) Prescribe dapagliflozin, 5 mg daily

Based on several 2021 clinical practice guidelines and the 2022 American Diabetes Association Standard of Care, the SGLT-2 inhibitor drug class is considered first-line therapy for individuals with established atherosclerotic cardiovascular disease, heart failure, and/or diabetic kidney disease independent of the need to improve glycemic control. This patient has all 3 of these conditions. Therefore, the best answer is to prescribe dapagliflozin (Answer B). Recommending no change (Answer E) is incorrect.

The results of several cardiovascular outcome trials and dedicated trials targeting heart failure and kidney disease have collectively shown an approximate 25% to 30% reduction in hospitalization due to heart failure, 40% reduction in kidney disease progression (with DAPA-CKD using dapagliflozin showing considerable reduction in all-cause mortality in those with chronic kidney disease at baseline), modest efficacy (approximately 10%) for the composite major adverse cardiac events outcome, and variable reductions in cardiovascular death.

While increasing the lisinopril dosage to 10 mg daily (Answer A) could improve albuminuria, so would dapagliflozin but with additional benefits as described.

Although the mineralocorticoid receptor antagonist finerenone (Answer C) has recently been found to reduce mortality in individuals at high risk for progressive kidney disease in the Fidelio-DKD study, this benefit was seen in more advanced stages of nephropathy (urinary albumin-to-creatinine ratio ≥300 mg/g creat) or in those with both microalbuminuria (urinary albumin-to-creatinine ratio <300 mg/g creat) and retinopathy, and would not be expected to have specific heart failure–related benefits.

In the large cardiovascular outcome PIONEER trial, oral semaglutide (Answer D) was not shown to have a significant benefit on major adverse cardiac events, and because this patient's hemoglobin A_{1c} value is in goal range, this additional therapy would have limited benefit and significant expense.

EDUCATIONAL OBJECTIVE

Identify SGLT-2 inhibitors as the drug class indicated for patients with established atherosclerotic cardiovascular disease, heart failure, and/or diabetic kidney disease independent of the need to improve glycemic control.

REFERENCE(S)

American Diabetes Association Professional Practice Committee, Drazin B, Aroda VR, et al. 11. Chronic kidney disease and risk management: standards of medical care in diabetes-2022. *Diabetes Care.* 2022;45(Suppl 1):S175-S184. PMID: 34964873

Schnell O, Cos X, Cosentino F, et al. Report from the CVOT Summit 2020: new cardiovascular and renal outcomes. *Cardiovasc Diabetol.* 2021;20(1):75. PMID: 33789663

Braunwald E. Gliflozins in the management of cardiovascular disease. *N Engl J Med.* 2022;386(21):2024-2034. PMID: 35613023

34 ANSWER: A) Add finerenone, 10 mg daily

Given her relative youth and current estimated glomerular filtration rate, this patient is at very high risk of progressing to end-stage kidney disease requiring renal replacement therapy in her lifetime. Since there are few interventions other than kidney transplant that can restore lost nephron function in classic diabetes-related kidney disease, the therapeutic goal is to stabilize the estimated glomerular filtration rate and modify the risk of cardiovascular death, which accompanies progressive kidney disease. Recently, SGLT-2 inhibitors and the mineralocorticoid receptor agonist finerenone (Answer A) have been found to effectively lower the risk of kidney failure. In the Fidelio-DKD study, 5734 patients with type 2 diabetes and chronic kidney disease with microalbuminuria and diabetic retinopathy or macroalbuminuria and an estimated glomerular filtration rate of 25 to 75 mL/min per 1.73 m^2 already taking an ACE inhibitor were randomly assigned to the nonsteroidal mineralocorticoid antagonist finerenone (10 mg daily for estimated glomerular filtration rate <60 mL/min per 1.73 m^2 and 20 mg daily if the estimated glomerular filtration rate is higher) or placebo. There was an 18% reduction in the primary composite endpoint of time to kidney failure (eg, sustained decrease of ≥40% in baseline estimated glomerular filtration rate or death of kidney causes) and a 14% lowering of the secondary composite endpoint of time to death of cardiovascular cause, nonfatal myocardial infarction, nonfatal stroke, or hospitalization due to heart failure.

While her losartan dosage is low, it was most likely reduced after weight loss due to reduced blood pressure. Increasing the dosage (Answer D) is unlikely to have a major effect on kidney outcomes. In addition, her blood pressure appears to be well controlled.

Statin therapy (Answer E) does benefit microvascular disease, but it has not been shown to reduce the risk of kidney failure. Additionally, her LDL-cholesterol concentration is at goal, and switching to a moderate- or high-dosage statin (atorvastatin or rosuvastatin), which could be considered, is not a listed option.

Adding insulin (Answer B) would most likely be excessive given that her current hemoglobin A_{1c} level is already below 7.0% (<53 mmol/mol) and she is on only 1 glucose-lowering agent. On its own, insulin would not be expected to affect kidney outcomes.

Dulaglutide, 1.5 mg, has been shown to modestly reduce progression to kidney failure in a cardiovascular outcomes trial, and it is unlikely that an increase in the dosage (Answer C) would augment this risk reduction.

EDUCATIONAL OBJECTIVE
Explain the relative benefit of agents in the treatment of diabetes-related kidney disease.

REFERENCE(S)
Bakris GL, Agarwal R, Anker SD, et al; FIDELIO-DKD Investigators. Effect of finerenone on chronic kidney disease outcomes in type 2 diabetes. *N Engl J Med.* 2020;383(23):2219-2229. PMID: 33264825

35 ANSWER: B) Relocate the glucose sensor

Several studies of continuous glucose monitors have observed aberrant sleep position–related readings where sudden decreases in reported glucose values are spontaneously resolved with repositioning. This compression artifact or compression hypoglycemia occurs when direct external pressure on a continuous glucose monitoring sensor leads to decreased perfusion and, usually, falsely low sensor glucose values. This most classically occurs during sleep when a sensor is worn on the arm, and removing the external pressure quickly normalizes the sensor glucose values. Users should be mindful of where the sensor is worn so as to avoid false alerts for hypoglycemia. The sensor's location should be changed (Answer B) if the sleep position is consistent.

Ciprofloxacin has been associated with hypoglycemia, but because this is not a new medication for the patient, it would not be expected to suddenly cause this pattern. Thus, replacing ciprofloxacin (Answer A) is not indicated.

Reducing his basal insulin dosage (Answer C) is important to consider, but excess 24-hour duration basal insulin would be expected to produce a more consistent pattern of overnight hypoglycemia and occasional daytime hypoglycemia as well.

Reducing the predinner lispro dose (Answer D) is not indicated because he appears to begin his evening meal at 8:30 PM and the hypoglycemia reading as shown occurred at 4:30 AM. Since the duration of action of lispro is not expected to exceed 6 hours, it is not the likely culprit.

EDUCATIONAL OBJECTIVE
Recognize compression artifact when interpreting continuous glucose monitoring output.

REFERENCE(S)
Mensh BD, Wisniewski NA, Neil BM, Burnett DR. Susceptibility of interstitial continuous glucose monitor performance to sleeping position. *J Diabetes Sci Technol.* 2013;7(4):863-870. PMID: 23911167

Marks BE, Williams KM, Sherwood JS, Putman MS. Practical aspects of diabetes technology use: continuous glucose monitors, insulin pumps, and automated insulin delivery systems. *J Clin Transl Endocrinol.* 2021;27:100282. PMID: 34917483

36 ANSWER: C) Reduce all insulin doses by 10% to 20%

This patient has entered an early phase of type 1 diabetes often called the "honeymoon period," which is characterized by reduced exogenous insulin requirements in the face of well-maintained glycemic control. It may develop relatively soon after the diagnosis and is a transient phase of "partial remission," thought to be due either to adaptive immune tolerance or to some improvement in β-cell function. Improved residual insulin secretory function reduces the need for all exogenous insulin, not only basal insulin (thus, Answer C is correct and Answer D is incorrect).

Although in the remote past, insulin was often discontinued entirely for some time (Answer A), this was during an era when glucose monitoring was imprecise and directed insulin therapy based on the presence of urinary glucose levels consistent with plasma glucose values generally higher than 200 mg/dL (>11.1 mmol/L). Current practice includes continuation of insulin at reduced dosages to maintain excellent glycemic control, which may potentially prolong the honeymoon period.

Increasing his carbohydrate intake to at least 50 g with each meal (Answer B) is not the best choice, as it does not correct the problem of excessive insulin at mealtimes, requires that the patient ingest extra calories, and would not address overnight hypoglycemia.

While hybrid closed-loop insulin pump therapy (Answer E) will be a reasonable option in time, this type of change is often best initiated when insulin needs are relatively stable; moreover, reducing current insulin doses is a higher priority.

EDUCATIONAL OBJECTIVE
Develop a strategy to manage glycemic levels during the "honeymoon" phase of type 1 diabetes.

REFERENCE(S)
Aly H, Gottlieb P. The honeymoon phase: intersection of metabolism and immunology. *Curr Opin Endocrinol Diabetes Obes.* 2009;16(4):286-292. PMID: 19506474

Akirav E, Kushner JA, Herold KC. Beta-cell mass and type 1 diabetes: going, going, gone? *Diabetes.* 2008;57(11):2883-2888. PMID: 18971435

37 ANSWER: C) She has excessive hyperglycemia

The current American Diabetes Association guidelines recommend the following for glycemic targets when continuous glucose monitoring is used in nonpregnant adults:

- Time in range >70%
- Time below range <4%
- Time below 54 mg/dL (<3.0 mmol/L) <1%

This patient's percentage of time in range is lower than the general time-in-range target because of excessive hyperglycemia (Answer C). The percentage of time she has hypoglycemia is acceptable (thus, Answer D is incorrect).

Acceptable variability is considered to be below a coefficient of variation of 36% (thus, Answer B is incorrect).

Her overall glycemic control does not meet recommended targets (thus, Answer A is incorrect.)

Empirical evidence from the A1C-Derived Average Glucose study showed that a hemoglobin A_{1c} value of 7.0% (53 mmol/mol) correlated approximately to a mean plasma glucose concentration of 155 mg/dL (8.6 mmol/L), and a hemoglobin A_{1c} value of 6.0% (42 mmol/mol) correlated to a mean plasma glucose concentration of 126 mg/dL (7.0 mmol/L). Therefore, this patient's hemoglobin A_{1c} should produce a mean glucose value well below 162 mg/dL (<9/0 mmol/L) (thus, Answer E is incorrect). She has polycythemia, typically requiring intermittent phlebotomy. As this therapy is expected to increase red blood cell turnover, hemoglobin A_{1c} is unlikely to provide an accurate and/or precise assessment of average blood glucose for the expected 60 to 90 days. For this reason, as clearly demonstrated in this patient's case, either frequent blood glucose monitoring or a continuous glucose monitoring profile has considerable potential for optimizing glycemic management.

EDUCATIONAL OBJECTIVE

Select appropriate premeal glucose targets for managing type 2 diabetes mellitus.

REFERENCE(S)

Nathan DM, Kuenen J, Borg R, Zheng H, Schoenfeld D, Heine RJ; A1c-Derived Average Glucose Study Group. Translating the A1C assay into estimated average glucose values [published correction appears in *Diabetes Care.* 2009;32(1):207]. *Diabetes Care.* 2008;31(8):1473-1478. PMID: 18540046

American Diabetes Association Professional Practice Committee; Draznin B, Aroda VR, Bakris G, et al. 6. Glycemic targets: standards of medical care in diabetes-2022. *Diabetes Care.* 2022;45(Suppl 1):S83-S96. PMID: 34964868

Lundholm MD, Emanuele MA, Ashraf A, Nadeem S. Applications and pitfalls of hemoglobin A1C and alternative methods of glycemic monitoring. *J Diabetes Complications.* 2020;34(8):107585. PMID: 32553575

38 ANSWER: B) Ask him to demonstrate how he self-administers insulin injections

This patient is taking 288 units of insulin daily, corresponding to 3.4 units/kg per day. This is an excessive amount of insulin, even in the setting of common insulin resistance as indicated by a BMI of 32 kg/m² and hypertension. Increasing the insulin doses by 30% is the rule of thumb that his endocrinologist has been following when making relatively aggressive insulin adjustments. However, in view of the patient's body size and the high number of units of insulin per kg body weight—and yet still no response in terms of blood glucose lowering—it is important to consider other causes, including administration error, of the apparently high insulin requirement. Therefore, increasing the insulin dosage (Answer C) is incorrect.

In some patients with marked insulin resistance, U500 insulin (Answer E) can be very beneficial, and it is often introduced at lower total doses given potentially improved absorption characteristics. However, before this is done, more investigation is warranted to understand this patient's apparent and unexpected increased insulin requirement.

When the patient was asked to demonstrate how he self-administers an injection of insulin aspart (Answer B), he dialed the dose into the pen correctly and administered the shot into his abdomen by twisting down the dose knob to the top of the pen, rather than pushing down on the dose knob to engage the spring and allow insulin release from the pen needle. Many patients with diabetes do not receive adequate diabetes self-management education to support optimal self-care outcomes. This has been even more concerning during the COVID-19 pandemic when much of the education administered was virtual. Despite evidence that diabetes self-management education reduces the number of emergency department visits and hospitalizations, lowers hemoglobin A_{1c}, and improves other outcomes, less than 55% of US patients with diabetes receive this type of education over the course of their illness and less than 7% receive it within the first year of diagnosis.

In this case, with proper assessment and education and guidance to increase oral hydration, a visit to the emergency department (Answer A) can be avoided, especially because he is ambulatory without signs of significant hypovolemia.

Lastly, stopping sulfonylurea therapy suddenly when replacing with another antidiabetes agent can lead to temporarily challenging hyperglycemia as the new drug is titrated, and tapering is often more advisable. However, combination sulfonylurea with basal-bolus insulin therapy would place him at high risk of hypoglycemia and would not resolve the current problem of insulin deficiency. Thus, restarting glipizide (Answer D) is incorrect.

EDUCATIONAL OBJECTIVE
Evaluate the need for diabetes self-management and skills education in patients with suboptimally controlled diabetes mellitus.

REFERENCE(S)
Powers MA, Bardsley J, Cypress M, et al. Diabetes self-management education and support in type 2 diabetes: a joint position statement of the American Diabetes Association, the American Association of Diabetes Educators, and the Academy of Nutrition and Dietetics. *Diabetes Care.* 2015;38(7):1372-1382. PMID: 26048904

Bari B, Corbeil M-A, Farooqui H, et al. Insulin injection practices in a population of Canadians with diabetes: an observational study. *Diabetes Ther.* 2020;11(11):2595-2609. PMID: 32893337

39 ANSWER: B) Avoiding sugar-sweetened beverages

The provided options have all been the subject of investigations focused on addressing risk factors for developing diabetes (either type 1 or type 2). Only avoiding sugar-sweetened beverages (Answer B) has adequate evidence that it lowers the risk of developing diabetes (type 2) by decreasing the risk of rapid childhood growth and childhood obesity. There is also some evidence that this approach may decrease the risk of developing type 1 diabetes, which is less of a concern overall in this case given that the patient herself has type 2 diabetes.

There has been great interest in identifying factors that lower the risk of type 1 diabetes. Overall, the evidence is poor for direct causal relationships between type 1 diabetes and environmental factors, but there are many studies that have clear directionality on risk. For example, vaccines (Answer C) do not increase risk of type 1 diabetes, and omega-3 fatty acids (Answer A) may be protective. Additionally, it has been proposed that some component of albumin in cow milk (Answer E) (bovine serum albumin), the basis for most infant milk formulas, may trigger the autoimmune response characteristic of type 1 diabetes; however, this has not been verified in larger studies.

EDUCATIONAL OBJECTIVE
Identify perinatal and early childhood environmental factors known to increase the risk of developing diabetes mellitus.

REFERENCE(S)
Rewers M, Ludvigsson J. Environmental risk factors for type 1 diabetes. *Lancet.* 2016;387(10035):2340-2348. PMID: 27302273

Malik VS, Pan A, Willett WC, Hu FB. Sugar-sweetened beverages and weight gain in children and adults: a systematic review and meta-analysis. *Am J Clin Nutr.* 2013;98(4):1084-1102. PMID: 23966427

Bennett AM, Murray K, Ambrosini GL, Oddy WH, Walsh JP, Zhu K. Prospective associations of sugar-sweetened beverage consumption during adolescence with body composition and bone mass at early adulthood. *J Nutr.* 2022;152(2):399-407. PMID: 34791346

40 ANSWER: B) Basal rate = 0.6 units/h; carbohydrate ratio = 1 units/15 g; sensitivity factor = 1 unit/55 mg/dL

Understanding how to convert a regimen of multiple daily injections to continuous subcutaneous insulin infusion is very important. Many articles explain the conversion, all summarized nicely in the 2014 American Association of Clinical Endocrinologists/American College of Endocrinology Consensus Statement specifically on insulin pump management. References may vary slightly regarding the conversion numbers. For example, the pump total daily dose (TDD) can be 0.75 to 1 x prepump TDD depending on the patient's glycemic control. The carbohydrate ratio is 450 to 500 divided by the TDD, and the insulin sensitivity factor is 1700 to 1800 divided by the TDD. Thus, the optimal parameters are listed in Answer B.

EDUCATIONAL OBJECTIVE

Convert a regimen of multiple daily insulin injections to insulin pump therapy in a patient with type 1 diabetes mellitus.

REFERENCE(S)

Grunberger C, Abelseth JM, Bailey TS, et al. Consensus statement by the American Association of Clinical Endocrinologists/American College of Endocrinology Insulin Pump Management Task Force. *Endocr Pract.* 2014;20(5):463-489. PMID: 24816754

Bode BW, Kyllo J, Kaufman ER. *Pumping Protocol: A Guide to Insulin Pump Initiation.* Medical Education Academia. Northridge, CA: Medtronic, 2013.

41 ANSWER: D) Tissue transglutaminase antibodies

About 5% of patients with type 1 diabetes mellitus develop celiac disease (gluten-sensitive enteropathy diagnosed by a positive small-bowel biopsy sample), and 7% to 10% have tissue transglutaminase antibodies (Answer D). The 2022 American Diabetes Association guidelines state that adults with type 1 diabetes should be screened for celiac disease in the presence of gastrointestinal symptoms, signs, or laboratory manifestations suggestive of celiac disease. However, for children and adolescents (defined by the World Health Organization to include individuals aged 10 to 19 years), the recommendation is to screen with antibodies soon after diagnosis given the higher prevalence in persons with youth-onset type 1 diabetes.

Although 15% to 30% of patients with type 1 diabetes have positive antithyroid antibodies (TPO and/or thyroglobulin antibodies) (Answer E), the preferred screening test for hypothyroidism in adults and adolescents is measurement of TSH rather than TPO antibodies. This is in part due to the fact that studies have shown a TPO positivity rate between 12% and 15% in the general healthy euthyroid population, and even higher rates in older women. An abnormal TSH value is also required for diagnosis and treatment of hypothyroidism.

Measurement of antinuclear antibodies (Answer B) is done to identify rheumatologic conditions such as systemic lupus erythematosus in those presenting with consistent symptoms, and it should not be used as a general screening test.

Less than 1% to 2% of children and adolescents with type 1 diabetes have autoimmune adrenalitis with circulating antibodies to steroid 21-hydroxylase (Answer A). Overall, the prevalence of Addison disease is relatively low. Testing should be driven by signs and symptoms of a low cortisol state, and antibodies should only be measured after a confirmed diagnosis of primary adrenal insufficiency.

Glutamic acid decarboxylase 65 antibodies (Answer C) are the most prevalent of several β islet cell–associated autoantibodies. Therefore, this assessment was most likely already part of the diagnostic tests confirming this young man's type 1 diabetes.

EDUCATIONAL OBJECTIVE

Recommend appropriate screening for autoimmune conditions in persons with type 1 diabetes mellitus.

REFERENCE(S)

American Diabetes Association Professional Practice Committee; Draznin B, Aroda VR, Bakris G, et al. 14. Children and adolescents: standards of medical care in diabetes-2022. *Diabetes Care.* 2022;45(Suppl 1):S208-S231. PMID: 34964865

Kahaly GJ, Hansen MP. Type 1 diabetes associated autoimmunity. *Autoimmun Rev.* 2016;15(7):644-648. PMID: 26903475

Janovsky CCPS, Bittencourt MS, Goulart AC, et al. Prevalence of antithyroperoxidase antibodies in a multiethnic Brazilian population: the ELSA-Brasil Study. *Arch Endocrinol Metab.* 2019;63(4):351-357. PMID: 31038589

Amouzegar A, Gharibzadeh S, Kazemian E, Mehran L, Tohidi M, Azizi F. The prevalence, incidence and natural course of positive antithyroperoxidase antibodies in a population-based study: Tehran Thyroid Study. *PLoS One.* 2017;12(1):e0169283. PMID: 28052092

42

ANSWER: A) Eat breakfast, take insulin glargine (14 units) and insulin lispro with an insulin-to-carbohydrate ratio of 1:20

With an adequate concentration of insulin on board, aerobic activities are associated with reductions in blood glucose concentrations. By contrast, anaerobic activities usually do not reduce blood glucose concentrations, and may be associated with elevations in glycemia in certain circumstances. Aerobic exercise is associated with a more modest rise (2- to 4-fold) in catecholamines, while anaerobic exercise is associated with a much higher increase in catecholamine release (14- to 18-fold rise). It is also well established that exercise increases muscle glucose uptake through insulin-dependent and insulin-independent mechanisms. Glycemia during exercise is also affected by substrate availability, as well as insulin concentrations. The net balance effect varies among individuals. However, in general, assuming insulin is present and the blood glucose level is within the normal range, aerobic activity can lead to hypoglycemia, usually during or immediately after exercise, although in some patients, delayed hypoglycemia hours after exercise can be seen.

In the presented scenario, the best way to prevent hypoglycemia is to cut back on the mealtime bolus by 50%, just an hour before playing tennis (Answer A).

Skipping lispro insulin entirely and drinking a high–glycemic index beverage (Answer D) is not recommended because the insulin-deficient state is likely to lead to postexercise hyperglycemia.

Taking the full bolus at breakfast but reducing the basal dose (Answer C) would most likely lead to hypoglycemia during exercise and to hyperglycemia later in the day.

Delaying the 24-hour basal insulin for 12 hours (Answer B) would lead to late hyperglycemia and possibly diabetic ketoacidosis due to an insulin-deficient state.

EDUCATIONAL OBJECTIVE
Manage insulin therapy during exercise.

REFERENCE(S)

Riddell MC, Gallen IW, Smart CE, et al. Exercise management in type 1 diabetes: a consensus statement. *Lancet Diabetes Endocrinol.* 2017;5(5):377-390. PMID: 28126459

Thabit H, Leelarathna L. Basal insulin delivery reduction for exercise in type 1 diabetes: finding the sweet spot. *Diabetologia.* 2016;59(8):1628-1631. PMID: 27287376

Basu R, Johnson ML, Kudva YC, Basu A. Exercise, hypoglycemia, and type 1 diabetes. *Diabetes Technol Ther.* 2014;16(6):331-337. PMID: 24811269

43

ANSWER: A) 1.5 L of 0.9% NaCl over the first hour, and intravenous insulin bolus of 10 units then 10 units per hour

This patient meets the criteria for the hyperosmolar hyperglycemic state (also known as hyperosmotic hyperglycemic nonketotic state). The diagnostic criteria are a plasma glucose concentration greater than 600 mg/dL (>33.3 mmol/L), effective serum osmolality greater than 320 mOsm/kg (>320 mmol/kg), arterial pH greater than 7.30, serum bicarbonate greater than 18 mEq/L (>18 mmol/L), and severe dehydration with absence of or minimal ketoacidosis.

The most common precipitating factors for hyperosmolar hyperglycemic state are infection (often pneumonia or urinary tract infection) and discontinuation of or inadequate insulin therapy. Compromised water intake due to underlying medical conditions, particularly in older patients, can promote the development of severe dehydration and the hyperosmolar hyperglycemic state. Other conditions and factors associated with the hyperosmolar hyperglycemic state include acute major illnesses such as myocardial infarction, cerebrovascular accident, sepsis, or pancreatitis, etc.

The hyperosmolar hyperglycemic state is treated with fluids and insulin. Because of severe dehydration, isotonic 0.9% NaCl is initiated at a rate of 15 to 20 mL/kg over the first hour (thus, Answers C, D, and E are incorrect). A decision is then made as to whether to continue the 0.9% NaCl or switch to 0.45% NaCl depending on volume status and corrected serum sodium. In fact, in this patient, the corrected serum sodium was

145 mEq/L (145 mmol/L) (serum sodium may be corrected by adding 1.6 mg/dL to the measured serum sodium for each 100 mg/dL of glucose above 100 mg/dL [>5.6 mmol/L]). Administration of hypertonic saline at 3.0% (Answer E) might worsen the hypernatremia and hyperosmolarity.

Intravenous insulin treatment can be initiated with an intravenous bolus of regular insulin (0.1 units/kg body weight) followed within 5 minutes by a continuous infusion of regular insulin of 0.1 units/kg per hour (bolus of 10 units and 10 units as a drip in this patient who weighs 220 lb [100 kg]) (thus, Answer B is incorrect). Alternatively, the bolus dose can be omitted if a higher dose of continuous intravenous regular insulin (0.14 units/kg per hour) is initiated.

The best approach for this patient is to administer 1.5 L of 0.9% NaCl over the first hour, and then an intravenous insulin bolus of 10 units followed by 10 units per hour (Answer A).

EDUCATIONAL OBJECTIVE
Manage the hyperosmolar hyperglycemic state.

REFERENCE(S)
French EK, Donihi AC, Korytkowski MT. Diabetic ketoacidosis and hyperosmolar hyperglycemic syndrome: review of acute decompensated diabetes in adult patients. *BMJ.* 2019;365:l1114. PMID: 31142480

44 **ANSWER: D) Start treatment with a statin**

The American College of Cardiology/American Heart Association Blood Cholesterol and the National Lipid Association Guidelines recommend statin treatment (Answer D) for patients such as the one described in this vignette (ie, individuals with diabetes aged 40 to 75 years with LDL-cholesterol levels between 70 and 189 mg/dL [1.81-4.90 mmol/L] and without clinical atherosclerotic cardiovascular disease).

After 19 years of diabetes, it is not clear whether a relatively minor reduction in hemoglobin A_{1c} from 7.2% to less than 7.0% (Answer A) would have any effect on his cardiovascular disease risk. His previous degree of glycemic control is much more important.

Without clinical albuminuria, adding an ACE inhibitor (Answer E) would not be expected to result in a cardiovascular disease benefit in a normotensive, normoalbuminuric patient with type 1 diabetes.

His BMI of 28 kg/m² is modestly elevated, thus much benefit from any weight loss (Answer B) is not expected.

Lastly, aspirin (Answer C) is no longer recommended for primary prevention of cardiovascular disease in patients at lower overall risk because of excess potential harm (eg, bleeding) and minimal benefit.

EDUCATIONAL OBJECTIVE
Recommend statin use as part of cardiovascular risk reduction in patients with type 1 diabetes mellitus.

REFERENCE(S)
American Diabetes Association Professional Practice Committee. 10. Cardiovascular disease and risk management: standards of medical care in diabetes-2022. *Diabetes Care.* 2022;45(Suppl 1):S144-S174. PMID: 34964815

Grundy SM, Stone NJ, Bailey AL, et al. 2018 AHA/ACC/AACVPR/AAPA/ABC/ACPM/ADA/AGS/APhA/ASPC/NLA/PCNA guideline on the management of blood cholesterol: a report of the American College of Cardiology/American Heart Association Task Force on Clinical Practice Guidelines. *Circulation.* 2019;139(25):e1082-e1143. PMID: 30586774

Nathan DM, Cleary PA, Backlund J-YC, et al; Diabetes Control and Complications Trial/Epidemiology of Diabetes Interventions and Complications (DCCT/EDIC) Study Research Group. Intensive diabetes treatment and cardiovascular disease in patients with type 1 diabetes. *N Engl J Med.* 2005;353(25):2643-2653. PMID: 16371630

ASCEND Study Collaborative Group, Bowman L, Mafham M, et al. Effects of aspirin for primary prevention in persons with diabetes mellitus. *N Engl J Med.* 2018;379(16):1529-1539. PMID: 30146931

45 ANSWER: D) Rosuvastatin, 20 mg daily

According to the ASCVD Risk Estimator, this patient's lifetime estimated risk for atherosclerotic cardiovascular disease is approximately 40%.

The correct answer is to switch her regimen to a high-potency statin to achieve an LDL cholesterol–lowering effect greater than 50% to offer maximal benefit for reducing risk of major cardiovascular events. The current guidelines recommend a high-potency statin for those with clinical evidence of atherosclerotic cardiovascular disease, LDL-cholesterol concentration greater than 190 mg/dL (>4.92 mmol/L), or a 10-year risk greater than 7.5%. According to multiple guidelines and results of several randomized controlled trials, rosuvastatin (Answer D) and atorvastatin, but not simvastatin, are the 2 statins that can be dosed for high potency.

Recently, a large randomized controlled trial compared aspirin, 100 mg daily (Answer A), vs placebo in patients with diabetes but no evident cardiovascular disease. The primary efficacy outcome was the first serious vascular event (ie, myocardial infarction, stroke, or transient ischemic attack, or death of any vascular cause, excluding any confirmed intracranial hemorrhage). The primary safety outcome was the first major bleeding event (ie, intracranial hemorrhage, sight-threatening bleeding event in the eye, gastrointestinal bleeding, or other serious bleeding). Secondary outcomes included gastrointestinal tract cancer. A total of 15,480 participants were included. During a mean follow-up of 7.4 years, serious vascular events occurred in a significantly lower percentage of participants in the aspirin group than in the placebo group (658 participants [8.5%] vs 743 [9.6%]; rate ratio, 0.88; 95% CI, 0.79-0.97; P = .01). In contrast, major bleeding events occurred in 314 participants (4.1%) in the aspirin group, compared with 245 (3.2%) in the placebo group (rate ratio, 1.29; 95% CI, 1.09-1.52; P = .003), with most of the excess being gastrointestinal bleeding and other extracranial bleeding. There was no significant difference between the aspirin group and the placebo group in the incidence of gastrointestinal tract cancer (157 [2.0%] and 158 [2.0%] participants, respectively) or all cancers (897 [11.6%] and 887 [11.5%] participants, respectively). Long-term follow-up of these outcomes is planned. Aspirin use prevented serious vascular events in persons who had diabetes and no evident cardiovascular disease at trial entry, but it also caused major bleeding events. The absolute benefits were largely counterbalanced by the bleeding hazard. As a result, while aspirin therapy (75-162 mg daily) may be considered a primary prevention strategy in those with diabetes who are at increased cardiovascular risk, based on available evidence, this strategy should be considered only in those with optimized risk factors, including LDL cholesterol, blood pressure, and triglycerides.

Neither lixisenatide (Answer C) nor sitagliptin (Answer E) has been shown to significantly lower the 3-point major adverse cardiovascular events in their respective cardiovascular outcome trials, ELIXA (Evaluation of Lixisenatide in Acute Coronary Syndrome) and TECOS (Trial Evaluating Cardiovascular Outcomes with Sitagliptin).

Empagliflozin (Answer B) did significantly lower major adverse cardiovascular events in the EmpaReg trial, but more than 99% of the patients had established cardiovascular disease (secondary prevention) as opposed to the patient in this vignette who is not known to have cardiovascular disease (primary prevention). In addition, most SGLT-2 inhibitor trials indicate that benefit lies mainly in heart failure–related events.

EDUCATIONAL OBJECTIVE
Prioritize strategies to lower atherosclerotic cardiovascular disease risk in patients with diabetes mellitus.

REFERENCE(S)

American Diabetes Association. 10. Cardiovascular disease and risk management: standards of medical care in diabetes-2022. *Diabetes Care*. 2022;545(Suppl 1):S144-S174. PMID: 34964815

The ASCEND Study Collaborative Group, Bowman L, Mafham M, et al. Effects of aspirin for primary prevention in persons with diabetes mellitus. *N Engl J Med*. 2018;379(16):1529-1539. PMID: 30146931

Cefalu WT, Kaul S, Gerstein HC, et al. Cardiovascular outcomes trials in type 2 diabetes: where do we go from here? Reflections from a *Diabetes Care* Editors' Expert Forum. *Diabetes Care*. 2018;41(1):14-31. PMID: 29263194

46 ANSWER: E) >90%

The annual incidence of diabetic retinopathy ranges from 2.2% to 12.7%, and the incidence of progression ranges from 3.4% to 12.3%. Progression to proliferative diabetic retinopathy is higher in individuals with mild disease than in those with no disease at baseline. Understanding the available treatment options for persons with diabetic retinopathy is key because targeted glycemic control, blood pressure, and lipid control has been shown to reduce both the incidence and progression of retinopathy.

The American Diabetes Association recommends retinopathy screening by an eye specialist within 5 years of the diagnosis of type 1 diabetes in adults. Patients with type 2 diabetes should have an initial dilated and comprehensive eye examination by an ophthalmologist or optometrist at the time of the diabetes diagnosis, because microvascular changes can begin before diagnosis if prediabetes has been present. Female patients should be advised to have a dilated eye exam before conception or during the first trimester of pregnancy, and then every trimester and for 1 year postpartum. If any level of diabetic retinopathy is present, subsequent dilated retinal examinations for patients with type 1 (or type 2) diabetes should be repeated at least annually by an ophthalmologist or optometrist. If retinopathy is progressive or sight-threatening, examinations are required more frequently.

Management recommendations call for optimizing glycemic control, blood pressure, and lipids to reduce the risk or slow the progression of retinopathy. It is important to emphasize to the patient that attention to lifestyle and pharmacotherapeutic measures to optimize blood glucose, blood pressure, and lipids can be highly effective and would indeed reduce risk of vision loss due to retinopathy by more than 90% (Answer E). Effective metabolic control would significantly reduce her risk of progression to proliferative retinopathy, macular edema, and the need for laser or alternative treatments, thus protecting sight.

If retinopathy does advance, current therapeutic options can be remarkably effective at preventing severe vision loss when administered in an appropriate and timely manner.

EDUCATIONAL OBJECTIVE
Counsel patients regarding the effect of appropriate medical care on the risk of vision loss in type 1 diabetes.

REFERENCE(S)

American Diabetes Association. 11. Microvascular complications and foot care: standards of medical care in diabetes-2020. *Diabetes Care*. 2020;43(Suppl 1):S135-S151. PMID: 31862754

Sabanayagam C, Banu R, Chee ML, et al. Incidence and progression of diabetic retinopathy: a systematic review. *Lancet Diabetes Endocrinol*. 2019;7(2):140-149. PMID: 30005958

Bloomgarden ZT. Screening for and managing diabetic retinopathy: current approaches. *Am J Health Syst Pharm*. 2007;64(17 Suppl 12):S8-S14. PMID: 17720893

47 ANSWER: A) Disseminated granuloma annulare

Granuloma annulare (Answer A) is an inflammatory dermatosis largely seen in women; it is associated with systemic illnesses, including dyslipidemia and diabetes mellitus, although the linkage has not been clearly established. There are 4 types: (1) localized, representing 75% of cases, occurring primarily in those younger than age 30 years, and self-limited; (2) generalized such as disseminated, occurring in 10% to 15% of cases and primarily affecting adults; (3) subcutaneous, most often seen in children aged 2 to 5 years; and (4) perforating, which is the least common type and also predominantly seen among children and young adults. Disseminated granuloma annulare most often occurs on the fingers and ears, and some patients report mild itching. While the etiology of this condition is unknown, possible pathogenic mechanisms include cell-mediated immunity, immune complex vasculitis, and an abnormality of tissue monocytes. Lesions range from widespread papules to annular plaques to large, discolored patches with a variety of coloration from yellow to purple. Treatment includes intralesional steroids for localized disease, but disseminated disease is not very responsive to steroids although antitumor necrosis factor-α therapies have been successful.

Lichen planus (Answer B) is a pruritic eruption commonly associated with hepatitis C virus. Lesions are characteristically papular, purple, polygonal, and located on the distal extremities. Lichen planus may also affect the genitalia or mucous membranes.

Tinea corporis (Answer D) is a superficial dermatophyte infection characterized by either inflammatory or noninflammatory lesions on skin normally lacking hair. The lesion typically begins as a red, scaly plaque that may rapidly worsen as inflammation results in the development of scales, crust, papules, vesicles, and bullae.

Necrobiosis lipoidica (Answer C) is a disorder that results from collagen degeneration with a granulomatous response, thickening of blood vessel walls, and fat deposition. However, patients with necrobiosis lipoidica typically present with shiny, asymptomatic patches in the pretibial area that slowly enlarge and progress to yellow, depressed, atrophic plaques over time.

EDUCATIONAL OBJECTIVE
Identify dermopathies common to type 2 diabetes mellitus.

REFERENCE(S)
Thornsberry LA, English JC 3rd. Etiology, diagnosis, and therapeutic management of granuloma annulare: an update. *Am J Clin Dermatol.* 2013;14(4):279-290. PMID: 23696233

Murdaca G, Colombo BM, Barabino G, Caiti M, Cagnati P, Puppo F. Anti-tumor necrosis factor-a treatment with infliximab for disseminated granuloma annulare. *Am J Clin Dermatol.* 2010;11(6):437-439. PMID: 20515080

48 **ANSWER: E) Insufficient potency**

This patient has established type 2 diabetes and has had loss of glycemic control with monotherapy that is all too common in these patients. However, she is relatively young, generally healthy, and has no evidence of diabetes end-organ complications. Thus, a reasonable treatment goal for her is a hemoglobin A_{1c} value less than 7.0% (<53 mmol/mol). Sitagliptin is unlikely to help her achieve this goal, even when combined with metformin. In most clinical trials, monotherapy with DPP-4 inhibitors such as sitagliptin generally reduces hemoglobin A_{1c} by 0.6% to 0.9%, and when used as add-on therapy to metformin, the reduction is 0.5% to 0.7%. Thus, this single addition would most likely have insufficient potency (Answer E), and another, possibly less expensive drug could be used.

Although there is some question about the relative potency of DPP-4 inhibitors relative to other oral agents, there is no question regarding their safety and tolerability. These agents have no clearly defined adverse effects and few drug-drug interactions (thus, Answers A, B, C, and D are incorrect). Single reports have noted increased rates of infections, headache, and rash with DPP-4 inhibitors, but when the data from clinical trials are evaluated in total, the overall rates of these complications do not differ from those observed in placebo-treated patients. Sitagliptin is renally excreted and dosages must be adjusted in patients with reduced glomerular filtration rates. However, neither sitagliptin, nor any other DPP-4 inhibitor, is a known nephrotoxin.

EDUCATIONAL OBJECTIVE

Identify insufficient potency as a potential concern with the use of DPP-4 inhibitors in the treatment of hyperglycemia.

REFERENCE(S)

Amori RE, Lau J, Pittas AG. Efficacy and safety of incretin therapy in type 2 diabetes: systematic review and meta-analysis. *JAMA.* 2007;298(2):194-206. PMID: 17622601

Drucker DJ, Nauck MA. The incretin system: glucagon-like peptide-1 receptor agonists and dipeptidyl peptidase-4 inhibitors in type 2 diabetes. *Lancet.* 2006;368(9548):1696-1705. PMID: 17098089

49   ANSWER: B) Clozapine

The key features in this case are rapid weight gain and development of hypertriglyceridemia since initiation of an antipsychotic drug. Atypical antipsychotic agents, such as clozapine, came into favor to treat thought disorders because of a lower risk of extrapyramidal adverse effects than with traditional antipsychotic drugs. However, several compounds in this drug class were noted to have metabolic consequences, including weight gain, hyperlipidemia, insulin resistance, and impaired glucose metabolism. The drugs most frequently implicated are clozapine (Answer B) and olanzapine. Although definitive epidemiologic data are not available, up to 30% to 40% of patients treated with clozapine and olanzapine are reported to gain weight and develop associated metabolic disorders.

Other antipsychotic drugs have lesser metabolic effects. Risperidone (Answer D) and quetiapine (Answer C) have intermediate effects and would not be expected to result in the dramatic metabolic changes described in this vignette. Aripiprazole (Answer A), ziprasidone, and amisulpride have little or no association with metabolic abnormalities.

EDUCATIONAL OBJECTIVE

Explain the metabolic complications of atypical antipsychotic medications.

REFERENCE(S)

De Hert M, Detraux J, van Winkel R, Yu W, Correll CU. Metabolic and cardiovascular adverse effects associated with antipsychotic drugs. *Nat Rev Endocrinol.* 2011;8(2):114-126. PMID: 22009159

Newcomer JW. Metabolic considerations in the use of antipsychotic medications: a review of recent evidence. *J Clin Psychiatry.* 2007;68(Suppl 1):20-27. PMID: 17286524

50   ANSWER: D) Ezetimibe

Multiple large randomized controlled trials have investigated the benefits of adding nonstatin agents to statin therapy, including those that have evaluated further lowering of LDL cholesterol with ezetimibe and PCSK9 inhibitors.

For secondary prevention in adults with diabetes and atherosclerotic cardiovascular disease who are at very high risk, if the LDL-cholesterol concentration is 70 mg/dL or greater (≥1.81 mmol/L) on the maximally tolerated statin dosage, additional LDL-cholesterol–lowering therapy should be added. The American College of Cardiology Cholesterol Guideline for secondary prevention in patients with clinical atherosclerotic cardiovascular disease recommends adding ezetimibe (Answer D) as the next step. As noted in the American Diabetes Association 2020 Standards of Medical Care in Diabetes, an additional consideration is the fact that ezetimibe costs less than a PCSK9 inhibitor.

Evolocumab (Answer C) is a PCSK9 inhibitor antibody. In adults with established cardiovascular disease, PCSK9 inhibitors are indicated to reduce the risk of myocardial infarction, stroke, and coronary revascularization. Addition of a PCSK9 inhibitor is deemed reasonable when the maximal tolerated dosage of statin plus ezetimibe does not result in an LDL-cholesterol concentration less than 70 mg/dL (<1.81 mmol/L).

On the basis of evidence from the REDUCE-IT trial, icosapent ethyl (Answer E) is indicated as an adjunct to maximally tolerated statin therapy to reduce the risk of myocardial infarction, stroke, coronary revascularization, and unstable angina requiring hospitalization in adults with hypertriglyceridemia (>150 mg/dL

[>1.70 mmol/L]) and established cardiovascular disease or diabetes mellitus and 2 or more additional risk factors for cardiovascular disease. This patient does not have hypertriglyceridemia, so icosapent ethyl is incorrect.

Coenzyme Q10 (Answer A) is one of the most commonly used dietary supplements in the United States. Because of its antioxidant and antiinflammatory effects, coenzyme Q10 has been studied extensively for possible use in managing coronary heart disease. One of the most common applications of coenzyme Q10 is to mitigate statin-associated muscle symptoms based on the theory that statin-associated muscle symptoms are caused by statin depletion of coenzyme Q10 in the muscle. Although previous studies of coenzyme Q10 for statin-associated muscle symptoms have produced mixed results, coenzyme Q10 appears to be safe. Current evidence does not support routine use of coenzyme Q10 in patients with coronary heart disease.

Compared with placebo, use of colchicine (Answer B), 0.5 mg daily, among patients with recent myocardial infarction has been shown to lead to a significantly lower risk of ischemic cardiovascular events. However, this woman has not had a myocardial infarction, so there is no evidence base for adding colchicine to her regimen. It also is not an LDL-cholesterol–lowering agent.

EDUCATIONAL OBJECTIVE
Discuss agents that may alter cardiovascular disease outcomes in adults with type 2 diabetes and established high risk for cardiovascular disease.

REFERENCE(S)

American Diabetes Association Professional Practice Committee. 10. Cardiovascular disease and risk management: standards of medical care in diabetes-2022. *Diabetes Care.* 2022;43(Suppl 1):S144-S174. PMID: 34964815

Grundy SM, Stone NJ, Bailey AL, et al. 2018 AHA/ ACC/AACVPR/AAPA/ABC/ACPM/ADA/AGS/ APhA/ASPC/NLA/PCNA guideline on the management of blood cholesterol: executive summary: a report of the American College of Cardiology/American Heart Association Task Force on Clinical Practice Guidelines. *J Am Coll Cardiol.* 2019;73(24):3168-3209. PMID: 30423391

Ayers J, Cook J, Koenig RA, Sisson EM, Dixon DL. Recent developments in the role of coenzyme Q10 for coronary heart disease: a systematic review. *Curr Atheroscler Rep.* 2018;20(6):29. PMID: 29766349

Tardif JC, Kouz S, Waters DD, et al. Efficacy and safety of low-dose colchicine after myocardial infarction. *N Engl J Med.* 2019;381(26):2497-2505. PMID: 31733140

Bhatt DL, Steg PG, Miller M, et al; REDUCE-IT Investigators. Cardiovascular risk reduction with icosapent ethyl for hypertriglyceridemia. *N Engl J Med.* 2019;380(1):11-22. PMID: 30415628

51 ANSWER: D) Pioglitazone
Nonalcoholic fatty liver disease (NAFLD) is observed worldwide and is the most common liver disorder in Western industrialized countries, where the major risk factors are common (central obesity, type 2 diabetes mellitus, dyslipidemia, and metabolic syndrome). One of the management options for NAFLD includes optimization of blood glucose control in those with diabetes. In addition, certain antidiabetes agents have been shown to improve liver histology such as steatosis, lobular inflammation, hepatocellular ballooning, and fibrosis.

The effect of thiazolidinediones on histologic parameters in nonalcoholic steatohepatitis (NASH) was examined in a meta-analysis of 4 randomized controlled trials that compared thiazolidinediones with placebo in 334 patients with NASH. The analysis found that compared with placebo, thiazolidinediones were more likely to improve hepatic histologic parameters such as ballooning degeneration, lobular inflammation, and steatosis. Improvement in fibrosis was not seen when all thiazolidinediones were examined, but when the analysis was limited to 3 studies that used pioglitazone (Answer D), there was a significant improvement in fibrosis among patients treated with pioglitazone compared with placebo.

The effectiveness of metformin (Answer C) for the treatment of NASH was evaluated in a meta-analysis that included 3 randomized trials of metformin with histologic data available both before and after treatment. There was no difference between the patients who received metformin and control patients regarding histologic response (steatosis, ballooning, inflammation, or fibrosis) or changes in ALT levels.

There are no available data on changes in liver histology in patients with NASH and type 2 diabetes regarding dulaglutide (Answer B), dapagliflozin (Answer A), or sitagliptin (Answer E).

Another option to treat NASH is liraglutide. In a randomized controlled trial, 52 patients with NASH (one-third had type 2 diabetes) were assigned to either receive liraglutide or placebo for 48 weeks. An end-of-treatment biopsy was performed in 23 patients in the liraglutide arm and in 22 patients in the placebo arm. NASH resolved in 9 patients (39%) who received liraglutide and in 2 patients (9%) who received placebo. Regarding fibrosis progression, patients who received liraglutide were less likely to have progression of fibrosis.

EDUCATIONAL OBJECTIVE
Explain the effect of various antidiabetes agents on nonalcoholic steatohepatitis.

REFERENCE(S)

Portillo-Sanchez P, Cusi K. Treatment of nonalcoholic fatty liver disease (NAFLD) in patients with type 2 diabetes mellitus. *Clin Diabetes Endocrinol.* 2016;2(9):1-9. PMID: 28702244

Rakoski MO, Singal AG, Rogers MA, Conjeevaram H. Meta-analysis: insulin sensitizers for the treatment of non-alcoholic steatohepatitis. *Aliment Pharmacol Ther.* 2010;32(10):1211-1221. PMID: 20955440

Armstrong MJ, Gaunt P, Aithal GP, et al. Liraglutide safety and efficacy in patients with non-alcoholic steatohepatitis (LEAN): a multicentre, double-blind, randomised, placebo-controlled phase 2 study. *Lancet.* 2016;387(10019):679-690. PMID: 26608256

52 ANSWER: B) Low-carbohydrate diet

Gastric bypass surgery has a dramatic effect on carbohydrate metabolism. Eighty percent of patients who had diabetes preoperatively do not require medication for diabetes after surgery. Diabetes resolves in many of these individuals within weeks of the operation. It appears that the exposure of distal bowel to food results in exaggerated secretion of GLP-1, which may facilitate the improvement in glucose control seen after surgery.

Postprandial hypoglycemia is an uncommon late complication of gastric bypass surgery that is increasingly recognized. It appears that in some individuals, perhaps in response to ongoing stimulation by GLP-1, β-cell proliferation occurs, resulting in nesidioblastosis, which is a state of islet hyperplasia associated with excessive insulin secretion and endogenous hyperinsulinemic hypoglycemia. Some patients develop multiple small insulinomas. The management of this condition is controversial. While partial pancreatectomy (Answer D) was suggested in the initial series, other authors have suggested that many of these patients can be managed by reducing carbohydrate intake (Answer B), consuming low–glycemic index carbohydrates, and always eating carbohydrates in the context of a mixed meal. While acarbose, octreotide (Answer C), calcium channel blockers, and diazoxide (Answer A) have all been used as treatments, diet alone alleviates symptoms in 50% to 70% of affected individuals, so it is the initial treatment of choice. It appears that the condition recurs in many individuals who have subtotal pancreatectomy, and those who have more aggressive pancreatic surgery can develop pancreatic diabetes. For this reason, pancreatectomy is a treatment that is currently used only if other treatments fail and the patient remains debilitated by frequent episodes of hypoglycemia that limit functional capacity.

EDUCATIONAL OBJECTIVE
Select the appropriate evaluation for patients with hyperinsulinemic hypoglycemia.

REFERENCE(S)

Service GJ, Thompson GB, Service FJ, Andrews JC, Collazo-Clavell ML, Lloyd RV. Hyperinsulinemic hypoglycemia with nesidioblastosis after gastric-bypass surgery. *N Engl J Med.* 2005;353(3):249-254. PMID: 16034010

Kellogg TA, Bantle JP, Leslie DB, et al. Postgastric bypass hyperinsulinemic hypoglycemia syndrome: characterization and response to a modified diet. *Surg Obes Relat Dis.* 2008;4(4):492-499. PMID: 18656831

Cui Y, Elahi D, Andersen DK. Advances in the etiology and management of hyperinsulinemic hypoglycemia after Roux-en-Y gastric bypass. *J Gastrointest Surg.* 2011;15(10):1879-1888. PMID: 21671112

Female Reproduction Board Review

Kathryn A. Martin, MD

1 **ANSWER: C) Add LH**

Women with congenital GnRH deficiency (without anosmia [idiopathic hypogonadotropic hypogonadism] or with anosmia [Kallmann syndrome]) or functional hypothalamic amenorrhea have anovulatory infertility due to hypogonadotropic hypogonadism. With appropriate therapy, rates of ovulation and live birth are very high in this population. Unlike women with polycystic ovary syndrome who respond to the antiestrogen clomiphene citrate with an increase in LH and FSH, women with functional hypothalamic amenorrhea or idiopathic hypogonadotropic hypogonadism/Kallmann syndrome do not. An exception would be women with functional hypothalamic amenorrhea who are recovering and whose ovaries are beginning to secrete estradiol. In the past, pulsatile GnRH was the treatment of choice because it was associated with the lowest rate of multiple gestations, but it is no longer available. Most women with idiopathic hypogonadotropic hypogonadism/functional hypothalamic amenorrhea require ovulation induction with gonadotropin therapy with *both* LH and FSH. Administering FSH alone results in the growth of follicles that do not make estrogen. Thus, the best next step is to add LH (Answer C) to stimulate theca-cell androgen production; the androgens are then aromatized to estrogen in the granulosa cells. LH and FSH can be administered separately, but there are also combination preparations.

Administering a higher dosage of FSH (Answer D) does not provide additional benefit.

Given her low gonadotropins and hypoestrogenemia, she is unlikely to benefit from the addition of either clomiphene citrate (Answer A) or letrozole (Answer B), an aromatase inhibitor, as both medications require circulating endogenous estrogen for a response.

Recommending in vitro fertilization (Answer E) is probably not appropriate now unless there is a known male factor contributing to infertility.

EDUCATIONAL OBJECTIVE

Explain the specific challenges of ovulation induction in women with hypogonadotropic hypogonadism.

REFERENCE(S)

Lunenfeld B. Historical perspectives in gonadotrophin therapy. *Hum Reprod Update.* 2004;10(6):453-467. PMID: 15388674

Gordon CM, Ackerman KE, Berga SL, et al. Functional hypothalamic amenorrhea: an Endocrine Society clinical practice guideline. *J Clin Endocrinol Metab.* 2017;102(5):1413-1439. PMID: 28368518

2 **ANSWER: C) No differences**

Obesity increases the metabolic rate and clearance of hepatically metabolized drugs. Although concerns have been raised that women with obesity could take longer to achieve therapeutic levels of contraceptive hormones, higher rates of contraceptive failure (Answer A) have not been observed. Contraceptive outcomes and adverse effect profiles are similar in women with and without obesity (thus, Answer C is correct).

Other outcomes such as impaired glucose tolerance (Answer B), weight gain (Answer E), or unscheduled bleeding (Answer D) do not appear to be more common in women with obesity taking combined oral contraceptives. Both obesity and combined oral contraceptives are risk factors for venous thromboembolism, but given her age and absence of a personal or family history of venous thromboembolism, her absolute risk of venous thromboembolism is lower than the risk of pregnancy-associated venous thromboembolism.

In general, healthy, young individuals with obesity can safely use any contraceptive method following appropriate counseling regarding potential risks and benefits.

EDUCATIONAL OBJECTIVE
Counsel young women with obesity regarding hormonal contraceptive options.

REFERENCE(S)

Lopez LM, Bernholc A, Chen M, et al. Hormonal contraceptives for contraception in overweight or obese women. *Cochrane Database Syst Rev.* 2016;(8):CD008452. PMID: 27537097

ACOG Practice Bulletin No. 206: Use of hormonal contraception in women with coexisting medical conditions. *Obstet Gynecol.* 2019;133(2):e128-e150. PMID: 30681544

3 **ANSWER: B) Female-pattern hair loss**
Female-pattern hair loss (Answer B) (formerly referred to as androgenetic alopecia) is the most likely cause of this patient's hair loss. She has polycystic ovary syndrome. The most common symptoms of hyperandrogenism in women with polycystic ovary syndrome are hirsutism and acne. Alopecia is less common, but it does occur. Patterned hair loss refers to the finding that some areas of the scalp are more affected than others. Female-pattern hair loss is common, affecting up to 40% of women by age 50 years. Of note, most women with female-pattern hair loss do not have hyperandrogenism.

Telogen effluvium (Answer D) is also common, but compared with female-pattern hair loss, it results in more rapid and diffuse hair loss. Shedding from telogen effluvium takes 3 to 6 months to stop, and regrowth can take 12 to 18 months.

With alopecia areata (Answer A), physical examination would show additional areas of hair loss such as the eyelashes and eyebrows.

Traction alopecia (Answer E) is unlikely in this patient with short hair, as it occurs primarily in women with a history of pulling their hair back in ponytails or braids.

Frontal fibrosing alopecia (Answer C) is incorrect because it is associated with scarring, and it is almost always seen in postmenopausal women older than 50 years.

EDUCATIONAL OBJECTIVE
Diagnose female-pattern hair loss.

REFERENCE(S)

Carmina E, Azziz R, Bergfeld W, et al. Female pattern hair loss and androgen excess: a report from the multidisciplinary Androgen Excess and PCOS Committee. *J Clin Endocrinol Metab.* 2019;104(7):2875-2891. PMID: 30785992

Grymowicz M, Rudnicka E, Podfigurna A, et al. Hormonal effects on hair follicles. *Int J Mol Sci.* 2020;21(15):5342. PMID: 32731328

Starace M, Orlando G, Alessandrini A, Piraccini BM. Female androgenetic alopecia: an update on diagnosis and management. *J Clin Dermatol.* 2020;21(1):69-84. PMID: 31677111

Ramos PM, Miot HA. Female pattern hair loss: a clinical and pathophysiological review. *An Bras Dermatol.* 2015;90(4):529-543. PMID: 26375223

Iamsumang W, Leerunyakul K, Suchonwanit P. Finasteride and its potential for the treatment of female pattern hair loss: evidence to date. *Drug Des Devel Ther.* 2020;14:951-959. PMID: 32184564

4 **ANSWER: B) Low-dosage vaginal estrogen**
Starting testosterone therapy (Answer E) is incorrect. The Global Consensus Position Statement on the Use of Testosterone Therapy for Women suggests that the only indication for testosterone therapy in women is female sexual interest/arousal disorder (this includes the former categories hypoactive sexual desire disorder [HSDD] and female sexual arousal disorder), defined by the lack of, or significantly reduced, sexual interest/arousal). Most women with these diagnoses have undergone total abdominal hysterectomy–bilateral salpingo-oophorectomy. They experience a precipitous decline in all gonadal steroids (estradiol and

testosterone) compared with women who undergo natural menopause (estrogen secretion ceases from the ovary, but testosterone secretion continues). Libido in women is less well understood/studied than in men, but supplementation with testosterone alone (Answer E) is not adequate.

Even for women with these defined disorders, one major challenge is the lack of availability of approved testosterone preparations. Testosterone preparations for women are unavailable in most countries except Australia, and the use of compounded testosterone or male formulations is discouraged. In addition, serum testosterone concentrations in postmenopausal women do not correlate well with libido.

This patient describes vaginal dryness, so the best answer is to start low-dosage vaginal estrogen (estradiol tablets, creams, or ring) (Answer B). Clinical trials have reported improvements in sexual function with this approach.

There is no indication to increase this patient's dosage of systemic estrogen (Answer A), as her vasomotor symptoms are well controlled.

Sex therapy (Answer D) may be useful but starting vaginal estrogen would be the best initial step.

Oral DHEA therapy (Answer C) has not been shown to effectively improve libido in women who have undergone natural menopause.

EDUCATIONAL OBJECTIVE
Identify the indications for exogenous testosterone therapy in women.

REFERENCE(S)
Davis SR, Baber R, Panay N, et al. Global consensus position statement on the use of testosterone therapy for women. *J Clin Endocrinol Metab.* 2019;104(10):4660-4666. PMID: 31498871

Nanette Santoro, Roisin Worsley, Miller KK, Parisk SJ, Davis SR. Role of estrogens and estrogen-like compounds in female sexual function and dysfunction. *J Sex Med.* 2016;13(3):305-316. PMID: 26944462

5 ANSWER: E) 5-Year breast cancer risk calculation

The most important evaluation before starting menopausal hormone therapy is a 5-year breast cancer risk calculation (Answer E). Women at higher risk (>3% over 5 years) are not good candidates and should be offered nonhormonal alternatives. Unfortunately, the currently available breast cancer risk calculators that are most commonly used have limitations, as they do not include mammographic density or a detailed family history.

A hypercoagulability profile (Answer D) is not indicated unless the patient has a personal or family history of venous thromboembolism.

Hemoglobin A_{1c} measurement (Answer C) might be part of her routine medical care but not part of her evaluation to determine eligibility for menopausal hormone therapy. Menopausal hormone therapy lowers the risk of new-onset type 2 diabetes mellitus.

Breast MRI (Answer A) is also not part of the routine premenopausal hormone therapy evaluation, and genetic testing for *BRCA1* and *BRCA2* (Answer B) would not be indicated given her family history of late-onset breast cancer in a single family member.

EDUCATIONAL OBJECTIVE
Recommend a 5-year breast cancer risk calculation as the most important evaluation to determine whether a patient is a candidate for menopausal hormone therapy.

REFERENCE(S)
Stuenkel CA, Davis SR, Gompel A, et al. Treatment of symptoms of the menopause: an Endocrine Society Clinical Practice Guideline. *J Clin Endocrinol Metab.* 2015;100(11):3975-4011. PMID: 26444994

de Villiers TJ, Hall JE, Pinkerton JV, et al. Revised global consensus statement on menopausal hormone therapy. *Maturitas.* 2016;91:153-155. PMID: 27389038

The NAMS 2017 Hormone Therapy Position Statement Advisory Panel. The 2017 hormone therapy position statement of The North American Menopause Society. *Menopause.* 2017;24(7):728-753. PMID: 28650869

6 ANSWER: C) Start a low-dosage continuous estrogen-progestin oral contraceptive (20 mcg ethinyl estradiol; 1 mg norethindrone acetate)

Approximately 40% to 50% of perimenopausal women experience depression and/or anxiety symptoms during the menopausal transition. The symptoms are responsive to estrogen, but many women need both estrogen and an antidepressant (a selective serotonin reuptake inhibitor). This patient has hot flashes and perimenopausal depression, which often coexist in this population. She also has irregular menstrual cycles (likely anovulatory) with heavy bleeding. Her psychopharmacologist has prescribed a selective serotonin reuptake inhibitor, citalopram, and her dosage has been titrated to 30 mg daily. However, she still does not feel like herself. She has vasomotor symptoms, but she has persistent depression symptoms as well. Although not FDA-approved for the treatment of perimenopausal depression, estrogen therapy has been shown to be effective in this population. Of note, estrogen is not effective for postmenopausal women with depression. Given her vasomotor symptoms, some form of estrogen would be the best option; a low-dosage oral contraceptive (Answer C) would suppress her hypothalamic-pituitary-ovarian axis and decrease her heavy bleeding. A physiologic dosage of estrogen would not do this.

Increasing the citalopram dosage further (Answer A) is not the best next step, and neither is referring her for cognitive behavioral therapy (Answer B). Both could help her depression symptoms but not her other menopausal symptoms.

Oral estradiol with cyclic micronized progesterone (Answer D) would relieve her hot flashes, but the cyclic progesterone could exacerbate her mood symptoms. In addition, the dosage is too low to suppress the hypothalamic-pituitary-ovarian axis and provide bleeding control. Therefore, the best option is a low-dosage oral contraceptive. This provides the estrogen, which will treat her vasomotor symptoms. It must be given *continuously*, however, or her vasomotor symptoms will recur during the pill-free interval. In addition, she may have premenstrual mood symptoms on a cyclic pill regimen; a continuous regimen would preclude this.

EDUCATIONAL OBJECTIVE
Identify and treat depression during the menopausal transition.

REFERENCE(S)
Maki PM, Kornstein SG, Joffe H, et al; Board of Trustees for The North American Menopause Society (NAMS) and the Women and Mood Disorders Task Force of the National Network of Depression Centers. Guidelines for the evaluation and treatment of perimenopausal depression: summary and recommendations. *Menopause.* 2018;25(10):1069-1085. PMID: 30179986

Stuenkel CA, Davis SA, Gompel A, et al. Treatment of symptoms of the menopause: an Endocrine Society clinical practice guideline. *J Clin Endocrinol Metab.* 2015;100(11):3975-4011. PMID: 26444994

Gordon JL, Girdler SS. Hormone replacement therapy in the treatment of perimenopausal depression. *Curr Psychiatry Rep.* 2014;16(12):517. PMID: 25308388

7 ANSWER: E) No testing required

Women older than 45 years who present with characteristic menopausal signs and symptoms are more likely to be in the menopausal transition than to have a new endocrine problem such as hyperprolactinemia or thyroid disease. Pregnancy must always be ruled out, but this patient's hCG was negative. Although she has no hot flashes, poor sleep and musculoskeletal symptoms are suggestive of perimenopause, as these symptoms occur in up to 40% to 50% of women during the transition. While most perimenopausal women's sleep disturbances are related to hot flashes, others have poor sleep because of new-onset primary sleep disorders. Depression and anxiety can also contribute.

Therefore, for women older than 45 years who present with irregular menstrual cycles and menopausal symptoms such as hot flashes, mood changes, joint aches, or sleep disturbances, biochemical evaluation or imaging is not necessary to make the diagnosis. Thus, no further testing is required (thus, Answer E is correct and Answers A, B, C, and D are incorrect). In fact, serum FSH measurement can be misleading because it is often normal (if measured after ovulation or when serum estradiol is high). An endocrine evaluation should be performed for women younger than 45 years who present with oligomenorrhea, with or without menopausal symptoms.

EDUCATIONAL OBJECTIVE
Guide the evaluation and diagnosis of the menopausal transition.

REFERENCE(S)
Harlow SD, Gass M, Hall JE, et al; STRAW + 10 Collaborative Group. Executive summary of the Stages of Reproductive Aging Workshop + 10: addressing the unfinished agenda of staging reproductive aging. *J Clin Endocrinol Metab.* 2012;97(4):1159-1168. PMID: 22344196

Randolph JF Jr, Crawford S, Dennerstein L, et al. The value of follicle-stimulating hormone concentration and clinical findings as markers of the late menopausal transition. *J Clin Endocrinol Metab.* 2006;91(8):3034-3040. PMID: 16720656

8 **ANSWER: A) Daily prospective symptom diary for 2 cycles**

This patient appears to have premenstrual dysphoric disorder. However, it is necessary to have prospective documentation of the timing of her symptoms to confirm the diagnosis (Answer A). Unlike other mood disorders, premenstrual dysphoric disorder symptoms should resolve in the follicular phase. In some cases, perimenopause must be ruled out with a cycle day 3 measurement of serum FSH (Answer B) and serum antimullerian hormone (Answer D), as there can be some overlap in clinical mood symptoms. Patients with thyroid disease may also have similar mood changes, but their symptoms would not be cyclic. Thus, TSH

measurement (Answer E) is not the best next step. Unipolar depression that worsens before menses is not considered to be premenstrual dysphoric disorder. Therefore, depression screening (Answer C) is not the best next step.

EDUCATIONAL OBJECTIVE
Identify the symptoms of premenstrual dysphoric disorder and diagnose this condition.

REFERENCE(S)
Cohen LS, Soares CN, Otto MW, Sweeney BH, Liberman RF, Harlow BL. Prevalence and predictors of premenstrual dysphoric disorder (PMDD) in older premenopausal women. The Harvard Study of Moods and Cycles. *J Affect Disord.* 2002;70(2):125-132. PMID: 12117624

Freeman EW, Halberstadt SM, Rickels K, Legler JM, Lin H, Sammel MD. Core symptoms that discriminate premenstrual syndrome. *J Womens Health (Larchmt).* 2011;20(1):29-35. PMID: 21128818

Endicott J, Nee J, Harrison W. Daily record of severity of problems (DRSP): reliability and validity. *Arch Womens Ment Health.* 2006;9(1):41-49. PMID: 16172836

9 **ANSWER: D) Hemoglobin A_{1c} measurement, liver enzymes, thyroid function tests**

Turner syndrome occurs in 1 in 2500 live births and is associated with growth failure, pubertal delay, and cardiac abnormalities. In addition, affected patients are at risk for a number of comorbidities, including type 2 diabetes, elevated liver enzymes, autoimmune thyroid disease, celiac disease, hearing loss, orthodontic problems, and psychosocial disorders. Cardiac MRI is the most important test because congenital cardiac abnormalities are present in up to 50% of patients and include coarctation of the aorta, bicuspid aortic valve, and partial anomalous pulmonary venous return. Echocardiography is also sometimes used as part of the routine follow-up of women with Turner syndrome (but it is not performed annually).

Current practice guidelines recommend annual visits for women with Turner syndrome. In addition to measuring blood pressure, calculating

BMI, and performing a full skin examination, the following assessments are recommended: thyroid function tests, hemoglobin A_{1c} measurement, and liver enzymes (AST, ALT, γ-glutamyl transferase, alkaline phosphatase) (Answer D). Screening for other comorbidities (eg, celiac disease [Answer B] or kidney disorders [Answer E]) is performed at less frequent intervals. Complete blood cell count (Answer C) is not recommended routinely. Serum antimullerian hormone (a marker of ovarian reserve) and transvaginal ultrasonography (Answer A) are not needed. Her diagnosis of hypogonadism due to Turner syndrome is already established, and she has no current indications for pelvic imaging.

EDUCATIONAL OBJECTIVE
Recommend appropriate evaluation for girls with gonadal dysgenesis.

REFERENCE(S)

Gravholt CH, Andersen NH, Conway GS, et al; International Turner Syndrome Consensus Group. Clinical practice guidelines for the care of girls and women with Turner syndrome: proceedings from the 2016 Cincinnati International Turner Syndrome Meeting. *Eur J Endocrinol.* 2017;177(3):G1-G70. PMID: 28705803

Shankar RK, Backeljauw PF. Current best practice in the management of Turner syndrome. *Ther Adv Endocrinol Metab.* 2018;9(1):33-40. PMID: 29344338

10 ANSWER: E) Transvaginal ultrasonography

Postmenopausal hirsutism or virilization of recent onset with a serum testosterone concentration greater than 150 ng/dL (>5.2 nmol/L) or a serum DHEA-S level greater than 700 to 800 µg/dL (18.9 to 21.7 µmol/L) suggests a neoplastic source of hyperandrogenism. Signs of virilization include deepening of the voice, increased muscle mass, and clitoromegaly. Clitoromegaly is defined by a clitoral length greater than 10 mm or a clitoral index (length × width) greater than 35 mm². Virilization is only seen with more severe hyperandrogenemia (serum testosterone >150 ng/dL [>5.2 nmol/L]). Postmenopausal women with polycystic ovary syndrome do not have serum testosterone levels in this range, nor are they virilized.

Women with ovarian hyperthecosis typically develop symptoms gradually, but some with severe hyperthecosis have a more rapid course with severe hyperandrogenemia that mimics androgen-secreting tumors. Women with androgen-secreting adrenal tumors often present with symptoms of Cushing syndrome in addition to virilization. Unlike ovarian tumors, adrenal androgen-secreting tumors often, but not always, cause elevation in serum DHEA-S. However, DHEA-S can be normal in androgen-secreting adrenal tumors. Androgen-secreting ovarian tumors include Sertoli-Leydig–cell tumors, arrhenoblastomas, or hilus-cell tumors.

The first step in the evaluation of severe hyperandrogenism in postmenopausal women is transvaginal ultrasonography (Answer E) to look for a tumor or asymmetry of the ovaries, as the tumors are typically very small. If findings on ultrasonography are normal, adrenal CT (Answer A) should be performed, because there are occasional cases of adrenal tumors that secrete only testosterone. However, adrenal CT would not be the first test one would do. In addition, ultrasonography is a better imaging choice than abdominal CT for visualizing the ovaries.

Dexamethasone-suppression testing (Answer B) is used in the workup of Cushing syndrome and might be indicated if an adrenal mass were detected. With adrenal Cushing syndrome, the presentation would be different from this patient's and the testosterone level would not be as high as it is in this vignette.

Serum inhibin (Answer D) is a marker for some ovarian tumors, including granulosa-cell tumors and sex-cord stromal tumors, but ultrasonography is the more important next step.

Serum 17-hydroxyprogesterone (Answer C) would be measured when there are concerns for nonclassic congenital adrenal hyperplasia due to 21-hydroxylase deficiency (which is associated with hirsutism, but not virilization).

EDUCATIONAL OBJECTIVE
Evaluate postmenopausal hyperandrogenism.

REFERENCE(S)

Alpañés M, González-Casbas JM, Sánchez J, Pián H, Escobar-Morreale HF. Management of postmenopausal virilization. *J Clin Endocrinol Metab.* 2012;97(8):2584-2588. PMID: 22669303

Meczekalski B, Szeliga A, Maciejewska-Jeske M, et al. Hyperthecosis: an underestimated nontumorous cause of hyperandrogenism. *Gynecol Endocrinol.* 2021;37(8):677-682. PMID: 33759685

Pugeat M, Déchaud H, Raverot V, Denuzière A, Cohen R, Boudou P; French Endocrine Society. Recommendations for investigation of hyperandrogenism. *Ann Endocrinol (Paris).* 2010;71(1):2-7. PMID: 20096825

Carmina E, Dewailly D, Escobar-Morreale HF, et al. Non-classic congenital adrenal hyperplasia due to 21-hydroxylase deficiency revisited: an update with a special focus on adolescent and adult women. *Hum Reprod Update.* 2017;23(5):580-599. PMID: 28582566

11 ANSWER: C) Reassurance; no evaluation needed

Amenorrhea is a common occurrence in women taking certain oral contraceptives. It is due to the development of an atrophic endometrium (progestin effect). Amenorrhea eventually develops in most women on continuous preparations (hormone pills only, no placebos), but it also can occur in women using cyclic preparations, most commonly the 20-mcg pills, which are more progestin-dominant than the 30- to 35-mcg preparations. Women should be reassured that the pill is effective and that no further evaluation is needed (Answer C).

As long as they have not missed pills or started medications that interfere with estrogen's metabolism, monthly pregnancy tests (Answer B) are unnecessary.

Some women prefer to switch to a different preparation with a higher dosage of estrogen that is less likely to result in an atrophic endometrium in order to restore menstrual bleeding each month. Many clinicians worry that a new endocrine disorder has developed when amenorrhea occurs in this setting, but the amenorrhea is a reflection of the endometrial response to exogenous estrogen and progestin. Thus, neither serum prolactin measurement (Answer E) nor endometrial biopsy (Answer A) is necessary.

EDUCATIONAL OBJECTIVE

Recommend the best course of action for women who develop amenorrhea on low-dosage oral estrogen-progestin contraceptives.

REFERENCE(S)

Hillard PA. Menstrual suppression: current perspectives. *Int J Womens Health.* 2014;6:631-637. PMID: 25018654

Archer DF. Menstrual-cycle-related symptoms: a review of the rationale for continuous use of oral contraceptives. *Contraception.* 2006;74(5):359-366. PMID: 17046376

Gallo MF, Nanda K, Grimes DA, Lopez LM, Schulz KF. 20 μg versus >20 μg estrogen combined oral contraceptives for contraception. *Cochrane Database Syst Rev.* 2013;2013(8):CD003989. PMID: 23904209

12 ANSWER: A) No treatment

No treatment is necessary for this patient now (Answer A) because it appears that she is recovering from functional hypothalamic amenorrhea. Her laboratory values are consistent with recent ovulation (she appears to be in the mid to late luteal phase and will have a period soon). The serum progesterone concentration of 7.0 ng/mL (22.3 nmol/L) confirms that she has ovulated. Progesterone levels are also high in pregnancy, but they are considerably higher than 7 ng/mL (>22.3 nmol/L). Serum LH and FSH vary across the cycle but are relatively low in the late luteal phase (just before the important small rise in serum FSH that is responsible for the recruitment of the cohort of follicles for the subsequent menstrual cycle). Serum estradiol concentrations peak just before the midcycle surge, but there is also a secondary rise in the luteal phase that corresponds with the rise in serum progesterone (both hormones secreted by the corpus luteum). The best option is to reassure her that she is recovering and will likely have a period.

If there were no evidence of recovery, the next step would be to start a physiologic dosage of estrogen (Answer E), rather than an oral contraceptive (Answer D), which contains a pharmacologic dose.

Bisphosphonates (Answer C) should not be given in this setting.

Isoflavone supplements (Answer B) are unlikely to change the course of her recovery.

EDUCATIONAL OBJECTIVE
Identify a postovulatory pattern of gonadotropin and gonadal steroid levels.

REFERENCE(S)
Perkins RB, Hall JE, Martin KA. Aetiology, previous menstrual function and patterns of neuro-endocrine disturbance as prognostic indicators in hypothalamic amenorrhoea. *Hum Reprod.* 2001;16(10):2198-2205. PMID: 11574516

Filicori M, Santoro N, Merriam GR, Crowley WF Jr. Characterization of the physiological pattern of episodic gonadotropin secretion throughout the human menstrual cycle. *J Clin Endocrinol Metab.* 1986;62(6):1136-1144. PMID: 3084534

13   ANSWER: E) Levonorgestrel-releasing intrauterine device

Contraceptive options for women after their childbearing years are evolving. The levonorgestrel-releasing intrauterine device (Answer E) is a good option for perimenopausal women who desire both contraception and management of bleeding. In addition, it is now often used as the progestin for women taking menopausal hormone therapy.

Cyclic progestin (Answer C) can help regulate menses in women who are anovulatory, but it does not provide contraception.

In healthy nonsmoking women, low-dosage (ethinyl estradiol, 20 mcg) combined oral contraceptives can be used until menopause. Higher dosages of ethinyl estradiol (Answer A) are not appropriate given the potential for increased cardiovascular risks. Both older age and higher BMI increase the risk for venous

thromboembolism, so this patient is not a good candidate for combined oral contraceptives.

A copper intrauterine device (Answer B) would be an effective contraceptive, but it is associated with increased menstrual bleeding, so it is not an optimal choice in this patient who is anemic.

Depo-medroxyprogesterone injections (Answer D) are not an optimal choice because they are associated with more adverse effects and complications (including bone loss) than other options.

EDUCATIONAL OBJECTIVE
Explain the treatment options for contraception in perimenopausal women with anemia due to heavy menses.

REFERENCE(S)
Long ME, Faubion SS, MacLaughlin KL, Pruthi S, Casey PM. Contraception and hormonal management in the perimenopause. *J Womens Health (Larchmt).* 2015;24(1):3-10. PMID: 24773233

Kaunitz AM. Clinical practice. Hormonal contraception in women of older reproductive age. *N Engl J Med.* 2008;358(12):1262-1270. PMID: 18354104

14   ANSWER: B) Leuprolide, 3.75 mg intramuscularly, plus estradiol, 50 mcg by transdermal patch

As is the case in postmenopausal women, use of estrogen in transgender patients is associated with an increased risk of venous thromboembolism. In this vignette, the patient is already at increased risk of venous thromboembolism by virtue of having an inherited thrombophilia. Therefore, the priority when selecting the most appropriate hormone regimen is to identify the one with the lowest thrombogenic potential.

Risk of venous thromboembolism from estrogen depends on the dosage, formulation, and route of administration. Incorporating a GnRH agonist into the hormone regimen for a transgender female patient has the advantage of causing profound suppression of endogenous testosterone, so that only physiologic doses of estrogen need to be administered. Of the 2 hormone regimens that include a GnRH agonist, the option with the estrogen patch (Answer B) is correct, as transdermal estrogen is associated with a lower clotting risk than oral formulations (Answer A) because it bypasses the liver and therefore leads to less of an increase in clotting factors.

Unlike GnRH analogues, use of antiandrogens such as spironolactone causes more modest suppression of testosterone, so higher estrogen dosages are needed to achieve the desired degree of testosterone suppression. Therefore, a regimen consisting of spironolactone without estrogen would not be potent enough to suppress testosterone even if combined with a 5α-reductase inhibitor such as finasteride (Answer D).

Of the different types of estrogen available, ethinyl estradiol (Answer C) has the highest risk of venous thromboembolism and should therefore be avoided.

EDUCATIONAL OBJECTIVE
Guide the initiation of hormone therapy in a transgender woman at increased risk of venous thromboembolism.

REFERENCE(S)
Hembree WC, Cohen-Kettenis PT, Gooren L, et al. Endocrine treatment of gender dysphoric/gender incongruent persons: an Endocrine Society clinical practice guideline. *J Clin Endocrinol Metab.* 2017;102(11):3869-3903. PMID: 28945902

T'Sjoen G, Arcelus J, Gooren L, Klink DT, Tangpricha V. Endocrinology of transgender medicine. *Endocr Rev.* 2019;40(1):97-117. PMID: 30307546

Safer JD, Tangpricha V. Care of transgender persons. *N Engl J Med.* 2019;381(25):2451-2460. PMID: 31851801

15 **ANSWER: B) 46,XX**
This patient most likely has mullerian agenesis. Mullerian agenesis or hypoplasia leads to variable uterine development and congenital absence of the vagina, termed the Mayer-Rokitansky-Kuster-Hauser syndrome. The uterus may be underdeveloped or absent. Affected persons have a normal female phenotype at birth, functioning ovaries, normal external genitalia, and

a 46,XX karyotype (Answer B). These individuals are raised as girls. Breast development and pubic hair growth are also normal.

Patients with complete androgen insensitivity who are diagnosed during their teenage years present with primary amenorrhea, absence of axillary or pubic hair, serum testosterone within or above the normal range for boys and men, high LH, and normal FSH. Mullerian structures are absent (blind vaginal pouch and absent uterus and cervix), and the karyotype is 46,XY (Answer C). This disorder is due to a defect in the androgen receptor that results in complete resistance to androgens.

Women with Turner syndrome have short stature, primary hypogonadism, a high rate of cardiovascular anomalies, a number of comorbidities, and a 45,X karyotype (Answer A). Women with Turner mosaicism often have a 45,X/46,XX karyotype (Answer D).

A 47,XXY karyotype (Answer E) is seen in patients with Klinefelter syndrome and such individuals have a male, not female, phenotype.

EDUCATIONAL OBJECTIVE
Distinguish between complete androgen insensitivity syndrome and mullerian agenesis in young women who present with primary amenorrhea.

REFERENCE(S)
Doehnert U, Bertelloni S, Werner R, Dati E, Hiort O. Characteristic features of reproductive hormone profiles in late adolescent and adult females with complete androgen insensitivity syndrome. *Sex Dev.* 2015;9(2):69-74. PMID: 25613104

Grimbizis GF, Gordts S, Di Spiezio Sardo A, et al. The ESHRE/ESGE consensus on the classification of female genital tract congenital anomalies. *Hum Reprod.* 2013;28(8):2032-2044. PMID: 23771171

16 **ANSWER: B) 21-Hydroxylase antibodies**
This patient has spontaneous primary ovarian insufficiency (POI). Additional evaluation is needed once this condition is diagnosed. Although the etiology of POI remains unknown in most cases, a

number of tests should be ordered once a diagnosis of POI is established. These investigations include karyotype analysis (primarily to diagnose Turner syndrome) and genetic testing for the fragile X premutation (approximately 6% of cases of POI are associated with premutations in the *FMR1* gene, the gene responsible for fragile X syndrome and fragile X–associated tremor/ataxia syndrome). Women with a premutation often have POI, but the main concern is expansion to a full mutation in male offspring, causing intellectual disability and a number of other features.

Approximately 3% of women with spontaneous POI have asymptomatic autoimmune adrenal insufficiency—the diagnosis of POI typically precedes that of adrenal insufficiency by several years. As a screen for the presence of asymptomatic autoimmune adrenal insufficiency, serum 21-hydroxylase antibodies (Answer B) should be measured in all women with a 46,XX karyotype at the time spontaneous POI is diagnosed. Women with adrenal autoimmunity detected by the presence of autoantibodies have a 50% risk of developing adrenal insufficiency. These women should then be evaluated for the presence of adrenal insufficiency by measuring 8-AM serum cortisol and plasma ACTH. Testing for 21-hydroxylase antibodies may serve the dual purpose of screening for autoimmune adrenal insufficiency and diagnosing autoimmune oophoritis. Autoimmune oophoritis is characterized by theca-cell destruction; granulosa cells are preserved.

Inhibin B levels (Answer D) are normal in women with autoimmune POI but are low in women with other types of POI. Therefore, affected women present with serum LH concentrations that are higher than FSH concentrations.

Measurement of serum ovarian antibodies (Answer E) (with an indirect immunofluorescence assay using cynomolgus monkey ovary) has poor predictive value for autoimmune POI. The prevalence of ovarian antibodies is similar (30%-50%) in normal cycling women and women with spontaneous POI.

IGF-1 measurement (Answer C) would not provide useful clinical information about POI.

GAD-65 antibodies (Answer A) would provide insight into her potential risk for type 1 diabetes, but the most important first step is evaluation for adrenal insufficiency and autoimmune oophoritis.

EDUCATIONAL OBJECTIVE
Diagnose the etiology of primary ovarian insufficiency.

REFERENCE(S)

Bakalov VK, Anasti JN, Calis KA, et al. Autoimmune oophoritis as a mechanism of follicular dysfunction in women with 46,XX spontaneous premature ovarian failure. *Fertil Steril.* 2005;84(4):958-965. PMID: 16213850

Welt CK, Hally JE, Adams JM, Taylor AE. Relationship of estradiol and inhibin to the follicle-stimulating hormone variability in hypergonadotropic hypogonadism or premature ovarian failure. *J Clin Endocrinol Metab.* 2005;90(2):826-830. PMID: 15562017

Novosad JA, Kalantaridou SN, Tong ZB, Nelson LM. Ovarian antibodies as detected by indirect immunofluorescence are unreliable in the diagnosis of autoimmune premature ovarian failure: a controlled evaluation. *BMC Womens Health.* 2003;3(1):2. PMID: 12694633

Male Reproduction Board Review

Stephanie Page, MD, PhD

1 ANSWER: C) Refer for mammography
Although breast cancer is rare in men, individuals with Klinefelter syndrome have a greater than 20-fold increased risk for breast cancer and greater than 50-fold increased risk for breast cancer mortality. In addition, on physical examination, this patient has findings that should raise suspicion for malignancy, including more breast tissue on one side and immobility of the right-sided mass. The more acute course of his gynecomastia also signals that further imaging (ie, mammography [Answer C]) is indicated.

The midinjection testosterone concentration in this patient is on the low end, but it is not below the lower limit of the reference range. Thus, attributing his gynecomastia to hypogonadism is incorrect and increasing his testosterone dosage (Answer B) or switching to transdermal delivery (Answer D) is unlikely to improve his gynecomastia or libido. His estradiol concentration is slightly above normal, but treatment with anastrozole (Answer A) is inappropriate given his physical examination findings and the long-term risk to his bone health.

While long-term opioid use can cause secondary hypogonadism and lead to gynecomastia due to low testosterone, this patient is on testosterone replacement and thus reduction in his pain medication dosage (Answer E) is unlikely to improve gynecomastia.

EDUCATIONAL OBJECTIVE
Identify elements of the medical history and physical examination that increase the risk of male breast cancer and require further evaluation.

REFERENCE(S)
Brinton LA. Breast cancer risk among patients with Klinefelter syndrome. *Acta Paediatr.* 2011;100(6):814-818. PMID: 21241366

2 ANSWER: B) Initiate intramuscular testosterone enanthate injections, 200 mg every 2 weeks
Twenty to twenty-five percent of men taking highly active antiretroviral therapy for HIV have low total or free testosterone concentrations. Highly active antiretroviral therapy is often associated with increases in SHBG. In men with HIV on highly active antiretroviral therapy, free testosterone should be measured when a borderline total testosterone concentration is noted and free testosterone should be used as a basis for biochemical hypogonadism. For a trial of testosterone therapy in men with suboptimally controlled hypertension, intramuscular testosterone (Answer B) is preferred over oral testosterone undecanoate (Answer D), which is associated with increases in blood pressure.

Low testosterone in men with HIV is associated with morbidity, and treatment with testosterone is associated with increases in body weight and lean body mass in 3 to 6 months. Dietary counseling alone (Answer E) is insufficient for this patient with hypogonadism.

On the basis of his low free testosterone concentration and persistent weight loss, he meets the threshold for therapy. While 5α-reductase inhibitors (Answer A) may slightly raise testosterone, this would be insufficient to treat his hypogonadism and weight loss.

Megestrol acetate (Answer C) primarily acts as an appetite stimulant and has been trialed in the setting of cancer and HIV cachexia with mixed results. This medication has numerous adverse effects. He is hypogonadal and reports a normal appetite; thus, megestrol should not be first-line therapy.

EDUCATIONAL OBJECTIVE
Recommend a trial of testosterone treatment to improve body composition in hypogonadal men with HIV and unexplained weight loss.

REFERENCE(S)
Pena Dias J, Haberlen SA, Dobs AS, et al. Longitudinal changes in sex hormone–binding globulin in men with HIV. *J Acquir Immune Defic Syndr.* 2021;87(5):1178-1186. PMID: 33990494

Bhasin S, Brito JP, Cunningham GR, et al. Testosterone therapy in men with hypogonadism: an Endocrine Society clinical practice guideline. *J Clin Endocrinol Metab.* 2018;103(5):1715-1744. PMID: 29562364

3 ANSWER: A) Increase metformin dosage to 1000 mg twice daily, refer to nutritionist, and encourage lifestyle modifications including weight-loss goals

This patient is overweight and has low total testosterone levels. Patients who are overweight have low SHBG levels, so in this setting free testosterone concentrations should be used to assess for biochemical hypogonadism. Moreover, he does not have concerns associated with low testosterone (he has normal libido and energy). Thus, neither testosterone therapy (Answer E) nor gonadotropin therapy (Answer D) is appropriate for this patient with obesity and normal free testosterone concentrations.

Weight loss and optimization of glucose management both increase testosterone concentrations, which is important for this patient's long-term fertility. Thus, increasing his metformin dosage to 1000 mg twice daily, referring to a nutritionist, and encouraging lifestyle modifications (Answer A) is the best option. His semen analysis shows sperm production within the reference range even though it is at the lower end of normal; sperm concentrations are highly variable from day to day in each individual.

Varicoceles may be associated with infertility, but data regarding the effect of varicocele repair (Answer B) on fertility are lacking. Surgical repair of grade 1 and 2 varicoceles is not recommended, even if this patient were to struggle with fertility in the future.

Similarly, administration of clomiphene citrate (Answer C) may mildly increase testosterone concentrations, but it has not been demonstrated to improve semen parameters in men with infertility. Moreover, long-term use of clomiphene citrate, an estrogen antagonist, is likely to have negative effects on bone health and is not recommended.

EDUCATIONAL OBJECTIVE
Interpret testosterone values in men with obesity and explain how weight loss can raise serum testosterone levels.

REFERENCE(S)
Helo S, Ellen J, Mechlin C, Feustel P, et al. A randomized prospective double-blind comparison trial of clomiphene citrate and anastrozole in raising testosterone in hypogonadal infertile men. *J Sex Med.* 2015;12(8):1761-1769. PMID: 26176805

Anawalt BD. Approach to male infertility and induction of spermatogenesis. *J Clin Endocrinol Metab.* 2013;98(9):3532-3542. PMID: 24014811

4 ANSWER: D) Maintain testosterone dosage as is and counsel the patient regarding the expected timeline for masculinizing effects

Transgender patients are often concerned regarding the time course and effectiveness of gender-normalizing hormone therapy. Setting patient expectations regarding the anticipated timeline for gender-normative characteristics is a key component of care delivery. In general, after 6 months of therapy, transgender men can expect cessation of menses, worsening or development of acne/skin oiliness, increased sexual desire, and perhaps some male-pattern hair growth. Voice deepening generally occurs 6 to 18 months into therapy and referrals for surgical procedures to deepen the voice (Answer E) should wait until maximal hormonal effects are observed. This patient should be advised to maintain testosterone dosing as is and be counseled regarding the expected timeline for masculinizing effects (Answer D).

When monitoring the effectiveness of gender-affirming hormone therapy, hormone concentrations also help guide therapy and should target the physiologic normal range for the transgender. When delivering hormone therapy via intramuscular injections, hormone concentrations may be assessed at the mid-dose time interval. In this case, mid-dose hormone levels were within the normal healthy male range, and the testosterone dosage should not be increased (Answer C).

Hemoglobin and hematocrit should be monitored every 3 months during the first year of hormone therapy in transgender men, and testosterone dosing should potentially be adjusted for polycythemia (Answer B), but this is not the case here.

GnRH antagonists (Answer A) are not indicated in transgender men who have ceased menses and have normal testosterone concentrations.

EDUCATIONAL OBJECTIVE
Set appropriate patient expectations for the timeline for physical changes during gender-affirming hormone therapy.

REFERENCE(S)
Hembree WC, Cohen-Kettenis PT, Gooren L, et al. Endocrine treatment of gender-dysphoric/gender-incongruent persons: an Endocrine Society clinical practice guideline. *J Clin Endocrinol Metab.* 2017;102(11):3869-3903. PMID: 28945902

5 **ANSWER: D) Increase the hCG dosage to 1500 IU 3 times weekly**
Men with secondary hypogonadism should be treated with exogenous testosterone therapy to achieve physiologic testosterone levels. However, men desiring fertility require gonadotropin therapy to provide stimulus to the testes to support spermatogenesis. In such men, exogenous testosterone therapy should be discontinued and not reintroduced (Answer A) until desired fertility outcomes are achieved.

Gonadotropin therapy is more likely to be successful in men with postpubertal secondary hypogonadism and normal testicular volumes. Gonadotropin therapy is initiated with hCG at dosages of 1000 to 2000 IU 3 times per week to achieve normal testosterone concentrations, although sometimes lower dosages of hCG are sufficient. In this man, testosterone concentrations are not within the normal range and the dosage of hCG should be increased (Answer D) to achieve normalization of serum testosterone.

The addition of recombinant FSH (Answer B) should not be considered until after 6 months of hCG therapy.

Initiation of spermatogenesis usually requires approximately 72 days (cycle of sperm maturation), but it requires adequate testosterone for effectiveness. Thus, waiting longer (Answer E) would be inappropriate in this case.

Opioids may cause or contribute to secondary hypogonadism, but in this case they are not the cause of his secondary hypogonadism which is being treated by the current gonadotropin therapy. Thus, gradually decreasing his methadone dosage (Answer C) is incorrect.

EDUCATIONAL OBJECTIVE
Explain the time course and treatment parameters needed to optimize gonadotropin therapy in patients with secondary hypogonadism.

REFERENCE(S)
Anawalt BD. Approach to male infertility and induction of spermatogenesis. *J Clin Endocrinol Metab.* 2013;98(9):3532-3542. PMID: 24014811

Liu PY, Baker HWG, Jayadev V, Zacharin M, Conway AJ, Handelsman DJ. Induction of spermatogenesis and fertility during gonadotropin treatment of gonadotropin-deficient infertile men: predictors of fertility outcome. *J Clin Endocrinol Metab.* 2009;94(3):801-808. PMID: 19066302

6 ANSWER: B) Total testosterone, high or high-normal; free testosterone, low or low-normal; estradiol, high; LH, normal

Gynecomastia is benign enlargement of the male breast due mainly to the proliferation of ductal tissue. Gynecomastia develops when there is an increase in the ratio of estrogen to androgens, with the former having a stimulatory effect on breast tissue, while the latter antagonize this effect. A small degree of breast enlargement is a relatively common finding, especially in older men, and generally does not require any workup when asymptomatic. However, breast enlargement that is prominent, painful, progressive, or of recent onset, as in this case, requires thorough evaluation.

The patient described is clinically and biochemically hyperthyroid, a condition known to cause gynecomastia. In men with hyperthyroidism, there is increased hepatic production of SHBG, which results in high levels of total but low or low-normal levels of free testosterone, high estradiol, and normal LH (Answer B). Because of the greater affinity of SHBG for testosterone than for estradiol, there is a relative increase in the amount of free estradiol compared with testosterone. There is also increased aromatization of testosterone to estradiol in extraglandular tissues.

Elevated serum estradiol with low testosterone and LH levels (Answer A) can be seen with exogenous estrogen use or with an estrogen-secreting testicular tumor of the Leydig or Sertoli cells.

High levels of testosterone, estradiol, and LH (Answer D) are typical of patients with partial androgen insensitivity.

A hormone profile characterized by normal testosterone levels, high estradiol, and low LH (Answer C) can be seen in patients with a testicular or extragonadal hCG-secreting tumor. In these patients, hCG stimulates production of both testosterone and estradiol, but because of its stimulatory effect on the aromatase enzyme, there is preferential estradiol production leading to a lower than normal testosterone-to-estradiol ratio.

EDUCATIONAL OBJECTIVE
Describe the presentation of gynecomastia due to hyperthyroidism.

REFERENCE(S)
Ali SN, Jayasena CN. Sam AH. Which patients with gynaecomastia require more detailed investigation? *Clin Endocrinol (Oxf).* 2018:88(3):360-363. PMID: 29193251

Narula HS, Carlson HE. Gynaecomastia-- pathophysiology, diagnosis and treatment. *Nat Rev Endocrinol.* 2014; 10(11):684-698. PMID: 25112235

Braunstein GD. Clinical practice. Gynecomastia. *N Engl J Med.* 2007;357(12):1229-1237. PMID: 17881754

7 ANSWER: C) Sperm cryopreservation before chemotherapy

After 1 year of follow-up, azoospermia is seen in 90% of men with Hodgkin lymphoma who are treated with more than 3 courses of chemotherapy that includes an alkylating agent. The most reliable option for the preservation of male fertility is cryopreservation of sperm before treatment (Answer C). Cryopreservation of human sperm does not decrease its capability for fertilization, and studies have demonstrated successful pregnancies with cryopreserved sperm. Optimal semen collection procedures for cryopreservation include obtaining at least 3 samples after abstinence for a minimum of 48 hours. However, in men with Hodgkin lymphoma, semen analysis is frequently abnormal even before treatment and only 20% to 30% of patients meet traditional criteria for sperm cryopreservation for intrauterine insemination.

Infertility related to chemotherapy is due to loss of spermatogonial stem cells, and the recovery of spermatogenesis occurs via recolonization of the seminiferous tubules by these stem cells. Currently, cryopreservation and subsequent transplant of spermatogonial stem cells (Answer B) is considered experimental.

It has been hypothesized that hormonal suppression and the resulting disruption of gametogenesis (Answer D) renders the gonad less sensitive to damage by the cytotoxic drugs. However, in clinical trials, hormonal suppression with GnRH agonists has not been shown to reliably afford gonadal protection and its use has led to recovery of spermatogenesis in only 20% of patients.

The combination of exogenous testosterone and a progestin (Answer A) has been used in male contraceptive trials but has not been evaluated in the setting of cytotoxic chemotherapy.

Although his testosterone is below normal without a compensatory rise in LH (a pattern often observed during illness), he has plenty of sperm for cryopreservation. Treatment with hCG (Answer E) to increase sperm numbers and increase serum testosterone would delay initiation of cryopreservation and is neither warranted nor beneficial.

EDUCATIONAL OBJECTIVE
Counsel men planning to undergo cytotoxic chemotherapy on the options for fertility preservation.

REFERENCE(S)
Oktay K, Harvey BE, Partridge AH, et al. Fertility preservation in patients with cancer: ASCO clinical practice guideline update. *J Clin Oncol.* 2018;36(19):1994-2001. PMID: 29620997

Ethics Committee of the American Society for Reproductive Medicine. Fertility preservation and reproduction in patients facing gonadotoxic therapies: an Ethics Committee opinion. *Fertil Steril.* 2018;110(3):380-386. PMID: 30098684

Jahnukainen K, Ehmcke J, Hou M, Schlatt S. Testicular function and fertility preservation in male cancer patients. *Best Pract Res Clin Endocrinol Metab.* 2011;25(2):287-302. PMID: 21397199

Levine J, Canada A, Stern CJ. Fertility preservation in adolescents and young adults with cancer. *J Clin Oncol.* 2010;28(32):4831-4841. PMID: 20458029

8 ANSWER: E) Trial of an oral phosphodiesterase inhibitor

Most experts recommend testing for hypogonadism in men who have erectile dysfunction. Eugonadism is necessary for normal male sexual function, including normal tumescence, but serum total testosterone concentrations must be very low (<150 ng/dL [<5.2 nmol/L]) to cause erectile dysfunction. In this man with normal libido and a mid-range, normal total testosterone concentration, it is very unlikely that hypogonadism is the cause of his erectile dysfunction. Thus, measurement of calculated free testosterone (Answer D) is unlikely to be useful in determining the cause of his erectile dysfunction even though many men with type 2 diabetes have low testosterone.

Optimizing his glycemic control (Answer C) and lipid control (Answer A) might provide microvascular benefits, and only his lipids are currently reasonably controlled. While there is evidence that optimal glycemic control may reduce the risk of erectile dysfunction in men with diabetes, there is no evidence that reversal of established erectile dysfunction occurs with improved glycemic control.

Once the diagnosis of erectile dysfunction is established, first-line therapy for men with and without diabetes is phosphodiesterase inhibitors (Answer E).

Erectile dysfunction is a strong marker of cardiovascular disease. Sexual intercourse is typically about 3 to 4 metabolic equivalents. Walking a mile in 20 minutes is about 4 metabolic equivalents. Thus, while this patient has cardiovascular risk factors, he is not taking nitrates and leads an active lifestyle. Thus, cardiac stress echocardiography (Answer B) is incorrect.

EDUCATIONAL OBJECTIVE
Recommend optimal treatment for a man with diabetes mellitus and erectile dysfunction.

REFERENCE(S)
Finkelstein JS, Lee H, Burnett-Bowie S-AM, et al. Gonadal steroids and body composition, strength, and sexual function in men. *N Engl J Med.* 369(11):1011-1022. PMID: 24024838

McVary KT. Clinical practice. Erectile dysfunction. *N Engl J Med.* 2007;357(24):2472-2481. PMID: 18077811

Miner M, Seftel AD, Nehra A, et al. Prognostic utility of erectile dysfunction for cardiovascular disease in younger men and those with diabetes. *Am Heart J.* 2012;164(1):21-28. PMID: 22795278

Wessells H, Penson DF, Cleary P, et al. Effect of intensive glycemic therapy on erectile function in men with type 1 diabetes. *J Urol.* 2011;185(5):1828-1834. PMID: 21420129

9 ANSWER: B) Start alprostadil injections

This man has normal total and free testosterone levels. He has well-controlled diabetes and other cardiovascular risk factors that contribute to a vascular cause of his erectile dysfunction. Starting alprostadil injections (Answer B) is the best next step.

Phosphodiesterase inhibitors have been shown to improve erectile function consistently in clinical trials. Low testosterone and erectile dysfunction are frequent comorbid conditions. Sexual symptoms are common in hypogonadal men, particularly in men with unequivocally low testosterone levels. Many studies have suggested a benefit to testosterone treatment in conjunction with the use of phosphodiesterase inhibitors, but blinded, randomized placebo-controlled trials have been lacking. A recent double-blind, randomized placebo-controlled trial treated middle-aged men (40-70 years) who had erectile dysfunction with low testosterone (total testosterone <330 ng/dL [<11.5 nmol/L] or free testosterone <5 ng/dL [<0.2 nmol/L]) with sildenafil and then randomly assigned them to an additional 14 weeks of sildenafil alone or sildenafil plus testosterone therapy (testosterone gel). No difference in erectile function was observed between the groups, and the investigators concluded that the addition of testosterone treatment to sildenafil did not improve erectile function. A second blinded, randomized controlled trial in middle-aged and older men (45-80 years) with mild hypogonadism found no difference in erectile function between men for whom phosphodiesterase treatment failed and were then randomly assigned to testosterone gel plus tadalafil compared with tadalafil alone. The investigators did observe some benefit from the addition of testosterone therapy to tadalafil in men with total testosterone concentrations less than 300 ng/dL (<10.4 nmol/L). On the basis of these recent trial findings, the addition of testosterone replacement (Answer E) to phosphodiesterase inhibitor therapy is unlikely to improve erectile function in this patient with mild, late-onset secondary hypogonadism.

Similarly, although hCG (Answer D) raises testosterone without suppressing spermatogenesis, he has a normal serum testosterone concentration.

Increasing his metformin dosage (Answer A) to improve his glycemic control is not likely to have an effect given that his hemoglobin A_{1c} value is 6.8% (51 mmol/mol).

A 5α-reductase inhibitor (Answer C) may mildly increase serum testosterone but has not been shown to improve erectile function.

EDUCATIONAL OBJECTIVE

Counsel patients about recent trials that do not show benefit from the addition of testosterone to phosphodiesterase inhibitor therapy for the treatment of erectile dysfunction in middle-aged to older men with mild hypogonadism.

REFERENCE(S)

Wu FCW, Tajar A, Beynon JM, et al; EMAS Group. Identification of late-onset hypogonadism in middle-aged and elderly men. *N Engl J Med.* 2010;363(2):123-135. PMID: 20554979

Spitzer M, Basaria S, Travison TG, et al. Effect of testosterone replacement on response to sildenafil citrate in men with erectile dysfunction: a parallel, randomized trial. *Ann Intern Med.* 2012;157(10):681-691. PMID: 23165659

Buvat J, Montorsi F, Maggi M, et al. Hypogonadal men nonresponders to the PDE5 inhibitor tadalafil benefit from normalization of testosterone levels with a 1% hydroalcoholic testosterone gel in the treatment of erectile dysfunction (TADTEST study). *J Sex Med.* 2011;8(1):284-293. PMID: 20704642

Isidori AM, Buvat J, Corona G, et al. A critical analysis of the role of testosterone in erectile function: from pathophysiology to treatment-a systematic review. *Eur Urol.* 2014;65(1):99-112. PMID: 24050791

Basaria S, Coviello AD, Travison TG, et al. Adverse events associated with testosterone administration. *N Engl J Med.* 2010;363(2):109-122. PMID: 20592293

10 **ANSWER: D) Schedule a sleep study**
Testosterone esters, including enanthate and cypionate, have been used to treat male hypogonadism for more than 7 decades. They have the advantage of being the least expensive of the testosterone replacement modalities, and they predictably restore testosterone levels to the normal range. However, they have unfavorable pharmacokinetics characterized by significant fluctuation in serum testosterone between peak and trough values. When administered by a deep intramuscular injection, testosterone is slowly released from this oily suspension into the circulation over a period of weeks. The esters are typically injected at 2-week intervals, with levels reaching peak concentrations 24 to 48 hours after the injection followed by a gradual decline to the low-normal range before the next injection is due. When the interval between injections is extended to every 3 weeks, peak concentrations tend to be supraphysiologic and testosterone levels may fall to the hypogonadal range by the time the next injection is administered. Such wide excursions in serum testosterone concentrations can, in turn, cause undesirable swings in mood, libido, and energy levels. Given the pharmacokinetics of testosterone esters, they also tend to increase hematocrit more than transdermal testosterone preparations, especially when high dosages are given at less frequent intervals.

Increasing the testosterone dosage (Answer C) in a patient whose hematocrit is already high is not appropriate, especially given that this patient's testosterone concentration is in the desired range for a trough level (namely, the lower end of the normal range). Markedly decreasing his testosterone dosage (Answer B) is likely to leave him hypogonadal throughout much of his dosing period and thus is unlikely to treat his symptoms of hypogonadism.

The pharmacokinetics of testosterone enanthate are similar to those of testosterone cypionate. Hence, switching esters (Answer E) will not address his problem.

Before initiating testosterone therapy, baseline hematocrit should be measured. Baseline hematocrit greater than 48% (and greater than 50%

for men living at higher altitudes) is a relative contraindication to testosterone therapy because these men are more likely to develop a hematocrit level greater than 54% when treated with testosterone. The baseline hematocrit of 50% for this hypogonadal, nonsmoking patient is high. The Endocrine Society clinical practice guidelines recommend investigating the underlying cause of erythrocytosis before androgen therapy is prescribed. Given the patient's obesity and history of daytime somnolence, the possibility of obstructive sleep apnea should be considered and a sleep study should be arranged (Answer D).

Occasionally, phlebotomy (Answer A) may be necessary to continue testosterone therapy in a hypogonadal patient, but it is important to exclude other causes of erythrocytosis such as sleep apnea, chronic obstructive pulmonary disease, or polycythemia rubra vera before doing so.

EDUCATIONAL OBJECTIVE
Describe the pharmacokinetics of injectable testosterone esters and manage potential adverse effects.

REFERENCE(S)
Bhasin S, Brito JP, Cunningham GR, et al. Testosterone therapy in men with hypogonadism: an Endocrine Society clinical practice guideline. *J Clin Endocrinol Metab.* 2018;103(5):1715-1744. PMID: 29562364

Dobs AS, Meikle AW, Arver S, Sanders SW, Caramelli KE, Mazer NA. Pharmacokinetics, efficacy, and safety of a permeation-enhanced testosterone transdermal system in comparison with bi-weekly injections of testosterone enanthate for the treatment of hypogonadal men. *J Clin Endocrinal Metab.* 1999;84(10):3469-3478. PMID: 10522982

11 **ANSWER: A) Cough and shortness of breath following the injection**
A long-acting intramuscular formulation comprising testosterone undecanoate was approved for the treatment of male hypogonadism in the United States in 2014. This preparation has the advantage of having a superior

pharmacokinetic profile compared with other injectable formulations such as enanthate and cypionate, and it has the ability to maintain testosterone levels more consistently in the normal range over a 10-week period. The absence of marked swings in serum testosterone levels means that fluctuations in mood and energy (Answer D) are not typical adverse effects.

The US FDA has stipulated that all injections of testosterone undecanoate must be administered in an office or hospital setting by a trained health care provider and that the patient be monitored for adverse effects for 30 minutes after the injection. The restrictions associated with use of this drug result from reported cases of pulmonary oil microembolism (1.5 cases/10,000 injections) and anaphylaxis (0.4 cases/10,000 injections). Symptoms of pulmonary oil microembolism include the urge to cough, dyspnea (Answer A), throat tightening, chest pain, dizziness, and syncope. These symptoms have been reported with all testosterone injections but are more common with testosterone undecanoate because of the larger injection volume (3 mL compared with 1 mL or less for the shorter-acting formulations).

Flu-like symptoms (Answer B) have not been reported with testosterone undecanoate injections.

Increased blood pressure (Answer E) has been observed with a newly approved daily oral form of testosterone undecanoate but is not reported with long-acting intramuscular formulation.

When ingested orally, methyltestosterone (an older formulation of oral testosterone) is broken down by the liver and has the potential to cause liver damage, including cholestatic jaundice, peliosis hepatis, and hepatomas. However, testosterone formulations administered intramuscularly are not hepatotoxic, so jaundice (Answer C) is incorrect.

EDUCATIONAL OBJECTIVE
Counsel patients about potential adverse effects of the long-acting intramuscular formulation of testosterone undecanoate.

REFERENCE(S)

Wang C, Harnett M, Dobs AS, Swerdloff RS. Pharmacokinetics and safety of long-acting testosterone undecanoate injections in hypogonadal men: an 84-week phase III clinical trial. *J Androl.* 2010;31(5):457-465. PMID: 20133964

Bhasin S, Brito JP, Cunningham GR, et al. Testosterone therapy in men with hypogonadism: an Endocrine Society clinical practice guideline. *J Clin Endocrinol Metab.* 2018;103(5):1715-1744. PMID: 29562364

12 **ANSWER: A) Anabolic steroid use**
The fact that this patient is asymptomatic and has elevated hematocrit despite having a hormone profile showing profound hypogonadotropic hypogonadism suggests that he is being exposed to androgens other than testosterone that are not being detected in the testosterone assay. Therefore, use of androgenic anabolic steroids (Answer A) is the most likely cause.

Hereditary hemochromatosis (Answer B), Kallmann syndrome (Answer C), opioid use (Answer D), and prolactinoma (Answer E) would be expected to be associated with symptoms of androgen deficiency given the degree of hypogonadism. In addition, the fact that the patient is normally virilized and has testes of 10 cc is not consistent with a diagnosis of Kallmann syndrome.

In patients with marked hyperprolactinemia due to a large macroadenoma, serum prolactin levels can be reported as normal unless serial dilution of serum is done to assess for the "hook effect." However, if a prolactinoma (Answer E) were responsible for this patient's hypogonadism, MRI would show a large pituitary adenoma as opposed to the 5-mm lesion seen in this case, which is most likely an incidentaloma.

While opioid use (Answer D) is an increasingly common cause of hypogonadism and could lead to the degree of gonadotropin suppression described in the vignette, it would not explain the patient's lack of symptoms or his elevated hematocrit.

Hereditary hemochromatosis (Answer B) is in the differential diagnosis for acquired hypogonadotropic hypogonadism, but it would not typically cause such profoundly low testosterone and gonadotropin levels. In addition, patients with this disorder are not asymptomatic and typically have other manifestations, including arthralgias, chondrocalcinosis, and hyperpigmentation. Later in the disease course, patients may experience heart failure, cirrhosis, and diabetes mellitus. Hemochromatosis is inherited in an autosomal recessive manner and has a prevalence of about 0.4% in populations of northern European descent, but it has much lower clinical penetrance and disease severity is highly variable. Pathogenic variants in the *HFE* gene are responsible, and the most common genotype is homozygosity for the Cys282Tyr (C282Y) variant.

EDUCATIONAL OBJECTIVE
Diagnose anabolic steroid use as a cause of secondary hypogonadism.

REFERENCE(S)
Anawalt BD. Diagnosis and management of anabolic androgenic steroid use. *J Clin Endocrinol Metab.* 2019;104(7):2490-2500. PMID: 30753550

13 ANSWER: E) Testosterone plus an aromatase inhibitor

The patient's estradiol concentration is low in the presence of a high testosterone level, which serves as the substrate for aromatase, and indicates that he must be taking an aromatase inhibitor (Answers A or E). The fact that his testosterone concentration is high rules out the possibility that he is taking an anabolic steroid (Answer A) because anabolic steroids are not detected in modern testosterone assays. While modest reductions in HDL cholesterol may be seen with testosterone administration, nonaromatizable anabolic androgens profoundly suppress HDL cholesterol, which is not observed here. This patient's hormone profile is best explained by testosterone plus an aromatase inhibitor (Answer E).

Exogenous testosterone, hCG, or anabolic steroids all suppress gonadotropins, so the degree of gonadotropin suppression does not help to differentiate among the hormone regimens. hCG increases serum testosterone, which in turn is aromatized to estradiol; thus, exogenous hCG (Answer C) would raise both serum estradiol and testosterone concentrations, which is not the case here.

Exogenous thyroid might mildly suppress TSH, but exogenous DHEA does not increase testosterone nor profoundly suppress gonadotropins (thus, Answer B is incorrect).

5α-Reductase inhibitors (Answer D) may mildly increase serum testosterone, but estradiol would be expected to increase in concert with testosterone, and profound gonadotropin suppression is not observed with 5α-reductase inhibitors.

EDUCATIONAL OBJECTIVE
Highlight the different hormonal profiles associated with testosterone and androgenic anabolic steroid use.

REFERENCE(S)
Pope HG Jr, Wood RI, Rogol A, Nyberg F, Bowers L, Bhasin S. Adverse health consequences of performance-enhancing drugs: an Endocrine Society scientific statement. *Endocr Rev.* 2014;35(3):341-375. PMID: 24423981

Anawalt BD. Diagnosis and management of anabolic androgenic steroid use. *J Clin Endocrinol Metab.* 2019;104(7):2490-2500. PMID: 30753550

14 ANSWER: D) Substitute dutasteride for tamsulosin

Ejaculation is the discharge of semen from the male reproductive tract usually accompanied by orgasm. Retrograde ejaculation occurs when semen, which would normally be ejaculated via the urethra, is instead redirected to the bladder. Normally, the sphincter of the bladder contracts before ejaculation, which acts to both inhibit the release of urine and prevent a reflux of seminal fluids into the bladder during ejaculation. Any condition, medication, or surgical procedure that interferes with central control of ejaculation or the autonomic innervation to the seminal tract can cause ejaculatory dysfunction. Use of α-adrenergic blockers such as tamsulosin to treat symptoms of benign prostatic hyperplasia is a common cause of retrograde ejaculation given that they relax the bladder sphincter. Other drug classes used to treat benign prostatic hyperplasia, such as 5α-reductase inhibitors, do not have this adverse effect, so substituting dutasteride for tamsulosin (Answer D) would be a helpful strategy for this patient.

While cross-sectional studies show an association between low testosterone levels and ejaculatory dysfunction, testosterone replacement (Answer A) has not been shown to be beneficial to such patients. In any case, the patient described does not meet criteria for hypogonadism given that his testosterone concentration is in the normal range.

This patient can get and sustain an erection adequate for intercourse, and phosphodiesterase-5 inhibitors have no effect on ejaculatory function. Therefore, initiating treatment with a phosphodiesterase-5 inhibitor (Answer C) would not be helpful. In addition, an agent such as tadalafil can interact with tamsulosin and result in hypotension.

Surgical treatment of benign prostatic hyperplasia (Answer B) is not indicated for treatment of retrograde ejaculation. Retrograde ejaculation is not uncommon following surgery for benign prostatic hyperplasia.

A diuretic might not be an ideal choice for a patient with benign prostatic hyperplasia. Nonetheless, hydrochlorothiazide is a safe, effective, and inexpensive agent that is doing a good job controlling this patient's blood pressure at a low dosage. While it may contribute to erectile dysfunction, it does not cause ejaculatory dysfunction. Therefore, substituting spironolactone for hydrochlorothiazide (Answer E) is not indicated, as it would not be expected to confer any additional benefit and could cause gynecomastia.

EDUCATIONAL OBJECTIVE
Explain the association between use of α-adrenergic blockers and retrograde ejaculation.

REFERENCE(S)
Mehta A, Sigman M. Management of the dry ejaculate: a systematic review of aspermia and retrograde ejaculation. *Fertil Steril.* 2015;104(5):1074-1081. PMID: 26432530

Paduch DA, Polzer PK, Ni X, Basaria S. Testosterone replacement in androgen-deficient men with ejaculatory dysfunction: a randomized controlled trial. *J Clin Endocrinol Metab.* 2015;100(8);2956-2962. PMID: 26158605

Marra G, Sturch P, Oderda M, Tabatabaei S, Muir G, Gontero P. Systematic review of lower urinary tract symptoms/benign prostatic hyperplasia surgical treatments on men's ejaculatory function: time for a bespoke approach? *Int J Urol.* 2016 Jan;23(1):22-35. PMID: 26177667

15 ANSWER: A) Reevaluate his hypothalamic-pituitary-gonadal axis in 6 months

Although the incidence of pituitary dysfunction after traumatic brain injury varies widely in published studies, it appears that pituitary dysfunction occurs commonly in men who experience moderate to severe traumatic brain injury. Low GH and testosterone concentrations are the most common abnormalities. Indeed, hypogonadism has been reported in up to 80% of men in the acute phase of posttraumatic brain injury. However, it is unclear whether treatment with GH and/or testosterone is beneficial. Furthermore, longitudinal follow-up has demonstrated that many men recover function of these axes within the first year after traumatic brain injury. In this man who appears to be recovering well, the best option is therefore to reassess his gonadal axis 6 months after the initial injury (Answer A).

Treatment with hCG (Answer D) would raise his testosterone concentration and stimulate spermatogenesis; however, he does not wish to start a family for at least 1 year, so there is no urgency in starting treatment until it is clear that his hypothalamic-pituitary-gonadal axis has not recovered.

Given that his libido is already beginning to improve and he has no problem with erections, there is no indication to start testosterone (Answer C).

A phosphodiesterase-5 inhibitor (Answer B) would not be appropriate for a patient with low libido but normal erectile function.

EDUCATIONAL OBJECTIVE

Counsel a patient regarding the time course of secondary hypogonadism following traumatic brain injury.

REFERENCE(S)

Schneider HJ, Schneider M, Saller B, et al. Prevalence of anterior pituitary insufficiency 3 and 12 months after traumatic brain injury. *Eur J Endocrinol.* 2006;154(2):259-265. PMID: 16452539

Tanriverdi F, Senyurek H, Unluhizarci K, Selcuklu A, Casanueva FF, Kelestimur F. High risk of hypopituitarism after traumatic brain injury: a prospective investigation of anterior pituitary function in the acute phase and 12 months after trauma. *J Clin Endocrinol Metab.* 2006;91(6):2105-2111. PMID: 16522687

Agha A, Thompson CJ. High risk of hypogonadism after traumatic brain injury: clinical implications. *Pituitary.* 2005;8(3-4):245-249. PMID: 16470352

16 ANSWER: D) *FGFR1*

Once congenital hypogonadotropic hypogonadism has been diagnosed, targeted genetic testing can be considered. In the last decade, considerable advances have been made in unraveling the genetic basis of congenital hypogonadotropic hypogonadism, and to date, pathogenic variants have been identified in approximately 40% of patients. While in familial cases the mode of inheritance can be used to guide genetic testing, most cases of congenital hypogonadotropic hypogonadism are sporadic, as in the patient described in this vignette. However, a careful clinical evaluation can be helpful in prioritizing genetic testing. In an analysis of 219 patients with congenital hypogonadotropic hypogonadism, the following clinical features were highly associated with specific gene defects: synkinesia (*ANOS1* [formerly known as *KAL1*]) (Answer A), dental agenesis (*FGF8/FGFR1*), digital bony abnormalities (*FGF8/FGFR1*), and hearing loss (*CHD7*). In the case described where the patient has evidence of syndactyly, genetic testing for an *FGFR1* pathogenic variant (Answer D) would be the appropriate next step.

Pathogenic variants in the *GNRHR* gene (Answer C) cause hypogonadism but not anosmia or syndactyly.

While pathogenic variants in *CHD7* (Answer B) cause Kallmann syndrome, the absence of deafness and the presence of syndactyly in this patient make it make more likely that the genetic basis for his disease is a pathogenic variant in *FGFR1* rather than in *CHD7*.

Pathogenic variants in *NR0B1* (Answer E) (formerly known as *DAX1*) cause congenital hypogonadotropic hypogonadism and adrenal insufficiency and do not cause anosmia.

EDUCATIONAL OBJECTIVE

Guide the appropriate workup in a patient with congenital hypogonadotropic hypogonadism.

REFERENCE(S)

Young J. Approach to the male patient with hypogonadotropic hypogonadism. *J Clin Endocrinol Metab.* 2012;97(3):707-718. PMID: 22392951

Costa-Barbosa FA, Balasubramanian R, Keefe KW, et al. Prioritizing genetic testing in patients with Kallmann syndrome using clinical phenotypes. *J Clin Endocrinol Metab.* 2013;98(5):E943-E953. PMID: 23533228

Obesity and Lipids Board Review

Sangeeta R. Kashyap, MD

1 ANSWER: A) Dietary modification and acarbose

Postbariatric hypoglycemia is a rare complication of bariatric surgery that is occurring more frequently. Patients present at least 6 months postoperatively with frequent postprandial episodes of hypoglycemia accompanied by adrenergic and/or neuroglycopenic signs and symptoms, including altered mental status, visual changes, motor incoordination, loss of consciousness, and seizures. While the underlying physiology is incompletely understood, the presence of inappropriately high insulin secretion after oral ingestion of nutrients is well established. Hyperinsulinemia occurs in response to oral but not intravenous glucose, pointing to enteroinsular axis overstimulation and an exaggerated incretin effect. Plasma concentrations of GLP-1 secreted by L-cells in response to luminal nutrient stimulation are markedly elevated after meal intake. GLP-1 hypersecretion and hyperinsulinemic hypoglycemia are fully reversible by restoring the original route of nutrient transit via gastrostomy tube feeding into the remnant stomach. This suggests that altered nutrient transit with foregut bypass and hindgut stimulation potentiates hypoglycemia via GLP-1 secretion.

In this case, the Whipple triad has been fulfilled and there is symptomatic hypoglycemia in response to a mixed-meal challenge. The initial treatment for hypoglycemia is dietary counseling that eliminates refined starches and replaces with high-fiber, low–glycemic index foods. However, dietary modification alone for this patient with frequent hypoglycemia is not sufficient, and the use of a glucosidase inhibitor such as acarbose would reduce glucose absorption and decrease the postprandial insulin response. Thus, recommending both dietary modification and acarbose (Answer A) would be the best initial treatment. Other agents such as diazoxide and octreotide have been used if initial treatment with acarbose is suboptimal.

There is no role for reversal of gastric bypass (Answer E) in treating this condition. Placement of a gastrostomy tube to reverse nutrient ingestion through the intact alimentary tract has been shown to reverse post–gastric bypass hypoglycemia.

A ketogenic diet (Answer B) has no role in the treatment of post–gastric bypass hypoglycemia.

Although liraglutide (Answer C) is a GLP-1 receptor agonist that slows the motility of the gastrointestinal tract and nutrient absorption and has been shown in small case reports to be beneficial in treating hypoglycemia in patients who have undergone bariatric surgery, there are no trials documenting its efficacy in patients with post–gastric bypass hypoglycemia.

Use of a β-adrenergic blocker such as propranolol (Answer D) may mask the adrenergic response to hypoglycemia and has no role in this case.

A multicenter trial of exendin 9-36 (GLP-1 antagonist) has shown that it reduces hypoglycemia, but it is not available for commercial use.

EDUCATIONAL OBJECTIVE
Treat post–gastric bypass hypoglycemia.

REFERENCE(S)
Kellogg TA, Bantle JP, Leslie DB, et al. Postgastric bypass hyperinsulinemic hypoglycemia syndrome: characterization and response to a modified diet. *Surg Obes Relat Dis.* 2008;4(4):492-499. PMID: 18656831

Suhl E, Anderson-Haynes S-E, Mulla C, Patti M-E. Medical nutrition therapy for post-bariatric hypoglycemia: practical insights. *Surg Obes Relat Dis.* 2017;13(5):888-896. PMID: 28392017

Craig CM, Lawler HM, Lee CJE, et al. PREVENT: a randomized, placebo-controlled crossover trial of avexitide for treatment of postbariatric hypoglycemia. *J Clin Endocrinol Metab.* 2021;106(8):e3235-e3248. PMID: 33616643

2 ANSWER: D) Paroxetine

The effect of antidepressants on weight depends on the specific medication prescribed and the length of treatment. Short-term treatment for 2 to 3 months with selective serotonin reuptake inhibitors (SSRIs) usually causes little or no weight change.

However, treatment with SSRIs for longer periods may result in significant weight gain. In some cases, it is not clear whether this is a true medication adverse effect or the result of recovery from depression and reversal of undesired weight loss. Evidence suggests that both bupropion (Answer B) and fluoxetine (Answer C) may be the least problematic SSRIs regarding undesired weight gain. Bupropion leads to weight loss and is used in combination with naltrexone for weight loss. Paroxetine (Answer D) may be the most problematic. In 6% of patients, paroxetine leads to weight gain ranging from 1.6% to 3.6% of baseline body weight. Venlafaxine (Answer E) and amitriptyline (Answer A) are considered to be weight neutral or to promote weight loss.

Most studies on this topic have evaluated patients who have major depressive disorder. It is not clear whether weight change caused by SSRIs differs according to demographic profiles such as age or sex. A review found that weight gain during treatment with SSRIs may be due to remission of major depression, improved appetite, increased carbohydrate craving, and changes in serotonin 2C receptor activity. Conversely, weight loss during acute SSRI treatment may be related to poor appetite at the beginning of treatment.

Weight gain due to long-term treatment with SSRIs may lead to diabetes mellitus. A nested case-control study of patients with depression found that use of moderate to high daily dosages of SSRIs for periods longer than 24 months is associated with a significant 2-fold increased risk of developing diabetes mellitus compared with not using antidepressants (incidence rate ratio: 2.06; 95% CI, 1.20-3.52). Analysis of individual antidepressants found an increased risk estimate for paroxetine (incidence rate ratio: 1.33; 95% CI, 1.02-1.73), suggesting the possibility that the increased risk for SSRIs might have primarily been due to paroxetine.

EDUCATIONAL OBJECTIVE
Identify antidepressant medications associated with weight gain.

REFERENCE(S)
Uher R, Farmer A, Henigsberg N, et al. Adverse reactions to antidepressants. *Br J Psychiatry.* 2009;195(3):202-210. PMID: 19721108

de Jonghe F, Ravelli DP, Tuynman-Qua H. A randomized, double-blind study of fluoxetine and maprotiline in the treatment of major depression. *Pharmacopsychiatry.* 1991;24(2):62-67. PMID: 1852793

Wade A, Michael Lemming O, Bang Hedegaard K. Escitalopram 10 mg/day is effective and well tolerated in a placebo-controlled study in depression in primary care. *Int Clin Psychopharmacol.* 2002;17(3):95-102. PMID: 11981349

3 ANSWER: A) Avoid pregnancy until she is weight stable (use a nonoral contraceptive agent)

More than 80% of bariatric procedures are performed in women, and approximately half of these procedures are performed in reproductive-aged women. Thus, it has become increasingly common for women who have undergone bariatric surgery to present for preconception counseling or prenatal care. A joint 2013 clinical practice guideline by the American Association of Clinical Endocrinologists, the Obesity Society, and the American Society for Metabolic and Bariatric Surgery recommends that women avoid conception for 12 to 18 months after bariatric surgery because this time frame is when women are actively losing the most weight. This delay is done in an effort to optimize weight loss and reduce the potentially adverse effect of postbariatric surgical nutritional deficiencies. Procedures that create malabsorption, such as biliopancreatic diversion, jejunoileal bypass, or Roux-en-Y bypass, may interfere with the absorption of oral contraceptives, thereby reducing their effectiveness. Thus, an intrauterine device (Answer A) is preferable.

As discussed, pregnancy during the time of active weight loss after bariatric surgery is not recommended (thus, Answers B, C, D, and E are incorrect). Breastfeeding is not contraindicated following bariatric surgery (thus, Answer D is incorrect). Monitoring nutritional status (ie, prealbumin levels) and micronutrient levels (especially iron, ferritin, vitamin B_{12}, calcium, PTH, 25-hydroxyvitamin D) is essential after gastric bypass, as well as prior to, during, and after pregnancy.

EDUCATIONAL OBJECTIVE
Provide pregnancy counseling to women who have undergone bariatric surgery.

REFERENCE(S)
Mechanick JI, Youdim A, Jones DB, et al, American Association of Clinical Endocrinologists, Obesity Society, American Society for Metabolic & Bariatric Surgery. *Endocr Pract.* 2013;19(2):337-372. PMID: 23529351

American College of Obstetricians and Gynecologists. ACOG practice bulletin No. 105: bariatric surgery and pregnancy. *Obstet Gynecol.* 2009;113(6):1405-1413. PMID: 19461456

4   **ANSWER: B) Refer him for nutritional counseling to reduce his intake of saturated fat and alcohol**

This patient has metabolic syndrome without diabetes. He is at intermediate risk for atherosclerotic cardiovascular disease with moderate hypertriglyceridemia in the range of 300 to 500 mg/dL (3.39 to 5.65 mmol/L) and an LDL-cholesterol level at target. Hypertriglyceridemia in this range is considered atherogenic and warrants attention. The initial approach should consist of general measures, which include diet, exercise, weight loss, and assessment of secondary causes of hypertriglyceridemia (ie, hypothyroidism, medications) (Answer B).

For moderate hypertriglyceridemia, targets include less than 6% calories from added sugar, less than 30% to 35% of calories from total dietary fat, and 2 or fewer alcoholic drinks per day for men and 1 or fewer per day for women. For moderate to severe hypertriglyceridemia, targets include less than 5% of calories from added sugar, less than 20% to 25% of calories from total dietary fat, and alcohol abstinence. For patients with glucose intolerance or diabetes and high risk of atherosclerotic cardiovascular disease risk, moderate hypertriglyceridemia should not be treated with niacin (Answer D), as it can worsen glucose tolerance.

Fenofibrate (Answer C) is recommended for patients with severe hypertriglyceridemia (>1000 mg/dL [>11.30 mmol/L]) to avoid pancreatitis.

Changing atorvastatin to rosuvastatin (Answer A) would not significantly lower this patient's triglyceride levels.

The efficacy of triglyceride lowering in decreasing risk of atherosclerotic cardiovascular disease has not been established, in contrast to the established risk reduction with lowering LDL cholesterol.

Also, LDL-cholesterol levels may underrepresent cardiovascular risk in patients with hypertriglyceridemia. High triglyceride levels are associated with small, dense cholesterol-depleted LDL particles that may not be captured by LDL-cholesterol measurement. Non-HDL cholesterol and apolipoprotein B concentrations are better measures of excess concentrations of atherogenic lipoproteins in patients with moderate and severe hypertriglyceridemia.

EDUCATIONAL OBJECTIVE
Manage hypertriglyceridemia in patients with moderate risk of atherosclerotic cardiovascular disease.

REFERENCE(S)

Virani SS, Morris PB, Agarwala A, et al. 2021 ACC expert consensus decision pathway on the management of ASCVD risk reduction in patients with persistent hypertriglyceridemia: a report of the American College of Cardiology Solution Set Oversight Committee. *J Am Coll Cardiol.* 2021;78(9):960-993. PMID: 34332805

Ballantyne CM, Grundy SM, Oberman A, et al. Hyperlipidemia: diagnostic and therapeutic perspectives. *J Clin Endocrinol Metab.* 2000;85(6):2089-2112. PMID: 10852435

Gotto AM Jr. Hypertriglyceridemia: risks and perspectives. *Am J Cardiol.* 1992;70(19):19H-25H. PMID: 1466313

5 ANSWER: B) Start bempedoic acid

This patient presents for treatment of secondary cardiovascular disease risk and has an elevated LDL-cholesterol level that does not meet target (<55 mg/dL [<1.42 mmol/L]). He is not tolerant of PCSK9 inhibitors. Bempedoic acid (Answer B) is an inhibitor of adenosine triphosphate citrate lyase, an enzyme upstream of 3-hydroxy-3-methylglutaryl-CoA reductase (the target of statins) in the cholesterol biosynthesis pathway.

Two randomized controlled trials that evaluated the safety and LDL-cholesterol–lowering efficacy of this drug have been published. In both trials, patients with either established cardiovascular disease or heterozygous familial hypercholesterolemia were randomly assigned to bempedoic acid (180 mg once daily) or placebo in a 2:1 ratio and followed up for 52 weeks. The CLEAR Harmony trial enrolled 2230 patients taking maximally tolerated dosages of a statin (6.6% taking low-intensity statin therapy, 43.5% taking moderate-intensity statin therapy, and 49.9% taking high-intensity statin therapy). The baseline LDL-cholesterol concentration had to be above 70 mg/dL (>1.81 mmol/L). The primary endpoint of safety (any adverse event) was similar in the 2 groups who were randomly assigned to placebo vs bempedoic acid (78.5% vs 78.7%, respectively), as was the endpoint of serious adverse events. At week 12, bempedoic acid reduced the mean LDL-cholesterol concentration by 19.2 mg/dL (0.50 mmol/L), representing a change of −16.5% from baseline (difference vs placebo in change from baseline, −18.1%; P < .001). There was a trend toward a greater LDL-cholesterol–lowering response of bempedoic acid in patients receiving a low- to moderate-intensity statin (−20.0%) compared with those receiving a high-intensity statin (−17.5%). The CLEAR Wisdom trial enrolled 779 patients receiving maximally tolerated lipid-lowering therapies and whose baseline LDL-cholesterol concentration was at least 100 mg/dL (≥2.59 mmol/L). The primary efficacy endpoint of the percentage change in LDL cholesterol from baseline to week 12 was significantly lower with bempedoic acid than with placebo (−15.1% vs −2.4%; 97.6 mg/dL vs 122.8 mg/dL, respectively). Adverse events included elevated uric acid in a higher percentage of patients receiving active treatment. Measuring serum uric acid and stabilizing patients with active gout before starting bempedoic acid is advised.

The other lipid-lowering agents listed—fenofibrate (Answer C), niacin (Answer D), and omega-3 fatty acids (Answer E)—have not been shown to reduce MACE outcomes in patients in secondary prevention.

Changing atorvastatin to rousouvastatin (Answer A) would not result in more incremental LDL-cholesterol lowering that is needed to achieve this patient's target concentration.

EDUCATIONAL OBJECTIVE

Explain the benefits of bempedoic acid in patients with familial hypercholesterolemia.

REFERENCE(S)

Ray KK, Bays HE, Catapano AL, et al; CLEAR Harmony Trial. Safety and efficacy of bempedoic acid to reduce LDL cholesterol. *N Engl J Med.* 2019;380(11):1022-1032. PMID: 30865796

Goldberg AC, Leiter LA, Stroes ESG, et al. Effect of bempedoic acid vs placebo added to maximally tolerated statins on low-density lipoprotein cholesterol in patients at high risk for cardiovascular disease: the CLEAR Wisdom Randomized Clinical Trial. *JAMA.* 2019;322(18):1780-1788. PMID: 31714986

6

ANSWER: D) Semaglutide

Semaglutide (Answer D) is a long-acting GLP-1 receptor agonist with structural modifications to reduce renal clearance and decrease degradation by DPP-4, resulting in slower degradation and allowing for once-weekly subcutaneous or once-daily oral dosing. Semaglutide results in significant weight loss compared with placebo and confers benefits in terms of diabetes and lowering cardiovascular disease risk. Semaglutide also reduces liver injury from nonalcoholic fatty liver disease in overweight patients. All GLP-1 receptor agonists slow gastric emptying and can cause nausea. They are contraindicated in pregnancy, in patients with a personal or family history of medullary thyroid cancer, and in patients with a history of pancreatitis.

Orlistat (Answer B) induces some weight loss but has not been shown to alter cardiovascular disease risk or liver fat levels.

Phentermine (Answer C) is a stimulant and appetite suppressant that leads to weight loss without other benefits.

Bupropion (Answer A) reduces appetite and induces weight loss, but it does not have benefits with respect to cardiovascular disease or liver fat levels.

EDUCATIONAL OBJECTIVE

Explain the benefits of GLP-1 receptor agonists for weight loss.

REFERENCE(S)

Sorli C, Harashima S-I, Tsoukas GM, et al. Efficacy and safety of once-weekly semaglutide monotherapy versus placebo in patients with type 2 diabetes (SUSTAIN 1): a double-blind, randomised, placebo-controlled, parallel-group, multinational, multicentre phase 3a trial. *Lancet Diabetes Endocrinol.* 2017;5(4):251-260. PMID: 28110911

Seino Y, Terauchi Y, Osonoi T, et al. Safety and efficacy of semaglutide once weekly vs sitagliptin once daily, both as monotherapy in Japanese people with type 2 diabetes. *Diabetes Obes Metab.* 2018;20(2):378-388. PMID: 28786547

7

ANSWER: B) Calculate FIB-4 score and consider liver elastography

Nonalcoholic fatty liver disease commonly occurs in patients with type 2 diabetes, and approximately 15% of patients with type 2 diabetes in general endocrinology clinics have evidence of inflammation and fibrosis determined by liver biopsy. Screening for nonalcoholic steatohepatitis (Answer B) is critical in overweight patients with type 2 diabetes because liver steatosis can progress to liver cirrhosis and hepatocellular carcinoma. Liver scores to assess liver injury are validated, noninvasive screening measures. Several liver scores are used clinically; if the FIB-4 score is abnormal, then assessment with vibration-controlled transient elastography or other imaging can be recommended. FIB-4 uses the clinical parameters of age, AST, ALT, and platelets. A FIB-4 index greater than 3.25 indicates suspicion for liver scarring and warrants additional testing. A FIB-4 index less than 1.45 has a negative predictive value of 94.7% to exclude severe fibrosis with a sensitivity of 74.3%. A FIB-4 index higher than 3.25 has a positive predictive value of 82.1% for confirming the existence of significant fibrosis (F3-F4) with a specificity of 98.2%.

Nonalcoholic fatty liver disease/nonalcoholic steatohepatitis can be present even when liver transaminase levels are normal (thus, Answer C is incorrect).

Although it is important to check for secondary causes of liver fibrosis (Answer A), this choice does not best address direct assessment for nonalcoholic steatohepatitis. In patients with an abnormal liver score and/or imaging, secondary causes of liver disease should be evaluated.

Liver ultrasonography (Answer D) can detect steatosis but does not assess for fibrosis. Liver biopsy is the gold standard for diagnosing nonalcoholic steatohepatitis. There is insufficient evidence to recommend use of vitamin E in patients with diabetes. However, some antidiabetes agents (pioglitazone, liraglutide, and semaglutide) have been shown to reduce features of nonalcoholic steatohepatitis in patients with diabetes.

EDUCATIONAL OBJECTIVE
Assess for nonalcoholic steatohepatitis in patients with type 2 diabetes mellitus.

REFERENCE(S)
Angulo P, Keach JC, Batts KP, Lindor KD. Independent predictors of liver fibrosis in patients with nonalcoholic steatohepatitis. *Hepatology.* 1999;30(6):1356-1362. PMID: 10573511

Dixon JB, Bhathal PS, O'Brien PE. Nonalcoholic fatty liver disease: predictors of nonalcoholic steato-hepatitis and liver fibrosis in the severely obese. *Gastroenterology.* 2001;121(1):91-100. PMID: 11438497

Angulo P, Hui JM, Marchesini G, et al. The NAFLD fibrosis score: a noninvasive system that identifies liver fibrosis in patients with NAFLD. *Hepatology.* 2007;45(4):846-854. PMID: 17393509

8 ANSWER: A) DASH diet

The DASH diet (Answer A) is a healthy eating plan designed to help treat or prevent high blood pressure (hypertension). The DASH diet includes foods that are rich in potassium, calcium, and magnesium. These nutrients help control blood pressure. The diet limits foods that are high in sodium, saturated fat, and added sugars. The DASH diet has documented benefits to reduce mortality, hypertension, gout, prediabetes, and colorectal cancer but does not affect ulcerative colitis.

Ketogenic diets (Answer C) increase uric acid and may worsen gout in some patients. A vegan diet (Answer E), meal replacement shake plan (Answer D), and gluten-free diet (Answer B) have not demonstrated proven benefits with respect to all of this patient's comorbidities.

EDUCATIONAL OBJECTIVE
List expected benefits of the DASH diet.

REFERENCE(S)
Appel LJ, Moore TJ, Obarzanek E, et al. A clinical trial of the effects of dietary patterns on blood pressure. DASH Collaborative Research Group. *N Engl J Med.* 1997;336(16):1117-1124. PMID: 9099655

Sacks FM, Svetkey LP, Vollmer WM, et al; DASH-Sodium Collaborative Research Group. Effects on blood pressure of reduced dietary sodium and the Dietary Approaches to Stop Hypertension (DASH) diet. DASH-Sodium Collaborative Research Group. *N Engl J Med.* 2001;344(1):3-10. PMID: 11336953

Appel LJ, Champagne CM, Harsha DW, et al; Writing Group of the PREMIER Collaborative Research Group. Effects of comprehensive lifestyle modification on blood pressure control: main results of the PREMIER clinical trial. *JAMA.* 2003;289(16):2083-2093. PMID: 12709466

9 ANSWER: D) Lipoprotein lipase deficiency

This patient has marked hypertriglyceridemia. Lipoprotein lipase (LPL) is the enzyme that is responsible for the catabolism of triglyceride-rich lipoprotein particles. Deficiency of LPL (Answer D) therefore will produce this phenotype. LPL has a cofactor: apolipoprotein C2. Deficiency of apolipoprotein C2 can also produce this clinical picture. Individuals with severe hypertriglyceridemia develop eruptive xanthomas, which are the skin lesions described in this patient.

The apolipoprotein *E2/E2* phenotype (Answer A) is present in patients with dysbetalipoproteinemia, which is also referred to as type III hyperlipidemia, or broad-beta disease. Classic skin manifestations include tuberoeruptive lesions on the elbows and palmar xanthomas. The apolipoprotein *E2/E2* phenotype occurs in approximately 1 in 100 persons, but development of characteristic dyslipidemia is infrequent and usually appears later in life due to acquired medical conditions such as hypothyroidism, obesity, diabetes mellitus, or estrogen replacement therapy.

ATP-binding cassette A1 (ABCA1) is a protein involved in moving cholesterol from peripheral tissues onto HDL particles. Deficiency of this protein (Answer B) results in the condition known as Tangier disease, characterized by very low HDL-cholesterol levels and the classic physical examination finding of orange tonsils, which this patient does not have.

LDL-receptor deficiency (Answer C) results in the condition known as familial hypercholesterolemia. Patients with familial hypercholesterolemia have very high LDL-cholesterol levels, tendinous xanthomas, and premature coronary artery disease.

Overproduction of apolipoprotein B (Answer E) is the underlying problem in patients with familial combined hyperlipidemia. These individuals can have modest elevations in either triglycerides, LDL cholesterol, or both. This condition is associated with atherosclerotic cardiovascular disease; however, the degree of triglyceride elevation seen in this condition is not as high as it is in this patient, and it is not associated with eruptive xanthomas.

EDUCATIONAL OBJECTIVE
Identify the clinical features of genetic hyperlipidemias.

REFERENCE(S)
Garg A, Simha V. Update of dyslipidemia. *J Clin Endocrinol Metab.* 2007;92(5):1581-1589. PMID: 17483372

Berglund L, Brunzell JD, Goldberg AC, et al; Endocrine Society. Evaluation and treatment of hypertriglyceridemia: an Endocrine Society clinical practice guideline. *J Clin Endocrinol Metab.* 2012;97(9):2969-2989. PMID: 22962670

10 ANSWER: A) Ghrelin receptor antagonist

The discovery of leptin in 1994 expanded our understanding of the hypothalamic regulation of appetite and body weight. Studies over subsequent years identified 2 sets of neurons located in the arcuate nucleus of the hypothalamus. One group of neurons coproduces agouti-related protein (AGRP) and neuropeptide Y (NPY) that stimulate feeding. Another adjacent group of neurons synthesize pro-opiomelanocortin (POMC), which results in the secretion of α-melanocyte–stimulating hormone (α-MSH) that inhibits food intake by binding to and activating neuronal melanocortin 4 receptor (MCR4) on downstream neurons located in the paraventricular nucleus of the hypothalamus. Leptin, produced by adipose tissue, and ghrelin, produced by the gastrointestinal tract, act like the gas and brake pedals of a car to adjust food intake, with leptin inhibiting food intake and ghrelin stimulating it. Leptin acts by inhibiting AGRP neurons and stimulating POMC neurons, while ghrelin inhibits POMC neurons. Ghrelin is made in the stomach and small intestine but needs to be modified by the addition of a fatty acid (octanoate) to be active.

Ghrelin is an appetite stimulant, so a drug that is a ghrelin receptor antagonist (Answer A) would be predicted to inhibit appetite and produce weight loss. To become active, ghrelin undergoes a secondary modification by the addition of a fatty acid (octanoylation) by an enzyme called ghrelin O-acyltransferase (GOAT). Drugs are currently being developed that inhibit this enzyme as an alternative strategy to reduce ghrelin action.

One would predict that a medication that is an agonist of the appetite stimulant NPY (Answer E) would cause weight gain.

Since the function of MC4R is to reduce food intake, an antagonist of this peptide (Answer D) would also stimulate appetite and increase weight.

GLP-1 acts centrally to reduce appetite. One GLP-1 receptor agonist, liraglutide, is now FDA approved for weight loss. However, a GLP-1 receptor antagonist (Answer B) would be predicted to do the opposite: increase, not reduce, appetite.

Similarly, leptin induces satiety and facilitates weight loss, so a leptin antagonist (Answer C) would reduce satiety and may increase weight.

EDUCATIONAL OBJECTIVE
Explain the neurotransmitter and hormonal systems in the hypothalamus that regulate feeding.

REFERENCE(S)
Morton GJ, Meek TH, Schwartz MW. Neurobiology of food intake in health and disease. *Nat Rev Neurosci.* 2014;15(6):367-378. PMID: 24840801

Sohn JW, Elmquist JK, Williams KW. Neuronal circuits that regulate feeding behavior and metabolism. *Trends Neurosci.* 2013;36(9):504-512. PMID: 23790727

Al Massadi O, Tschöp MH, Tong J. Ghrelin acylation and metabolic control. *Peptides.* 2011;32(11):2301-2308. PMID: 21893140

11

ANSWER: C) Lecithin-cholesterol acyltransferase deficiency

The most striking feature of this patient's clinical presentation is his very low HDL-cholesterol level. His phenotype is typical of lecithin-cholesterol acyltransferase (LCAT) deficiency (Answer C). LCAT enzyme is responsible for converting the relatively polar free cholesterol in the developing HDL particle into nonpolar cholesterol esters. Cholesterol esters are then "trapped" in the HDL particle to be taken back to the liver. When LCAT is deficient, free cholesterol does not stay associated with the HDL particle, resulting in low circulating HDL-cholesterol levels. This condition is associated with cholesterol accumulation in the eyes resulting in corneal clouding. Affected patients also have proteinuria that develops in childhood, progressive kidney dysfunction leading eventually to end-stage kidney disease, and anemia due to red cell fragility secondary to abnormal membrane lipids.

ATP-binding cassette A1 (ABCA1) deficiency (Answer A), or Tangier disease, is also a cause of very low HDL cholesterol, but it is not associated with abnormal kidney function. Tangier disease is associated with accumulation of cholesterol in lymphoid tissue giving a classic physical finding: orange tonsils.

Surreptitious testosterone abuse (Answer E) can lower HDL-cholesterol levels—even dramatically. However, individuals abusing testosterone would be expected to exhibit findings of excess androgens (increased muscle mass, acne) that are not described here, and such individuals would not have the eye or kidney problems described in this patient.

Patients with defective apolipoprotein B (Answer B) are clinically similar to those with familial hypercholesterolemia with tendinous xanthomas and very high LDL-cholesterol levels.

Lipoprotein lipase deficiency (Answer D) results in very high triglyceride levels (>1000 mg/dL [>11.30 mmol/L]) and a more modest decrease in HDL cholesterol.

EDUCATIONAL OBJECTIVE

Describe the clinical features of conditions that cause very low HDL-cholesterol.

REFERENCE(S)

Rader DJ, deGoma EM. Approach to the patient with extremely low HDL-cholesterol. *J Clin Endocrinol Metab.* 2012;97(10):3399-3407. PMID: 23043194

Schaefer EJ, Anthanont P, Asztalos BF. High-density lipoprotein metabolism, composition, function, and deficiency. *Curr Opin Lipidol.* 2014;25(3):194-199. PMID: 24785961

Rader DJ, Hovingh GK. HDL and cardiovascular disease. *Lancet.* 2014;384(9943):618-625. PMID: 25131981

12

ANSWER: B) Cholesteryl ester transfer protein deficiency

This presentation is classic for cholesterol ester transfer protein (CETP) deficiency (Answer B). CETP catalyzes the exchange of triglyceride and cholesterol ester between triglyceride-rich lipoprotein particles and HDL particles. In normal individuals, the result is a net transfer of triglyceride to HDL, which leads to increased catabolism and reduced HDL-cholesterol concentrations. Persons with CETP deficiency have very high HDL cholesterol. This condition is more common in individuals of Asian ancestry. On the basis of this underlying physiology, pharmaceutical companies have developed a number of CETP inhibitors. Surprisingly, these medications to date have not been shown to reduce cardiovascular disease risk despite dramatically raising HDL-cholesterol concentrations.

Oral contraceptives (Answer E) can raise HDL-cholesterol levels but typically not to this degree. Their use is often associated with increased triglycerides.

Several medical conditions, including multiple myeloma and other paraproteinemias, can cause problems with the laboratory measurement of HDL cholesterol (Answer C), but in these cases, HDL cholesterol is low, not high.

Apolipoprotein A1 deficiency (Answer A) and lipoprotein lipase deficiency (Answer D) are associated with low, not high, HDL cholesterol.

EDUCATIONAL OBJECTIVE

Describe the function of the cholesteryl ester transfer protein and the clinical features of cholesteryl ester transfer protein deficiency.

REFERENCE(S)

de Grooth GJ, Klerkx AHEM, Stroes ESG, Stalenhoef AFH, Kastelein JJP, Kuivenhoven JA. A review of CETP and its relation to atherosclerosis. *J Lipid Res.* 2004;45(11):1967-1974. PMID: 15342674

Niesor EJ. Different effects of compounds decreasing cholesteryl ester transfer protein activity on lipoprotein metabolism. *Curr Opin Lipidol.* 2011;22(4):288-295. PMID: 21587074

Rader DJ, Hovingh GK. HDL and cardiovascular disease. *Lancet.* 2014;384(9943):618-625. PMID: 25131981

13 ANSWER: E) Any diet to which the patient can adhere

Despite years of study and numerous randomized controlled trials, confusion and controversy persist regarding the question of which diet is best for weight loss. However, the single most important factor predicting success in losing weight on any diet is the ability of the person to adhere to the diet (Answer E).

While there are studies suggesting that intermittent fasting (Answer B) and low-carbohydrate diets (Answer C) produce greater weight loss, especially over the short term, the extensive evidence review conducted as part of the 2013 American Heart Association, American College of Cardiology, Obesity Society Guideline for the Management of Overweight and Obesity in Adults concludes that one should "Prescribe a calorie-restricted diet for obese and overweight individuals who would benefit from weight loss, based on the patient's preferences and health status, and preferably refer to a nutrition professional" for counseling. A variety of dietary approaches can produce weight loss in overweight and obese adults. The guideline specifically comments on 15 different dietary approaches, including high-protein (Answer A), low-fat, low-carbohydrate, low-glycemic index, Mediterranean diet (Answer D), and others and concludes that all of these dietary approaches work if they result in restriction of energy intake. No one dietary approach is viewed as superior to the others when considered for their effectiveness in producing weight loss.

EDUCATIONAL OBJECTIVE

Summarize the dietary strategies advocated in the recent obesity guidelines.

REFERENCE(S)

Jensen MD, Ryan DH, Apovian CM, et al; American College of Cardiology/American Heart Association Task Force on Practice Guidelines; Obesity Society. 2013 AHA/ACC/TOS guideline for the management of overweight and obesity in adults: a report of the American College of Cardiology/ American Heart Association Task Force on Practice Guidelines and The Obesity Society. *Circulation.* 2014;129(25 Suppl 2):S102-S138. PMID: 24222017

Bazzano LA, Hu T, Reynolds K, et al. Effects of low-carbohydrate and low-fat diets: a randomized trial. *Ann Intern Med.* 2014;161(5):309-318. PMID: 25178568

14 ANSWER: A) Cerebrotendinous xanthomatosis

This patient's surprising feature is the presence of tendinous xanthomas with normal LDL-cholesterol levels. The degree of LDL-cholesterol elevation distinguishes familial hypercholesterolemia and heterozygous forms of familial hypercholesterolemia (in which there are moderate to marked elevations) from cerebrotendinous xanthomatosis (Answer A) and sitosterolemia (Answer E) (in which LDL-cholesterol levels are normal to modestly increased). Tendinous xanthomas occur in patients with cerebrotendinous xanthomatosis because of the deposition of a steroid metabolite, cholestanol not cholesterol. Clinical signs and symptoms of cerebrotendinous xanthomatosis include adult-onset progressive neurologic dysfunction (ie, ataxia, dystonia, dementia, epilepsy, psychiatric disorders, peripheral neuropathy, and myopathy) and premature nonneurologic manifestations, including tendon xanthomas, childhood-onset cataracts, diarrhea, premature atherosclerosis, osteoporosis, and respiratory insufficiency. The described patient has several of these findings, and the most likely diagnosis is cerebrotendinous xanthomatosis.

The classic cause of tendinous xanthomas is familial hypercholesterolemia (Answer D). In this condition, the xanthomas are due to the accumulation of cholesterol resulting from the high circulating levels of LDL cholesterol. Although the molecular defect is different, the pathophysiology of familial defective apolipoprotein B_{100} (Answer C) is the same—LDL-cholesterol levels are very high due to a defect in removal as the LDL receptor recognizes the LDL particle via apolipoprotein B. Tendinous xanthomas are seen in this condition as well. Familial defective apolipoprotein B_{100} occurs in about 1 in 1000, while the heterozygous form of familial hypercholesterolemia occurs in about 2 in 1000. The frequency of the heterozygous form of familial hypercholesterolemia and familial defective apolipoprotein B varies with ethnicity and geography. LDL-cholesterol levels are high in both conditions, but the levels overlap, so that it can be difficult to phenotypically distinguish the 2 disorders.

Tendinous xanthomas are also found in individuals with sitosterolemia (Answer E). Sitosterolemia has been associated with pathogenic variants in *ABCG8* and *ABCG5* that regulate sterol transport at the apical surface of hepatocytes and enterocytes. These transporters are necessary for the movement of sterols across membranes in the intestine and liver. This condition is associated with an increased risk of cardiovascular disease but responds well to dietary restriction of cholesterol and phytosterols. The clinical manifestations include xanthomas, premature atherosclerosis, hemolytic anemia, and macrothrombocytopenia due to abnormal membrane lipids. Neurologic signs and symptoms are not part of this condition. Ezetimibe may be useful in lowering serum levels of plant sterols.

Familial combined heterozygous hyperlipidemia (Answer B) is not associated with tendinous xanthomas.

EDUCATIONAL OBJECTIVE
Differentiate among the conditions that are associated with tendinous xanthomas.

REFERENCE(S)
Escolà-Gil JC, Quesada H, Julve J, Martín-Campos JM, Cedó L, Blanco-Vaca F. Sitosterolemia: diagnosis, investigation, and management. *Curr Atheroscler Rep.* 2014;16(7):424. PMID: 24821603

Nie S, Chen G, Cao X, Zhang Y. Cerebrotendinous xanthomatosis: a comprehensive review of pathogenesis, clinical manifestations, diagnosis, and management. *Orphanet J Rare Dis.* 2014;9(1):179. PMID: 25424010

Tsouli SG, Kiortsis DN, Argyropoulou MI, Mikhailidis DP, Elisaf MS. Pathogenesis, detection and treatment of Achilles tendon xanthomas. *Eur J Clin Invest.* 2005;35(4):236-244. PMID: 15816992

15 **ANSWER: A) 2% to 4%**

Studies of familial aggregation of weight have suggested that 40% to 70% of interindividual variability in BMI is attributable to genetic factors. Twins have a great deal of similarity in weight, as well as how they respond to controlled overfeeding and exercise. One of the most common methods used to discover the genes underlying this association are linkage studies linking BMI to single nucleotide polymorphisms across the entire genome (genome-wide association studies [GWAS]). Recently, the largest GWAS meta-analysis ever conducted for BMI was published and included 339,224 individuals. It demonstrated that there are 97 BMI-associated loci, 56 of which had never been described before. Surprisingly, these 97 loci accounted for only 2.7% of the BMI variation seen in the populations studied. The results suggest that there are complex gene-by-gene interactions that are not accounted for by simply identifying the loci in the GWAS. In addition, it may be that the genetic underpinnings of obesity relate to other factors such as epigenetic changes or gene-by-environment factors that are not captured in GWAS studies. Much more research is needed before genetic information is available that will inform clinical care of the typical patient with obesity.

EDUCATIONAL OBJECTIVE

Describe the role of genetics in determining BMI, as well as the degree to which we understand the contribution of single nucleotide polymorphisms to this genetic variation.

REFERENCE(S)

Locke AE, Kahali B, Berndt SI, et al. Genetic studies of body mass index yield new insights for obesity biology. *Nature*. 2015;518(7538):197-206. PMID: 25673413

16   ANSWER: C) Lipoprotein (a) measurement

This patient has a first-degree relative with premature heart disease who sustained a myocardial infarction at age 45 years before being treated with lipid-lowering therapy. This history puts the patient at risk of early cardiovascular disease, possibly due to familial hyperlipidemia. Familial hyperlipidemia is a relatively common genetic disorder affecting 1 in 250 to 500 persons depending on the population. The American Heart Association recommends high-intensity statin treatment for individuals with an LDL-cholesterol concentration greater than 190 mg/dL (>4.92 mmol/L) due to the very high likelihood that they have familial hyperlipidemia and are at very high cardiovascular risk. However, some patients with familial hyperlipidemia may have LDL-cholesterol concentrations less than 190 mg/dL (<4.92 mmol/L) as well, depending on their lifestyle habits in relation to diet and exercise. Even patients with familial hyperlipidemia can lower their LDL cholesterol through lifestyle changes, as this patient did by adopting a vegan diet. Although she lowered her LDL cholesterol by approximately 27%, her LDL-cholesterol concentration remains above 100 mg/dL (>2.59 mmol/L), and her triglycerides are also above target according to the 2018 American Heart Association/American College of Cardiology cholesterol management guidelines.

Other conditions can put patients at high risk of premature cardiovascular disease. Elevated lipoprotein (a) (Answer C), a highly atherogenic lipoprotein, is also associated with very high cardiovascular disease risk, as well as aortic stenosis. Lipoprotein (a) is produced by the liver, and levels are predominantly genetically inherited. Lipoprotein (a) is a large lipoprotein in which apolipoprotein (a) is attached covalently to apolipoprotein B. Lipoprotein (a) may be modestly elevated in familial hyperlipidemia, but it is an independent risk factor for atherosclerotic disease. Persons with a lipoprotein (a) level in the upper tertile have increased risk of cardiovascular disease (odds ratio, 1.7; 95% CI, 1.4-1.9) compared with persons whose concentration is in the lower tertile. Elevated lipoprotein (a) is a strong indication for aggressive lipid lowering through available pharmacologic options in addition to lifestyle medication and a low-cholesterol diet to target a non–HDL-cholesterol concentration less than 100 mg/dL (<2.59 mmol/L) (LDL cholesterol <70 mg/dL [<1.81 mmol/L]). New therapeutic agents are in development that target lipoprotein (a) and effectively lower it in a dose-dependent manner. However, longer trials are needed to demonstrate a reduction in cardiovascular events with these compounds.

Current guidelines recommend screening for lipoprotein (a) in individuals at very high cardiovascular risk and those with a history of premature cardiovascular disease, a first-degree relative with premature cardiovascular disease or known lipoprotein (a) elevation, progressive cardiovascular disease despite maximal LDL-cholesterol lowering, or borderline 10-year cardiovascular risk with need for additional information to inform treatment decisions.

The 2018 American Heart Association guidelines recommend intensified lifestyle modification if triglycerides are greater than 150 mg/dL (>1.70 mmol/L) and consideration of additional lipid-lowering therapy if triglycerides are persistently greater than 175 mg/dL (>1.98 mmol/L) in patients at high cardiovascular risk, particularly in the setting of diabetes, which this patient does not have. For triglycerides in this range, therapy would start with a statin.

Non-HDL cholesterol is considered a marker of cardiovascular risk that includes all atherogenic particles, including triglyceride-rich particles, but it would not add any additional information. Thus, measuring non-HDL cholesterol (Answer D) is incorrect. Similarly, measurement of apolipoprotein B (Answer A) would also provide a measure of additional atherogenic triglyceride-rich lipoproteins, as apolipoprotein B is a structural component of all of them. Its measurement would not add additional information to what is already available in her lipid profile since her LDL-cholesterol and triglyceride concentrations are listed. Her triglycerides could be a secondary target clinically as they are above target for optimal cholesterol profiles.

Circulating chylomicrons (Answer B) relate to dietary fat ingestion, and severe elevations increase risk for pancreatitis. This patient's triglyceride concentration is less than 400 mg/dL (<4.52 mmol/L), which makes chylomicronemia syndrome unlikely.

Nuclear magnetic resonance spectroscopy (Answer E) gives information about particle size and concentration. Nuclear magnetic resonance spectroscopy typically provides information on lipoprotein profiles notable for high concentrations of small, dense LDL particles that are typical of an insulin-resistant phenotype associated with type 2 diabetes. This patient does not have diabetes. Nuclear magnetic resonance spectroscopy is not likely to provide additional insight into her risk of cardiovascular disease beyond her cholesterol profile with elevated LDL cholesterol.

EDUCATIONAL OBJECTIVE
Determine when measurement of lipoprotein (a) is indicated in the assessment of cardiovascular risk.

REFERENCE(S)
Danesh J, Collins R, Peto R. Lipoprotein(a) and coronary heart disease. Meta-analysis of prospective studies. *Circulation.* 2000;102(10):1082-1085. PMID: 10973834

Ma L, Chan DC, Ooi EMM, Marcovina SM, Barrett PHR, Watts GF. Apolipoprotein(a) kinetics in statin-treated patients with elevated plama lipoprotein(a) concentration. *J Clin Endocrinol Metab.* 2019;104(12):6247-6255. PMID: 31393573

Tsimikas S, Karwatowska-Prokopczuk E, Gouni-Berthold I, et al; AKCEA-APO(a)-LRx Study Investigators. Lipoprotein(a) reduction in persons with cardiovascular disease. *N Engl J Metab.* 2020;382(3):244-255. PMID: 31893580

Grundy SM, Stone NJ, Bailey AL, et al. 2018 AHA/ACC/AACVPR/AAPA/ABC/ACPM/ADA/AGS/APhA/ASPC/NLA/PCNA guideline on the management of blood cholesterol. *Circulation.* 2019;139(25):e1082-e1143. PMID: 30586774

17 ANSWER: B) Hypothyroidism

When caring for a patient with hyperlipidemia, the clinician must consider and rule out secondary causes. This patient had relatively normal lipid levels 1 year ago and now has elevated total and LDL cholesterol without much change in triglycerides or HDL cholesterol. The change over the last year suggests that the lipid abnormalities are not entirely genetic but due to something that has changed during this period. The changes described in the vignette are typical of those seen with hypothyroidism (Answer B). LDL-cholesterol and total cholesterol levels increase as hypothyroidism worsens and are increased by 30% in frank hypothyroidism. Both subclinical hypothyroidism and overt hypothyroidism are associated with increased risk for cardiovascular disease.

Sleep apnea (Answer C) per se does not alter lipid levels unless it is a manifestation of another condition such as insulin resistance and type 2 diabetes.

Undiagnosed diabetes (Answer D) would typically be expected to increase triglyceride levels significantly and to reduce HDL-cholesterol levels without much change in LDL cholesterol. This is not the case in this vignette.

Alcohol intake (Answer A) is associated with increased triglycerides and has no effect on LDL-cholesterol concentrations.

EDUCATIONAL OBJECTIVE
Identify hypothyroidism as a secondary cause of lipid abnormalities.

REFERENCE(S)

Pearce EN. Update in lipid alterations in subclinical hypothyroidism. *J Clin Endocrinol Metab.* 2012;97(2):326-333. PMID: 22205712

Duntas LH, Wartofsky L. Cardiovascular risk and subclinical hypothyroidism: focus on lipids and new emerging risk factors. What is the evidence? *Thyroid.* 2007;17(11):1075-1084. PMID: 17900236

Pearce EN. Hypothyroidism and dyslipidemia: modern concepts and approaches. *Curr Cardiol Rep.* 2004;6(6):451-456. PMID: 15485607

18 ANSWER: C) Change from gabapentin to topiramate

Drug-induced weight gain is a common clinical problem. Several drug classes can cause this problem, including antidiabetes medications, antipsychotic agents, antidepressant agents, mood stabilizers, glucocorticoids, and progestational agents. Several management options are available for patients who have drug-induced weight gain. One strategy is to reduce the dosage of the offending medication or to reconsider the value of that medication and to potentially stop it. Alternatively, a behavioral weight-management program can be instituted. Finally, the problematic medication can be stopped and an alternative medication can be prescribed. For example, a GLP-1 agonist or an SGLT-2 inhibitor can be used in place of, or in addition to, a sulfonylurea.

Among available antidepressant medications, bupropion (Answer B) is the most likely to produce weight loss. The weight loss with bupropion is in the 3% to 5% range. Fluoxetine can produce weight loss in some patients, but the effect is inconsistent. Topiramate (Answer C) is a medication that is FDA approved for epilepsy and migraine headaches. Although there are a number of studies in which it was used specifically for weight loss, it is not FDA approved for weight loss. However, there is strong evidence that it produces a 6% to 8% weight loss that is sustained at 1 year. While both bupropion and topiramate can produce weight loss, topiramate produces more weight loss on average than does bupropion.

A number of clinical trials have examined the efficacy of low-carbohydrate diets (Answer A).

These studies show that although weight loss over the initial 6 months may exceed that seen with other diet types, weight loss at 1 year is no different than that seen with other diet types, averaging 3% to 4%.

EDUCATIONAL OBJECTIVE

Identify medications used for other conditions that can promote weight gain and suggest alternatives that are weight neutral or produce weight loss.

REFERENCE(S)

Rosenstock J, Hollander P, Gadde KM, Sun X, Strauss R, Leung A; OBD-202 Study Group. A randomized, double-blind, placebo-controlled, multicenter study to assess the efficacy and safety of topiramate controlled release in the treatment of obese type 2 diabetic patients. *Diabetes Care.* 2007;30(6):1480-1486. PMID: 17363756

Eliasson B, Gudbjörnsdottir S, Cederholm J, Liang Y, Vercruysse F, Smith U. Weight loss and metabolic effects of topiramate in overweight and obese type 2 diabetic patients: randomized double-blind placebo-controlled trial. *Int J Obes (London).* 2007;31(7):1140-1147. PMID: 17264849

Apovian CM, Aronne LJ, Bessesen DH, et al; Endocrine Society. Pharmacological management of obesity: an Endocrine Society clinical practice guideline. *J Clin Endocrinol Metab.* 2015;100(2):342-362. PMID: 25590212

19 ANSWER: B) Thiamine

The symptoms displayed by this patient are characteristic of Wernicke encephalopathy, which is caused by thiamine deficiency (Answer B). Thiamine deficiency causes neuronal death due to metabolic dysfunction of astrocytes within the central nervous system. The classic triad of this condition is confusion, ataxia, and nystagmus. A wide range of other abnormalities can be seen, including cranial nerve dysfunction, peripheral neuropathies, seizures, and psychosis. Because thiamine is a water-soluble vitamin, body stores can be depleted within days to weeks of inadequate intake. The condition typically presents 4 to 12 weeks after bariatric surgery but can occur as early as 2 weeks and as late as 18 months. Although Wernicke encephalopathy is most commonly reported following gastric bypass surgery, it can occur after any type of bariatric surgery. The most common antecedent is persistent vomiting, which then severely limits thiamine intake. Other less common precipitating factors are intravenous glucose or parenteral nutrition administration without thiamine supplementation. The condition is important to recognize, as treatment with parenteral thiamine (100 mg daily for 7 to 14 days, or 500 mg 3 times daily for 3 days) must be administered to prevent serious morbidity.

Although vitamin B$_{12}$ deficiency (Answer C) can cause neurologic symptoms and signs, body stores of B$_{12}$ are sizable, so deficiency does not usually occur until 6 to 24 months after bariatric surgery.

Folate deficiency (Answer A) is uncommon and typically presents as anemia.

Zinc deficiency (Answer D) is rare. It is associated with skin and hair findings and is primarily seen after biliary pancreatic diversion.

EDUCATIONAL OBJECTIVE
Differentiate among the vitamin deficiencies that can occur after gastric bypass surgery.

REFERENCE(S)

Aasheim ET. Wernicke encephalopathy after bariatric surgery, a systematic review. *Ann Surg.* 2008;248(5):714-720. PMID: 18948797

Serra A, Sechi G, Singh S, Kumar A. Wernicke encephalopathy after obesity surgery: a systematic review. *Neurology.* 2007;69(6):615. PMID: 17679686

Mechanick JI, Kushner RF, Sugerman HJ, et al; American Association of Clinical Endocrinologists; Obesity Society; American Society for Metabolic & Bariatric Surgery. American Association of Clinical Endocrinologists, The Obesity Society, and American Society for Metabolic & Bariatric Surgery medical guidelines for clinical practice for the perioperative nutritional, metabolic, and nonsurgical support of the bariatric surgery patient [published correction appears in *Obesity (Silver Spring).* 2010;18(3):649]. *Obesity (Silver Spring).* 2009;17(Suppl 1):S1-S70. PMID: 19319140

20 ANSWER: B) Familial combined hyperlipidemia

This vignette is typical of a person from a family with familial combined hyperlipidemia (Answer B), the most common lipid abnormality among patients with coronary artery disease. Familial combined hyperlipidemia was discovered from studies of families that had many individuals afflicted with coronary artery disease and high serum lipid concentrations. In a large percentage of patients, it is also associated with insulin resistance and metabolic syndrome. Although familial, the phenotype is typically not expressed until the third or later decades of life. Affected family members can have 1 of 3 lipid abnormalities: hypercholesterolemia, hypertriglyceridemia, or both. The lipid abnormality may change and vary from time to time in a given patient, probably because of nutritional factors (weight gain/weight loss). Familial combined hyperlipidemia is caused by an overproduction of apolipoprotein B by the liver. The variable serum lipid phenotype reflects individual differences in the metabolism of VLDL depending on diet composition and other genes present in a particular patient.

Individuals with lipoprotein lipase deficiency (Answer E) have very high triglyceride levels, often greater than 1000 mg/dL (>11.30 mmol/L).

Familial hypercholesterolemia (Answer D) and familial defective apolipoprotein B (Answer C) are characterized by very high LDL-cholesterol levels (200-300 mg/dL [5.18-7.77 mmol/L]) and specific physical features, including tendinous xanthomas.

Apolipoprotein A1 is the structural lipoprotein associated with HDL. Patients with apolipoprotein A1 deficiency (Answer A), also known as hypoalphalipoproteinemia, have very low HDL-cholesterol concentrations (<20 mg/dL [<0.52 mmol/L]).

EDUCATIONAL OBJECTIVE
List the features of familial combined hyperlipidemia.

REFERENCE(S)

Brunzell JD, Albers JJ, Chait A, Grundy SM, Groszek E, McDonald GB. Plasma lipoproteins in familial combined hyperlipidemia and monogenic familial hypertriglyceridemia. *J Lipid Res.* 1983;24(2):147-155. PMID: 6403642

Hopkins PN, Heiss G, Ellison RC, et al. Coronary artery disease risk in familial combined hyperlipidemia and familial hypertriglyceridemia: a case-control comparison from the National Heart, Lung, and Blood Institute Family Heart Study. *Circulation.* 2003;108(5):519-523. PMID: 12847072

21 ANSWER: A) Resume fenofibrate

Serum total cholesterol, HDL-cholesterol, LDL-cholesterol, and triglyceride concentrations increase during pregnancy (in normal women, the increases are by 75%, 40%, 70%, and 33%, respectively). The mean values for total cholesterol and triglycerides during pregnancy are 317 mg/dL (8.21 mmol/L) and 300 mg/dL (3.39 mmol/L), respectively. After delivery, lipid levels slowly return to prepartum levels. In women with underlying disorders of triglyceride metabolism, levels may rise during pregnancy to a degree that puts the mother at risk for pancreatitis, which could have serious implications for both the mother and the fetus. In addition, the development of gestational diabetes could increase the risk of marked hypertriglyceridemia.

Drugs used for the treatment of lipid disorders should generally be stopped before conception. Statins are teratogenic and contraindicated in pregnancy (thus, Answer B is incorrect). Ideally, all medications should be avoided during pregnancy, particularly during the first trimester when embryogenesis and tissue differentiation occur. This patient continued fenofibrate during the critical first trimester. Few data are available on the treatment of hypertriglyceridemia during pregnancy. Omega-3 fatty acids (Answer D) have been used to treat hypertriglyceridemia during pregnancy, but the available data suggest that they are not very effective. However, omega-3 fatty acids may be the treatment of choice in the first trimester. Observational studies and case reports suggest that fibrates may be used safely and effectively during pregnancy. Fenofibrate (Answer A) is more potent than omega-3 fatty acids, so it is most likely the best choice in the second and third trimesters and it should be resumed in this patient. Nicotinic acid (Answer C) is less effective than fenofibrate in reducing triglyceride levels.

When pancreatitis due to hypertriglyceridemia develops during pregnancy, a number of treatment approaches have been used. The standard approach of fasting, fluid administration, and pain control is the best first step. If hyperglycemia is present, then intravenous insulin can be administered. Other treatments that have been tried include intravenous heparin, plasma exchange, lipoprotein apheresis, and cesarean delivery if the pregnancy is far enough along.

EDUCATIONAL OBJECTIVE
Develop an approach to treating severe hypertriglyceridemia during pregnancy.

REFERENCE(S)

Amin T, Poon LCY, Teoh TG, et al. Management of hypertriglyceridaemia-induced acute pancreatitis in pregnancy. *J Matern Fetal Neonatal Med.* 2015:28(8):954-958. PMID: 25072837

Crisan LS, Steidl ET, Rivera-Alsina ME. Acute hyperlipidemic pancreatitis in pregnancy. *Am J Obstet Gynecol.* 2008;198(5):e57-e59. PMID: 18359475

Whitten AE, Lorenz RP, Smith JM. Hyperlipidemia-associated pancreatitis in pregnancy managed with fenofibrate. *Obstet Gynecol.* 2011;117(2 Pt 2):517-519. PMID: 21252809

Nakao J, Ohba T, Takaishi K, Katabuchi H. Omega-3 fatty acids for the treatment of hypertriglyceridemia during the second trimester. *Nutrition.* 2015;31(2):409-412. PMID: 25592021

22 ANSWER: B) Apolipoprotein E genotyping

Increased triglycerides commensurate with increased cholesterol occur in 2 situations: familial combined hyperlipidemia and dysbetalipoproteinemia. The former is due to an increase in both VLDL and LDL and is a relatively common dyslipidemia, especially in patients with diabetes. However, the cholesterol concentration in this patient and her lack of obesity or thyroid disorder suggest that she has a primary genetic abnormality. She has palmar xanthomas and cholesterol and triglyceride levels greater than 600 mg/dL (>15.54 mmol/L and >6.78 mmol/L, respectively) that are approximately equal. This finding occurs in dysbetalipoproteinemia, a disorder that is usually associated with an *APOE*E2/ APOE*E2* genotype (Answer B). This molecular defect is autosomal recessive, but it occurs in 1% of the population. However, only 1 in 10,000 patients presents with the phenotype of this disease. Therefore, it is assumed that there must be additional underlying factors that lead to its manifestation. Apolipoprotein E is needed to clear many lipoprotein particles by the liver, and presumably a high-fat diet leads to large numbers of circulating remnant lipoproteins that are not efficiently cleared. Unlike LDL, the shortened apolipoprotein B$_4$8 in chylomicrons is unable to serve as a ligand for liver lipoprotein receptors, and remnant lipoproteins produced in the intestine use apolipoprotein E as the primary ligand for receptor-mediated uptake by the liver. As an alternative to genotyping, centrifugation analysis of VLDL particles should show that they are cholesterol enriched. Patients with dysbetalipoproteinemia respond well to fibric acids. Untreated, the disorder is associated with a marked increase in both cardiovascular and peripheral vascular disease. Of note, this is the same genetic locus that is associated with risk for Alzheimer disease (*APOE*E4/ APOE*E4* genotype).

Apolipoprotein A1 (Answer A) is an important structural protein in HDL-cholesterol particles. Apolipoprotein A1 deficiency leads to very low HDL-cholesterol levels (<20 mg/dL [<0.52 mmol/L]), but not the cholesterol profile in dysbetalipoproteinemia. Measuring apolipoprotein A1 levels has been done for research purposes, and low levels are associated with cardiovascular disease. However, measuring apolipoprotein A1 would not be helpful in this setting.

Assessment of LDL particle size (Answer C) would not add any information to determine her diagnosis.

Lipoprotein (a) (Answer D) is highly atherogenic and is associated with increased risk of cardiovascular disease, particularly premature cardiovascular disease. Lipoprotein (a) is an LDL particle with a large protein, apo (a), attached covalently to apolipoprotein B that can incorporate into the arterial wall and contribute to atherosclerosis. Lipoprotein (a) may be modestly elevated in familial hyperlipidemia, but very high levels are associated with a significant increase in atherosclerotic disease. Persons with a lipoprotein (a) level in the upper tertile have an increased risk of cardiovascular disease (odds ratio, 1.7; 95% CI, 1.4-1.9) compared with persons whose level is in the lowest tertile. However, elevated lipoprotein (a) is not associated with specific skin findings. Lipoprotein (a) gene analysis would not help to discern the cause of her elevated total cholesterol and triglycerides.

EDUCATIONAL OBJECTIVE
Evaluate mixed hyperlipidemia and diagnose dysbetalipoproteinemia.

REFERENCE(S)

Chahil TJ, Ginsberg HN. Diabetic dyslipidemia. *Endocrinol Metab Clin North Am.* 2006;35(3):491-510. PMID: 16959582

Mahley RW, Huang Y, Rall SC Jr. Pathogenesis of type III hyperlipoproteinemia (dysbetalipoprotein-emia). Questions, quandaries, and paradoxes. *J Lipid Res.* 1999;40(11):1933-1949. PMID: 10552997

Berglund L, Brunzell JD, Goldberg AC, et al; Endocrine Society. Evaluation and treatment of hypertriglyceridemia: an Endocrine Society clinical practice guideline. *J Clin Endocrinol Metab.* 2012;97(9):2969-2989. PMID: 22962670

23 ANSWER: D) Nonalcoholic fatty liver disease

This patient has hypobetalipoproteinemia with a reduction in production of both LDL (cholesterol) and VLDL (triglyceride). This condition is most often due to a defect in liver production of apolipoprotein B–containing lipoproteins because of defective production of apolipoprotein B or microsomal triglyceride transfer protein. With apolipoprotein B, a defective protein is associated with lower than one-half normal LDL-cholesterol levels. This condition should be distinguished from abetalipoproteinemia in which LDL cholesterol is markedly lower and affected patients develop deficiencies of fat-soluble vitamins. The third cause of this syndrome is a defect in angiopoietin-like protein 3 production.

In hypobetalipoproteinemia, inability to efficiently secrete lipoproteins from the liver can lead to nonalcoholic fatty liver disease (Answer D). This is also the adverse effect of drugs that inhibit microsomal triglyceride transfer protein or antisense therapies to reduce apolipoprotein B secretion. The patient should be instructed in lifestyle approaches to prevent nonalcoholic fatty liver disease, such as maintaining normal body weight and avoiding alcohol.

None of the other conditions listed (Answers A, B, C, or E) is associated with low LDL cholesterol.

EDUCATIONAL OBJECTIVE
Identify nonalcoholic fatty liver disease as a complication of hypobetalipoproteinemia.

REFERENCE(S)

Musunuru K, Pirruccello JP, Do R, et al. Exome sequencing, ANGPTL3 mutations, and familial combined hypolipidemia. *N Engl J Med.* 2010;363(23):2220-2227. PMID: 20942659

Cuchel M, Bloedon LT, Szapary PO, et al. Inhibition of microsomal triglyceride transfer protein in familial hypercholesterolemia. *N Engl J Med.* 2007;356(2):148-156. PMID: 17215532

Tanoli T, Yue P, Yablonskiy D, Schonfeld G. Fatty liver in familial hypobetalipoproteinemia: roles of the APOB defects, intra-abdominal adipose tissue, and insulin sensitivity. *J Lipid Res.* 2004;45(5):941-947. PMID: 14967820

24 ANSWER: C) Persons with prediabetes treated with lifestyle intervention

Surprisingly, good data from randomized controlled trials on the benefits of weight loss with a reduction in overall mortality are very limited. However, data from long-term follow-up of a trial in China similar to the Diabetes Prevention Program show a mortality benefit resulting from weight loss through lifestyle intervention in persons with prediabetes (Answer C). Overall, these data are consistent with the idea that while weight loss consistently improves markers of metabolic health, mortality benefits are most likely the result of marked weight loss in patients with a greater degree of obesity or more modest weight loss earlier in the course of the development of metabolic disease.

No data are available that show mortality benefits with weight-loss medications (Answer B).

While several studies demonstrate a mortality benefit related to gastric bypass surgery (Answer A), none of these are randomized controlled trials, which raises the question of potential selection bias. However, these data are growing and are strong.

The Look AHEAD trial (Action for Health in Diabetes) was designed to test the idea that weight loss through lifestyle changes would reduce cardiovascular morbidity and mortality in persons with diabetes (Answer D). Participants in this trial lost more than 8% of their body weight over the first year of the study and sustained a 4.5% weight loss at 4 years. The effect of this weight loss was to improve a range of health parameters, including blood pressure, glucose levels, insulin levels, and serum lipid levels. Unfortunately, the trial was stopped early because of "futility." The statisticians determined that despite enrolling and retaining more than 5000 participants, the study did not have adequate power to show a beneficial effect of weight loss. The reason being that the observed event rates for prespecified cardiovascular endpoints were much lower than had been predicted, making the original power calculations inaccurate. The low event rates were most likely due to the high-quality medical care that the participants were receiving, including good blood pressure control, statin use, and generally high levels of physical activity, even in those randomly assigned to the control arm.

EDUCATIONAL OBJECTIVE
Summarize the data from randomized controlled trials regarding the effect of weight-loss interventions on mortality.

REFERENCE(S)

Look AHEAD Research Group, Wing RR, Bolin P, et al. Cardiovascular effects of intensive lifestyle intervention in type 2 diabetes [published correction appears in *N Engl J Med.* 2014;370(19):1866]. *N Engl J Med.* 2013;369(2):145-154. PMID: 23796131

Brancati FL, Evans M, Furberg CD, et al; Look AHEAD Study Group. Midcourse correction to a clinical trial when the event rate is underestimated: The Look AHEAD (Action for Health in Diabetes) Study. *Clin Trials.* 2012;9(1):113-124. PMID: 22334468

Wing RR, Lang W, Wadden TA, et al; Look AHEAD Research Group. Benefits of modest weight loss in improving cardiovascular risk factors in overweight and obese individuals with type 2 diabetes. *Diabetes Care.* 2011;34(7):1481-1486. PMID: 21593294

Li G, Zhang P, Wang J, et al. Cardiovascular mortality, all-cause mortality, and diabetes incidence after lifestyle intervention for people with impaired glucose tolerance in the Da Qing Diabetes Prevention Study: a 23-year follow-up study. *Lancet Diabetes Endocrinol.* 2014;2(6):474-480. PMID: 24731674

Arterburn DE, Olsen MK, Smith VA, et al. Association between bariatric surgery and long-term survival. *JAMA.* 2015;313(1):62-70. PMID: 25562267

25 ANSWER: D) Phentermine/topiramate

Selection of weight-loss medications should be based on a patient's individual characteristics and clinical profile. Polycystic ovary syndrome is associated with overweight and obesity and significant metabolic dysfunction, including insulin resistance, type 2 diabetes, metabolic syndrome, and fatty liver disease. Weight loss will improve this patient's metabolic and reproductive dysfunction. There are no data to suggest one medication works better than another for weight loss in patients with polycystic ovary syndrome specifically. However, her clinical picture should guide selection of a weight-loss medication, particularly her history of migraines and gallbladder disease.

Phentermine/topiramate (Answer D) is a combination medication containing phentermine (increasing dosages up to 15 mg daily) and topiramate (increasing dosages up to 92 mg daily). Topiramate is approved by the US FDA for use in patients with chronic migraines to reduce the frequency of migraines and for patients with seizure disorders to reduce the frequency of seizures. Topiramate itself is not approved for weight loss. Given this patient's chronic migraines, phentermine/topiramate is a good choice for her.

One of the most common adverse effects of naltrexone/bupropion (Answer B) is headache, which would make it a poor choice in a patient with chronic migraines.

Liraglutide, 3.0 mg daily, (Answer A) is associated with gallbladder disease, including cholecystitis and gallstone pancreatitis. Over 3 years, treatment with liraglutide, 3.0 mg daily, for weight loss was associated with gallbladder disease in 4.9% of patients with consistent risk of gallbladder problems throughout the 3-year observation period. Given this patient's recurrent abdominal pain and known gallstones, liraglutide is not a good choice for her, although it would most likely improve her insulin resistance. Weight loss itself is associated with increased gallbladder dysfunction believed to be due to decreased gallbladder contractility, and GLP-1 receptor agonists are associated with added risk of gallbladder disease irrespective of the degree of weight loss.

Orlistat (Answer C) is typically not associated with substantial weight loss and is associated with significant gastrointestinal adverse effects.

EDUCATIONAL OBJECTIVE

Select appropriate medical therapy for weight loss based on a patient's individual characteristics and risk profile.

REFERENCE(S)

Apovian CM, Aronne LJ, Bessesen DH, et al; Endocrine Society. Pharmacological management of obesity: an Endocrine Society clinical practice guideline. *J Clin Endocrinol Metab.* 2015;100(2):342-362. PMID: 25590212

Yanovski SZ, Yanovski JA. Long-term drug treatment for obesity: a systematic and clinical review. *JAMA.* 2014;311(1):74-86. PMID: 24231879

Garvey WT, Ryan DH, Look M, et al. Two-year sustained weight loss and metabolic benefits with controlled-release phentermine/topiramate in obese and overweight adults (SEQUEL): a randomized, placebo-controlled, phase 3 extension study. *Am J Clin Nutr.* 2012;95(2):297-308. PMID: 22158731

le Roux CW, Astrup A, Fujioka K, et al; SCALE Obesity Prediabetes NN8022-1839 Study Group. 3 years of liraglutide versus placebo for type 2 diabetes risk reduction and weight management in individuals with prediabetes: a randomised, double-blind trial. *Lancet.* 2017;389(10077):1399-1409. PMID: 28237263

26 ANSWER: A) Decreased energy expenditure

Weight regain after successful weight loss is very common. The body adapts to weight loss in several ways. There is a shift in the hormones that regulate appetite and satiety. The premeal hunger hormone ghrelin is higher and the satiety hormones such as GLP-1, cholecystokinin, and peptide YY are lower than before weight loss. This shift in appetite regulation favors weight regain. The shift in hormones stimulates the corresponding anorexigenic (satiety) and orexigenic (hunger) pathways differently, favoring increased appetite and weight regain. Although she is most likely experiencing increased appetite (Answer C) and decreased satiety (Answer B) after successful weight loss, her food diary shows she has been able to maintain her target caloric intake over time.

Total energy expenditure is linearly related to lean body mass. To maintain weight stability, total daily energy intake must be the same as total daily energy expenditure. The components of total energy expenditure include resting metabolic rate, the thermic effect of feeding, and energy expended in physical activity. In addition, total energy expenditure decreases (Answer A) with both a drop in resting energy expenditure and voluntary energy expenditure with physical activity, creating a state of improved "energy efficiency." Resting energy expenditure represents the majority of energy expenditure in a day at 50% to 70% of total energy expenditure. Thermic energy expenditure is about 10%, and voluntary physical activity energy expenditure can vary between 20% and 30% for most people. Although increases in physical activity initially result in increased energy expenditure (Answer D), over time the body becomes more energy efficient and uses less energy for the same amount of physical activity.

Resting energy expenditure and total energy expenditure will fall with weight loss because of a loss in lean body mass in addition to loss of fat mass. In part, a reduction in the energy expended in physical activity is the result of mechanically moving less weight. However, several studies have demonstrated that there is an even greater fall in total and resting energy expenditure than would be predicted from loss of lean body mass alone. Therefore, the decrease in resting energy expenditure has the greatest magnitude of effect in terms of tendency for weight regain if nutrient/energy intake has not increased.

EDUCATIONAL OBJECTIVE
Explain the changes in energy expenditure that occur with weight loss.

REFERENCE(S)
Sumithran P, Prendergast LA, Delbridge E, et al. Long-term persistence of hormonal adaptations to weight loss. *N Engl J Med.* 2011;365(17):1597-1604. PMID: 22029981

Leibel RL, Rosenbaum M, Hirsch J. Changes in energy expenditure resulting from altered body weight [published correction appears in *N Engl J Med.* 1995;333(6):399]. *N Engl J Med.* 1995;332(10):621-628. PMID: 7632212

Goldsmith R, Joanisse DR, Gallagher D, et al. Effects of experimental weight perturbation on skeletal muscle work efficiency, fuel utilization, and biochemistry in human subjects. *Am J Physiol Regul Integr Comp Physiol.* 2010;298(1):R79-R88. PMID: 19889869

Lichtman SW, Pisarska K, Berman ER, et al. Discrepancy between self-reported and actual caloric intake and exercise in obese subjects. *N Engl J Med.* 1992;327(27):1893-1898. PMID: 1454084

Pituitary Board Review

Laurence Katznelson, MD

1 ANSWER: E) Stereotactic radiotherapy

This patient has a nonfunctioning gonadotroph pituitary macroadenoma (SF-1 staining tumor, reflecting gonadotroph origin) with residual cavernous sinus disease following surgery. Given that the cavernous sinus portion has grown in a relatively short period, further intervention is needed to address the tumor.

Another surgery (Answer A) is unlikely to be helpful, as the tumor is in the cavernous sinus and is not likely surgically accessible.

Radiation therapy is indicated, and stereotactic radiotherapy (Answer E) is the best choice to control tumor growth, if not shrink the tumor. Because the tumor is not adjacent to the optic chiasm, stereotactic radiotherapy can be applied, as there is very low risk of chiasmal damage.

Cabergoline (Answer C) has been used in studies of nonfunctioning adenomas, but the overall response is modest. Similarly, studies with bromocriptine (Answer B) have shown a mixed response.

Some studies have used octreotide (Answer D) for management of nonfunctioning adenomas. However, the response is modest and somatostatin analogues are not currently thought to be sufficiently effective to warrant use in this setting.

EDUCATIONAL OBJECTIVE
Recommend a treatment strategy for nonfunctioning gonadotroph pituitary adenomas.

REFERENCE(S)
Even-Zohar N, Greenman Y. Management of NFAs: medical treatment. *Pituitary*. 2018;21(2):168-175. PMID: 29344905

Minniti G, Flickinger J, Tolu B, Paolini S. Management of nonfunctioning pituitary tumors: radiotherapy. *Pituitary*. 2018;21(2):154-161. PMID: 29372392

Farrell CJ, Garzon-Muvdi T, Fastenberg JH, et al. Management of nonfunctioning recurrent pituitary adenomas. *Neurosurg Clin N Am*. 2019;30(4):473-482. PMID: 31471054

2 ANSWER: D) Switch to pasireotide

This patient has a growing tumor and persistently elevated IGF-1 levels despite octreotide long-acting release at the highest dosage approved by the US FDA. The option with the most rapid response regarding tumor shrinkage and biochemical control is pasireotide (Answer D), the somatostatin receptor ligand. Pasireotide effectively normalizes IGF-1 in approximately 40% to 45% of patients and may result in tumor shrinkage. A common adverse event is hyperglycemia, which affects up to two-thirds of patients.

The oral octreotide capsule (Answer E) is indicated in patients with acromegaly who previously responded to and tolerated treatment with octreotide or lanreotide. However, this patient is not responding well to parenteral octreotide, so the oral octreotide capsule is not indicated, as it will not likely be effective.

Adding cabergoline (Answer A) is unlikely to improve biochemical control in a patient with significant biochemical activity and tumor growth.

Adding pegvisomant (Answer B) may result in biochemical control, but given that it is a GH receptor antagonist, it is unlikely to further control tumor growth.

Stereotactic radiotherapy (Answer C) may control both tumor growth and GH hypersecretion, but it could take years to be effective and is unlikely to be effective within the next 6 months.

EDUCATIONAL OBJECTIVE
Recommend the best management of persistent acromegaly.

REFERENCE(S)
Fleseriu M, Biller BMK, Freda PU, et al. A Pituitary Society update to acromegaly management guidelines. *Pituitary*. 2021;24(1):1-13. PMID: 33079318

Coopmans EC, van Meyel SWF, van der Lely AJ, Neggers SJCMM. The position of combined medical treatment in acromegaly. *Arch Endocrinol Metab*. 2019;63(6):646-652. PMID: 31939490

Coopmans EC, Muhammad A, van der Lely AJ, Janssen JAMJL, Neggers SJCMM. How to position pasireotide LAR treatment in acromegaly. *J Clin Endocrinol Metab*. 2019;104(6):1978-1988. PMID: 30608534

3 ANSWER: D) Switch from testosterone to hCG injections, 3 times weekly

This patient has hypogonadotropic hypogonadism (due to surgical resection of the tumor, as well as parenteral testosterone administration) with resultant infertility, as demonstrated by azoospermia documented on semen analysis. Treatment of this patient's infertility requires use of gonadotropin therapy. LH, using the substitute hormone hCG, is always replaced alone before FSH for the following reasons: (1) hCG stimulates Leydig cells to produce high levels of intratesticular testosterone, important to stimulate spermatogenesis, and (2) hCG alone may be sufficient to stimulate spermatogenesis. Thus, the best next step is to switch from transdermal testosterone to hCG injections, 3 times weekly (Answer D). If the sperm count has not reached 5 to 10 million/mL and/or pregnancy has not occurred in 6 months, then FSH should be added (Answer E). Combined hCG and FSH produce adequate sperm within 6 to 10 months, although time to pregnancy may be longer.

Clomiphene (Answer C), an estrogen receptor antagonist, would not be expected to be useful in

stimulating gonadotropin production in a patient with hypopituitarism.

An aromatase inhibitor (Answer A), through reduction in the estradiol concentration, would lead to increased gonadotropin concentrations in a patient with an intact hypothalamic pituitary gland, but it would not be expected to be useful in this patient.

Blockage in this patient's testicular duct system is unlikely to be the cause of his azoospermia, so microdissection testicular sperm extraction (Answer B) is not the first step.

EDUCATIONAL OBJECTIVE
Manage infertility in men with hypopituitarism.

REFERENCE(S)
Marques JVO, Boguszewski CL. Fertility issues in aggressive pituitary tumors. *Rev Endocr Metab Disord*. 2020;21(2):225-233. PMID: 31984458

Farhat R, Al-zidjali F, Alzahrani AS. Outcome of gonadotropin therapy for male infertility due to hypogonadotrophic hypogonadism. *Pituitary*. 2010;13(2):105-110. PMID: 19838805

4 ANSWER: C) Mifepristone

Mifepristone (Answer C) is a glucocorticoid receptor blocker that is effective in the treatment of patients with all forms of endogenous Cushing syndrome. Because it blocks the glucocorticoid receptor, cortisol and ACTH levels may actually rise during treatment, but these higher levels are biologically unimportant because of the receptor blockade. Mifepristone is indicated for use in patients with Cushing disease and hyperglycemia. In this patient, the presence of signs and symptoms of hypercortisolism, including hyperglycemia, improved with mifepristone treatment.

Pasireotide long-acting release (Answer E) is a somatostatin receptor ligand used in the management of Cushing disease, and it decreases ACTH and cortisol. Pasireotide can also result in hyperglycemia as an adverse effect. None of these findings were noted in this patient.

Osilodrostat (Answer D) and levoketoconazole (Answer B) reduce adrenal gland production of cortisol and lead to a concomitant increase in ACTH.

Cabergoline (Answer A) is not indicated for use in Cushing disease, but it does reduce ACTH and cortisol in a subset of patients.

EDUCATIONAL OBJECTIVE
Describe the clinical and biochemical effects of medical therapy for Cushing syndrome.

REFERENCE(S)
Fleseriu M, Molitch ME, Gross C, Schteingart DE, Vaughan TB 3rd, Biller BMK. A new therapeutic approach in the medical treatment of Cushing's syndrome: glucocorticoid receptor blockade with mifepristone. *Endocr Pract.* 2013;19(2):313-326. PMID: 23337135

Katznelson L, Loriaux DL, Feldman D, Braunstein GD, Schteingart DE, Gross C. Global clinical response in Cushing's syndrome patients treated with mifepristone. *Clin Endocrinol (Oxf).* 2014;80(4):562-569. PMID: 24102404

Hinojosa-Amaya JM, Cuevas-Ramos D, Fleseriu M. Medical management of Cushing's syndrome: current and emerging treatments. *Drugs.* 2019;79(9):935-956. PMID: 31098899

5 **ANSWER: E) Pituitary apoplexy**
Empty sella refers to the radiologic description of an enlarged sella turcica that is not entirely filled with pituitary tissue. By itself, this is not a clinical condition but a reflection of an underlying disorder. Primary empty sella is characterized by a defect in the diaphragma sellae that is thought to allow cerebrospinal fluid pressure to enlarge the sella. Hypopituitarism has been described in a subset of such patients. Secondary empty sella is characterized by association of the empty sella with identifiable disease of the pituitary gland. In this scenario, a remnant of a partially destroyed pituitary adenoma with an empty sella suggests that the remaining pituitary gland could have residual function, although the patient is at risk for hypopituitarism. This patient's laboratory tests show mostly adequate pituitary function, but the IGF-1 level is low, suggesting the presence of GH deficiency (this diagnosis requires confirmation by provocative testing). The progressive fatigue and increased abdominal girth could be explained by GH deficiency. One example of secondary empty sella is in the setting of apoplexy (infarction/hemorrhage) of a preexisting pituitary tumor, which may be associated with abrupt onset of headache and, depending on extent of the apoplexy and subsequent healing of the sellar contents, hypopituitarism. By history, apoplexy into a pituitary adenoma (Answer E) is the most likely diagnosis in this patient.

Metastasis to the sella (Answer C) is unlikely given lack of clear disease on MRI and diabetes insipidus, which are common in patients with metastasis to the sella.

There is no clinical, biochemical, or radiologic evidence to suggest craniopharyngioma (Answer A).

The presentation of lymphocytic hypophysitis (Answer B) is usually one of contrast-enhancing, homogeneous enlargement of the sella associated with adrenal insufficiency and diabetes insipidus.

Similarly, neurosarcoidosis (Answer D) usually presents with diabetes insipidus, and it is unusual for affected patients to have acute-onset headaches along with empty sella.

EDUCATIONAL OBJECTIVE
Determine the most likely etiology of empty sella.

REFERENCE(S)
Chiloiro S, Giampietro A, Bianchi A, Tartaglione T, Capobianco A, Anile C, De Marinis L. Diagnosis of endocrine disease: primary empty sella: a comprehensive review. *Eur J Endocrinol.* 2017;177(6):R275-R285. PMID: 28780516

Prodam F, Caputo M, Mele C, Marzullo P, Aimaretti G. Insights into non-classic and emerging causes of hypopituitarism. *Nat Rev Endocrinol.* 2021;17(2):114-129. PMID: 33247226

Montalbán J, Sumalla J, Fernandez JL, Molins A, Simó R, Codina A. Empty sella syndrome and pituitary apoplexy. *Lancet.* 1988;1(8588):774. PMID: 2895306

6 **ANSWER: D) Repeated clinical assessment and laboratory monitoring in 6 months**
This patient has hyperprolactinemia associated with a microlesion of the pituitary gland, consistent with

a microprolactinoma. Indications to treat prolactinoma include oligo/amenorrhea, bothersome galactorrhea, infertility, macroadenoma (particularly if associated with local mass effect), and headache. She has mild, nonbothersome galactorrhea, so this is not a clear indication to treat. If surgery were a listed answer option, then this could be considered, but the decision to proceed with surgery in this setting is debatable, as there is no clear indication for any treatment.

She has evidence of anovulatory menstrual cycles, but she is not currently interested in fertility, so administration of a dopamine agonist (Answer B) is not indicated now. This may be considered in the future to restore ovulatory function when she is interested in fertility.

Serial dilution of prolactin (Answer C) is performed in the setting of a macrosellar lesion and normal or mildly elevated serum prolactin concentration to rule out the hook effect (a falsely low serum prolactin in the setting of a macroprolactinoma). In patients with a microsellar lesion, assessment for the hook effect is not indicated.

In addition, there is no indication to treat with stereotactic radiotherapy (Answer E), as this may take up to 10 years for effect, there is a reasonable risk of hypopituitarism, and there is an approximately 1% risk of malignancy.

Repeating MRI in 6 months (Answer A) is not indicated unless the serum prolactin level increases significantly within that time. Microprolactinomas tend to grow slowly, and only a minority have significant growth over 5 to 10 years. Thus, MRI within 6 months is unlikely to identify findings that would alter therapy.

Given the presented scenario, following this patient with serial monitoring (Answer D) is the best strategy.

EDUCATIONAL OBJECTIVE
Manage microprolactinomas.

REFERENCE(S)
Molitch ME. Diagnosis and treatment of pituitary adenomas: a review. *JAMA.* 2017;317(5):516-524. PMID: 28170483

Chanson P, Maiter D. The epidemiology, diagnosis and treatment of prolactinomas: the old and the new. *Best Pract Res Clin Endocrinol Metab.* 2019;33(2):101290. PMID: 31326373

Honegger J, Nasi-Kordhishti I, Aboutaha N, Giese S. Surgery for prolactinomas: a better choice? *Pituitary.* 2020;23(1):45-51. PMID: 31853793

Petersenn S, Giustina A. Diagnosis and management of prolactinomas: current challenges. *Pituitary.* 2020;23(1):1-2. PMID: 31900881

7 ANSWER: C) Pathogenic variant in the POU1F1 gene

This patient has childhood-onset GH deficiency, recent-onset central hypothyroidism, and hypoprolactinemia. Her history and biochemical assessment are notable for the presence of menses, consistent with adequate gonadotropin function, as well as normal adrenal reserve. These findings suggest that she has a pathogenic variant in the gene encoding the transcription factor POU1F1 (*POU1F1* [formerly *PIT1*]) (Answer C). POU1F1 is important for the development of the somatotroph, lactotroph, and thyrotroph lineages, and *POU1F*1 pathogenic variants lead to deficiencies of their respective hormones. The secretion of ACTH, FSH, and LH is preserved.

In patients with pathogenic variants in *PROP1* (Answer D), which is the most common cause of congenital combined pituitary hormone deficiency, gonadotropin deficiency is usually present as well. This is not the case in this patient. POU1F1 is the transcription factor that acts temporally just after PROP1.

Patients with pathogenic variants in *TBX19* (*TPIT*) (Answer E) present with isolated ACTH deficiency (not present in this case), as the *TBX19* gene product is necessary for differentiation of corticotroph cells.

Histiocytosis (Answer A) is not the diagnosis in this patient, as she does not have diabetes insipidus and the imaging does not reveal an enhancing posterior sellar mass. Acute trauma causing pituitary infarction may result in hypopituitarism and scan may reveal subsequent empty sella, but this patient does not have a history of significant trauma and the hypopituitarism predated the concussion (Answer B).

EDUCATIONAL OBJECTIVE
Determine the cause of childhood-onset combined hypopituitarism.

REFERENCE(S)
Prince KL, Walvoord EC, Rhodes SJ. The role of homeodomain transcription factors in heritable pituitary disease. *Nat Rev Endocrinol.* 2011;7(12):727-737. PMID: 21788968

Bertko E, Klammt J, Dusatkova P, et al. Combined pituitary hormone deficiency due to gross deletions in the POU1F1 (PIT-1) and PROP1 genes. *J Hum Genet.* 2017;62(8):755-762. PMID: 28356564

Majdoub H, Amselem S, Legendre M, Rath S, Bercovich D, Tenenbaum-Rakover Y. Extreme short stature and severe neurological impairment in a 17-year-old male with untreated combined pituitary hormone deficiency due to POU1F1 mutation. *Front Endocrinol (Lausanne).* 2019;10:381. PMID: 31316460

Mendonca BB, Osorio MG, Latronico AC, Estefan V, Lo LS, Arnhold IJ. Longitudinal hormonal and pituitary imaging changes in two females with combined pituitary hormone deficiency due to deletion of A301,G302 in the PROP1 gene. *J Clin Endocrinol Metab.* 1999;84(3):942-945. PMID: 10084575

8 ANSWER: C) Metastasis
The key features in this vignette are the rapid growth of the mass and the presence of diabetes insipidus, and they are most consistent with metastasis (Answer C). Diabetes insipidus occurs because the metastasis involves the posterior pituitary gland. Common cancers that metastasize to the sella include breast cancer, renal cell cancer, and lung cancer. This patient's history of renal cell cancer makes metastasis the most likely diagnosis.

Clinically nonfunctioning pituitary adenomas (Answer A) are usually slow growing and are rarely associated with diabetes insipidus.

Histiocytosis (Answer B) is a sellar lesion that can cause diabetes insipidus, but histiocytosis is contrast-enhancing and is thus incorrect.

Nivolumab (Answer D) is an anti-PD-1 antibody that is used as immunotherapy, and it has been associated with hypophysitis. However, because this patient has a discrete mass and diabetes insipidus, and because hypophysitis is uncommon with PD-1 inhibitors (more common with CTLA-4 checkpoint inhibitors), nivolumab is an unlikely culprit. In addition, immunotherapy-induced hypophysitis is usually associated with a hyperenhancing—not a hypoenhancing—mass on imaging, although this is a variable finding.

Prolactinoma (Answer E) is unlikely given the modestly elevated serum prolactin concentration, rapid increase in tumor size, and presence of diabetes insipidus (rarely associated).

EDUCATIONAL OBJECTIVE
Differentiate metastasis from other pituitary mass lesions.

REFERENCE(S)
Al-Aridi R, El Sibai K, Fu P, Khan M, Selman WR, Arafah BM. Clinical and biochemical characteristic features of metastatic cancer to the sella turcica: an analytical review. *Pituitary.* 2014;17(6):575-587. PMID: 24337713

Ariel D, Sung H, Coghlan N, Dodd R, Gibbs IC, Katznelson L. Clinical characteristics and pituitary dysfunction in patients with metastatic cancer to the sella. *Endocr Pract.* 2013;19(6):914-919. PMID: 23757610

Barroso-Sousa R, Barry WT, Garrido-Castro AC, et al. Incidence of endocrine dysfunction following the use of different immune checkpoint inhibitor regimens: a systematic review and meta-analysis. *JAMA Oncol.* 2018;4(2):173-182. PMID: 28973656

9 ANSWER: B) Glucagon-stimulation test with measurement of GH
Given this patient's history of pituitary adenoma and subsequent surgery, he is at risk for hypopituitarism. He has normal thyroid and adrenal function. His serum testosterone concentration is slightly low, but this is unlikely to account for his more recent symptoms. He is at risk for GH deficiency, which can present with change in body composition with increased abdominal

girth, change in well-being with fatigue and worsening cognitive function (including reduced short-term memory), decreased bone density, and cardiovascular risk. He does have signs and symptoms of GH deficiency, so further testing is important. A glucagon-stimulation test (Answer B) is the best next step. This patient's erectile dysfunction is not likely related to GH deficiency.

Given the patient's adequate morning cortisol, a cosyntropin-stimulation test (Answer A) would not be useful to search further for adrenal insufficiency and would not add to the evaluation. The oral GH secretagogue, macimorelin, is an additional available option for GH-stimulation testing. IGF-1, a marker of GH levels, can be normal even if an acceptable stimulation test documents GH deficiency. In this case, the IGF-1 concentration is low-normal. If 3 or more axes are deficient, then no stimulation test is needed if the IGF-1 level is low. This patient has 1 deficient axis, so a stimulation test is necessary to determine whether he is GH deficient.

Measurement of gonadotropins (Answer C) would not be clinically useful in this patient, as it is not clear that he has symptomatic hypogonadism given his normal libido.

Measurement of IGFBP-3 (Answer D), an IGF-binding protein stimulated by GH, is not useful for the diagnosis of adult-onset GH deficiency.

Morning GH measurement (Answer E) is incorrect, as a random level is not useful in the diagnosis of GH deficiency.

EDUCATIONAL OBJECTIVE

Determine the most appropriate test to diagnose GH deficiency.

REFERENCE(S)

Tritos NA, Biller BMK. Current concepts of the diagnosis of adult growth hormone deficiency. *Rev Endocr Metab Disord.* 2021;22(1):109-116. PMID: 32959175

Yuen KC, Tritos NA, Samson SL, Hoffman AR, Katznelson L. American Association of Clinical Endocrinologists and American College of Endocrinology Disease State Clinical Review: update on growth hormone stimulation testing and proposed revised cut-point for the glucagon stimulation test in the diagnosis of adult growth hormone deficiency. *Endocr Pract.* 2016;22(10):1235-1244. PMID: 27409821

Molitch ME, Clemmons DR, Malozowski S, Merriam GR, Vance ML; Endocrine Society. Evaluation and treatment of adult growth hormone deficiency: an Endocrine Society clinical practice guideline. *J Clin Endocrinol Metab.* 2011;96(6):1587-1609. PMID: 21602453

Yuen KCJ, Biller BMK, Radovick S, et al. American Association of Clinical Endocrinologists and American College of Endocrinology guidelines for management of growth hormone deficiency in adults and patients transitioning from pediatric to adult care. *Endocr Pract.* 2019;25(11):1191-1232. PMID: 3176082

10 ANSWER: D) α-Subunit measurement

This patient has hyperthyroidism, a goiter with high iodine uptake, and the unexpected finding of a TSH value that is not suppressed—an indication that a TSH-secreting tumor is the cause of her hyperthyroidism. Pituitary MRI would be an appropriate next test to confirm an adenoma, but imaging was not listed as an answer choice. Elevation of α-subunit is present in up to 85% of patients with a TSH-secreting pituitary adenoma, and its measurement (Answer D) would be an appropriate next test in this patient's evaluation. The relative increase in serum α-subunit is greater than that of serum TSH, resulting in a high molar ratio of α-subunit to TSH.

Assessment for a pathogenic variant in the thyroid hormone receptor gene (Answer A) may be diagnostic in a patient with presumed resistance to thyroid hormone, but this patient does not have evidence of clinical thyroid hormone resistance despite the elevated free T_4 and inappropriately normal TSH.

In patients with TSH-secreting adenomas, the tumor and TSH secretion are relatively resistant to dopamine agonists, so a trial of cabergoline (Answer B) would not be effective.

A diagnostic trial of thyroid hormone (Answer C) to overcome a relative resistance may be necessary in the setting of thyroid hormone resistance, but it would not be appropriate in this patient with clinical and biochemical hyperthyroidism.

Although she has hyperthyroidism with an increased and diffuse iodine uptake consistent with Graves disease, she does not have Graves disease given the inappropriately normal TSH. Thus, measurement of thyroid-stimulating immunoglobulin (Answer E) is not warranted. Once a pituitary lesion is detected by MRI, surgery would be the best management option.

EDUCATIONAL OBJECTIVE
Confirm the diagnosis of a TSH-secreting tumor.

REFERENCE(S)
Teramoto A, Sanno N, Tahara S, Osamura YR. Pathological study of thyrotropin-secreting pituitary adenoma: plurihormonality and medical treatment. *Acta Neuropathol*. 2004;108(2):147-153. PMID: 15185102

Beck-Peccoz P, Persani L, Mannavola D, Campi I. TSH-secreting adenomas. *Best Pract Res Clin Endocrinol Metab*. 2009;23(5);597-606. PMID: 19945025

Dieu X, Sueur G, Moal V, et al. Apparent resistance to thyroid hormones: from biological interference to genetics. *Ann Endocrinol (Paris)*. 2019;80(5-6):280-285. PMID: 31590893

Tjörnstrand A, Nyström HF. Diagnosis of endocrine disease: diagnostic approach to TSH-producing pituitary adenoma. *Eur J Endocrinol*. 2017;177(4):R183-R197. PMID: 28566440

11 ANSWER: B) A need to increase the hydrocortisone dosage

A number of interactions can occur following initiation of GH replacement. Due to increased metabolism of cortisol by GH, relative adrenal insufficiency may result. Therefore, the hydrocortisone dosage may need to be increased (Answer B).

Similarly, GH may metabolize free T_4, leading to an increased levothyroxine requirement, not a decreased requirement (Answer D).

Oral estrogens can act on the liver to decrease its responsiveness to GH with respect to IGF-1 production. Therefore, higher GH dosages may be necessary to maintain a steady IGF-1 level in such patients. A change in the oral contraceptive dosage (Answer C) is not indicated in this case, although one could consider switching to transdermal estrogen to potentially reduce the impact of estrogen on the GH dosage.

GH replacement does not regulate prolactin secretion, thus increased serum prolactin (Answer E) is unlikely.

GH therapy may lead to hyperglycemia, not a decrease in blood glucose (Answer A).

EDUCATIONAL OBJECTIVE
Describe interactions among hormonal replacement therapies.

REFERENCE(S)
Cook DM, Ludlam WH, Cook MB. Route of estrogen administration helps to determine growth hormone (GH) replacement dose in GH-deficient adults. *J Clin Endocrinol Metab*. 1999;84(11):3956-3960. PMID: 10566634

Fleseriu M, Hashim IA, Karavitaki N, et al. Hormonal replacement in hypopituitarism in adults: an Endocrine Society clinical practice guideline. *J Clin Endocrinol Metab*. 2016;101(11):3888-3921. PMID: 27736313

Yuen KCJ, Biller BMK, Radovick S, et al. American Association of Clinical Endocrinologists and American College of Endocrinology guidelines for management of growth hormone deficiency in adults and patients transitioning from pediatric to adult care. *Endocr Pract*. 2019;25(11):1191-1232. PMID: 31760824

12 ANSWER: E) Start tolvaptan

This patient has severe hyponatremia following pituitary surgery, which is usually due to the syndrome of inappropriate antidiuretic hormone secretion (SIADH). This is the second phase of the triphasic response after pituitary surgery (the first phase is diabetes insipidus, which this patient did not have). Because the hyponatremia occurred rapidly, it is possible to increase the serum sodium rapidly. She has no evidence of cognitive dysfunction, but the serum sodium concentration is very low, so it is critical to manage this appropriately.

Tolvaptan (Answer E) is an oral vasopressin receptor antagonist that is administered daily for up to 4 days, and it is very effective in the treatment of moderate to severe hyponatremia following pituitary surgery. A vasopressin receptor antagonist may facilitate recovery from SIADH in this setting. Compared with the other listed options, tolvaptan administration (15 mg) will result in the most rapid normalization of sodium. Hypertonic saline can also be used in this setting, usually at a recommended dose and rate of 0.5 to 1.0 mL/kg body weight per hour, which, in a patient weighing 130 lb (59 kg), translates to 30 to 60 mL per hour. A rate of 5 mL/h (Answer C) is too low.

If fluid restriction is to be successful, it should be to less than 500 to 1000 mL/24 h. A 1500-mL limit (Answer A) is too high. In addition, the severity of this patient's hyponatremia dictates that fluid restriction alone would not be appropriate.

Demeclocycline (Answer B) causes partial nephrogenic diabetes insipidus and can be useful for patients with chronic, symptomatic hyponatremia, such as that associated with malignancy; it is generally not used when hyponatremia develops acutely.

Administration of normal saline (Answer D) is not appropriate for this patient, as she does not appear to be hypovolemic, and normal saline administration may further lower the sodium in a patient with SIADH.

EDUCATIONAL OBJECTIVE
Manage severe hyponatremia in the postoperative setting following transsphenoidal surgery.

REFERENCE(S)

Verbalis JG, Goldsmith SR, Greenberg A, et al. Diagnosis, evaluation, and treatment of hyponatremia: expert panel recommendations. *Am J Med.* 2013;126(10 Suppl 1):S1-S42. PMID: 24074529

Jahangiri A, Wagner J, Tran MT, et al. Factors predicting postoperative hyponatremia and efficacy of hyponatremia management strategies after more than 1000 pituitary operations. *J Neurosurg.* 2013;119(6):1478-1483. PMID: 23971964

Woodmansee WW, Carmichael J, Kelly D, Katznelson L; AACE Neuroendocrine and Pituitary Scientific Committee. American Association of Clinical Endocrinologists and American College of Endocrinology disease state clinical review: postoperative management following pituitary surgery. *Endocr Pract.* 2015;21(7):832-838. PMID: 26172128

13 ANSWER: C) Lanreotide depot monthly
Somatostatin analogues are effective in managing acromegaly and are often used as first-line medical therapy. Therefore, lanreotide depot, a somatostatin analogue, given monthly (Answer C) would be the initial treatment choice in this patient.

Pegvisomant (Answer D) is effective and, in the most recent Endocrine Society guidelines, was recommended to be considered as first-line medical therapy when administered as daily, not weekly, dosing. However, somatostatin analogues are likely more effective at controlling headaches associated with acromegaly. As this patient has persistent headaches, somatostatin analogues are more indicated than pegvisomant.

Cabergoline (Answer B) may be used to treat acromegaly, but this is usually most effective with more modest disease. She has persistent residual tumor, as well as a relatively high IGF-1 level, and cabergoline would not likely be effective in such a patient.

Repeated surgery (Answer A) is probably not indicated, as the initial operation was performed by an experienced neurosurgeon and if the residual tumor is within the cavernous sinus, it is most likely not surgically accessible.

Stereotactic radiosurgery (Answer E) could certainly be done if surgery or medical therapy is ineffective. However, radiation can take 5 to 10 years for effect, and she is currently symptomatic, so immediate therapy with medication is necessary.

EDUCATIONAL OBJECTIVE
Manage persistent acromegaly after transsphenoidal surgery.

REFERENCE(S)
Katznelson L, Laws ER Jr, Melmed S, et al. Acromegaly: an endocrine society clinical practice guideline. *J Clin Endocrinol Metab.* 2014;99(11):3933-3951. PMID: 25356808

Giustina A, Chanson P, Kleinberg D, et al; Acromegaly Consensus Group. Expert consensus document: a consensus on the medical treatment of acromegaly. *Nat Rev Endocrinol.* 2014;10(4):243-248. PMID: 24566817

14   ANSWER: B) Discuss surgery
Of concern in this patient is the discrepancy between her prolactin concentration of only 152 ng/mL (6.61 nmol/L) and the size of the adenoma—2.4 cm. Although this discrepancy could be due to inefficient production of prolactin by a prolactinoma, it is more likely due to stalk dysfunction caused by a nonfunctioning adenoma or some other mass lesion such as a meningioma or Rathke cleft cyst. A dopamine agonist could indeed reduce, if not normalize, prolactin levels and correct amenorrhea and galactorrhea but have minimal to no effect on the growth of a mass lesion that is not a prolactinoma. Given the size of the lesion and its proximity to the optic chiasm, transsphenoidal surgery should be strongly considered and discussed (Answer B). Visual field testing would be indicated to ascertain the effect on chiasmal function, but this was not an offered answer choice.

Given the fact that this lesion is most likely not a prolactinoma, increasing the bromocriptine dosage (Answer C) or switching from bromocriptine to cabergoline (Answer E) is not indicated, as neither option would be likely to shrink the tumor further.

Performing a pituitary-directed MRI in 6 months (Answer D) to assess for an increase in tumor size could be considered, but given the proximity of the tumor to the chiasm, surgery is the best next step.

The somatostatin analogues octreotide (Answer A) and lanreotide are not useful in the management of patients with prolactinoma.

EDUCATIONAL OBJECTIVE
Distinguish prolactinomas from clinically nonfunctioning adenomas and recommend appropriate management.

REFERENCE(S)
Melmed S, Casanueva FF, Hoffman AR, et al; Endocrine Society. Diagnosis and treatment of hyperprolactinemia: an Endocrine Society clinical practice guideline. *J Clin Endocrinol Metab.* 2011;96(2):273-288. PMID: 21296991

Karavitaki N, Thanabalasingham G, Shore HC, et al. Do the limits of serum prolactin in disconnection hyperprolactinaemia need re-definition? A study of 226 patients with histologically verified non-functioning pituitary macroadenoma. *Clin Endocrinol (Oxf).* 2006;65(4):524-529. PMID: 16984247

15   ANSWER: E) Temozolomide
This patient has a rapidly enlarging macroprolactinoma that has been unresponsive to cabergoline, surgery, and stereotactic radiosurgery. The tumor is certainly acting in a malignant fashion. However, distant metastases would have to be demonstrated for this to qualify as a true malignancy. About 75% of these very aggressive tumors, and some true pituitary carcinomas, respond to temozolomide (Answer E), an alkylating agent used primarily for the treatment of glioblastomas. However, even patients who respond to this agent for a while may have, over time, a bad outcome.

Additional radiotherapy (Answer B) within 2 years of prior radiation may lead to excessive radiation exposure to the local brain structures, so this would not be advised now.

Surgery (Answer A) is unlikely to help given the location of the tumor mass.

No data have been published regarding the use of pasireotide (Answer D) to treat prolactinomas, nor are there sufficient data on the use of octreotide long-acting release (Answer C) in this setting.

EDUCATIONAL OBJECTIVE

Recommend a treatment strategy for aggressive pituitary tumors and pituitary carcinomas.

REFERENCE(S)

Di Ieva A, Rotondo F, Syro LV, Cusimano MD, Kovacs K. Aggressive pituitary adenomas--diagnosis and emerging treatments. *Nat Rev Endocrinol.* 2014;10(7):423-435. PMID: 24821329

McCormack AI, Wass JA, Grossman AB. Aggressive pituitary tumours: the role of temozolomide and the assessment of MGMT status. *Eur J Clin Invest.* 2011;41(10):1133-1148. PMID: 21496012

Whitelaw BC, Dworakowska D, Thomas NW, et al. Temozolomide in the management of dopamine agonist-resistant prolactinomas. *Clin Endocrinol (Oxf).* 2012;76(6):877-886. PMID: 22372583

16 ANSWER: C) Oral contraceptives

Because this woman does not desire pregnancy in the near future, restoring ovulation now is not critical. However, she has had amenorrhea for 4 years, implying hypoestrogenemia and an increased risk for osteoporosis. Oral contraceptives (Answer C) would supply needed estrogen and simultaneously provide contraception. Studies have shown that oral contraceptive use is safe in women with microadenomas, and there is minimal risk of tumor enlargement.

If the patient's course were followed with observation only (Answer D), her hypoestrogenemic state would persist, putting her at even higher risk of osteoporosis. The dopamine agonists bromocriptine (Answer A) and cabergoline (Answer B) can restore ovulatory cycles in more than 80% of women, but an additional mode of contraception would be needed. Furthermore, oral contraceptives are much cheaper than either bromocriptine or cabergoline, an important consideration in this woman with poor insurance coverage. A dopamine agonist would be indicated if pregnancy were desired.

In this clinical setting, transsphenoidal surgery (Answer E) is less effective than dopamine agonists and carries with it considerably higher risk and cost.

EDUCATIONAL OBJECTIVE

Compare and contrast the treatment options for women with prolactin-secreting microadenomas.

REFERENCE(S)

Gillam MP, Molitch ME, Lombardi G, Colao A. Advances in the treatment of prolactinomas. *Endocr Rev.* 2006;27(5):485-534. PMID: 16705142

17 ANSWER: A) Another transsphenoidal surgery

In patients truly cured of Cushing disease, ACTH and cortisol levels are very low because they have been suppressed by the previously high cortisol levels. Although this patient's current cortisol level is considered normal, it is expected that adrenal insufficiency will be detected following curative surgery. This patient's cortisol concentration never fell to a level consistent with adrenal insufficiency. Therefore, she has residual disease. Repeated surgery (Answer A) should be considered.

She is not currently truly hypocortisolemic nor hypercortisolemic, so hydrocortisone replacement therapy (Answer C) is not indicated now.

Medical therapy could be considered for management of hypercortisolism, but mitotane (Answer D) is not generally used as first- or second-line medical therapy in this setting. Furthermore, an attempt should be made to cure her surgically before committing to medical therapy.

Stereotactic radiosurgery (Answer E) would be indicated only if repeated surgery, and perhaps medical therapy, has failed. Cortisol levels are usually less than 5 µg/dL (<137.9 nmol/L) when patients are surgically cured and hydrocortisone is generally needed for several months, initially for both maintenance therapy and stress management, and then later just for stress.

Cosyntropin-stimulation testing (Answer B) is not useful in the immediate postoperative period because the adrenal glands themselves are not suppressed and should respond vigorously to exogenous ACTH, thereby giving a falsely reassuring result.

EDUCATIONAL OBJECTIVE

Assess patients with Cushing disease postoperatively.

REFERENCE(S)

Esposito F, Dusick JR, Cohan P, et al. Clinical review: early morning cortisol levels as a predictor of remission after transsphenoidal surgery for Cushing's disease. *J Clin Endocrinol Metab.* 2006;91(1):7- 13. PMID: 16234305

Hameed N, Yedinak CG, Brzana J, et al. Remission rate after transsphenoidal surgery in patients with pathologically confirmed Cushing's disease, the role of cortisol, ACTH assessment and immediate reoperation: a large single center experience. *Pituitary.* 2013;16(4):452-458. PMID: 23242860

Salmon PM, Loftus PD, Dodd RL, et al. Utility of adrenocorticotropic hormone in assessing the response to transsphenoidal surgery for Cushing's disease. *Endocr Pract.* 2014;20(11):1159-1164. PMID: 24936567

18 **ANSWER: A) Craniopharyngioma**

The key feature in this vignette is that the patient has diabetes insipidus, which indicates a primarily hypothalamic origin of his tumor. One tends to think of craniopharyngiomas as occurring mainly in children, but there is a distinct second peak in older adults (age 50-74 years). Diabetes insipidus is very uncommon in patients with pituitary adenomas (Answers B, D, and E) and is common in patients with craniopharyngiomas (Answer A). Craniopharyngiomas are typically described on MRI as calcified, solid, and/or cystic lesions, usually with a lobular shape and diameter of 20 to 40 mm. The solid elements are often isointense or hypointense on T1-weighted images, exhibit inhomogeneous high intensity on T2-weighted images, and heterogeneously enhance after gadolinium administration. The cystic elements of adamantinomatous craniopharyngiomas typically display high intensity on T1-weighted images, high or mixed intensity on T2-weighted images, and contrast enhancement of the cyst wall. The squamous-papillary subtype is found in approximately one-third of adults with craniopharyngiomas, and it rarely shows calcification. Overall, the mortality is much higher for patients with craniopharyngiomas than for those with pituitary adenomas. Recent studies suggest that activating pathogenic variants in the gene encoding β-catenin may be involved in the pathogenesis of the adamantinomatous variety of craniopharyngiomas.

The very mild prolactin elevation in this patient is from stalk compression rather than from a prolactinoma (Answer D) and could accompany any of these other tumors/lesions.

Langerhans cell histiocytosis (Answer C) usually presents as an infiltrative disease of the hypothalamus and stalk with stalk thickening on MRI rather than as a mass lesion.

EDUCATIONAL OBJECTIVE
Differentiate among hypothalamic and pituitary mass lesions.

REFERENCE(S)

Mende KC, Kellner T, Petersenn S, et al. Clinical situation, therapy, and follow-up of adult cranio-pharyngioma. *J Clin Endocrinol Metab.* 2020;105(1):dgz043. PMID: 31589293

Zada G, Lin N, Ojerholm E, Ramkissoon S, Laws ER. Craniopharyngioma and other cystic epithelial lesions of the sellar region: a review of clinical, imaging, and histopathological relationships. *Neurosurg Focus.* 2010;28(4):E4. PMID: 20367361

Erfurth EM, Holmer H, Fjalldal SB. Mortality and morbidity in adult craniopharyngioma. *Pituitary.* 2013;16(1):46-55. PMID: 22961634

Andoniadou CL, Gaston-Massuet C, Reddy R, et al. Identification of novel pathways involved in the pathogenesis of human adamantinomatous craniopharyngioma. *Acta Neuropathol.* 2012;124(2):259-271. PMID: 22349813

19 **ANSWER: B) Lymphocytic hypophysitis**

This pregnant woman has pituitary enlargement presenting near term, and it is most likely to be lymphocytic hypophysitis (Answer B). MRI shows diffuse pituitary enlargement, which is more compatible with hypophysitis than a pituitary adenoma (Answer D). Had gadolinium been given, there would have been diffuse enhancement rather than focal enhancement. No data show adverse effects of performing MRI or giving gadolinium during pregnancy, although it is recommended to withhold gadolinium during pregnancy. One of the striking features of hypophysitis occurring during pregnancy is the high risk of ACTH deficiency, and the lab tests shown here suggest presence of central adrenal insufficiency. Thus, glucocorticoids should be administered.

Histiocytosis (Answer A) is not more common in pregnancy, and it usually presents with diabetes insipidus and a posterior sellar mass.

The radiographic characteristics of the lesion are not consistent with a Rathke cyst (Answer E).

Of note, enlarged sellar contents may be seen in normal pregnancy (Answer C). However, the presence of central hypoadrenalism and headaches argues against a normal pituitary gland.

EDUCATIONAL OBJECTIVE
Diagnose lymphocytic hypophysitis in a pregnant woman.

REFERENCE(S)

Zhu Q, Qian K, Jia G, et al. Clinical features, magnetic resonance imaging, and treatment experience of 20 patients with lymphocytic hypophysitis in a single center. *World Neurosurg.* 2019;127:e22-e29. PMID: 30790734

Molitch ME. Pituitary disorders during pregnancy. *Endocrinol Metab Clin North Am.* 2006;35(1):99-116. PMID: 16310644

Khare S, Jagtap VS, Budyal SR, et al. Primary (auto-immune) hypophysitis: a single centre experience. *Pituitary.* 2015;18(1):16-22. PMID: 24375060

20 ANSWER: C) Octreotide long-acting release

This patient has hyperthyroidism, a thyroid gland with increased iodine uptake, a pituitary lesion, and the unexpected finding of a TSH value that is not suppressed—an indication that a TSH-secreting tumor is the cause of her hyperthyroidism. Surgery would be the best option, but she prefers not to undergo this now.

Somatostatin inhibits both GH and TSH, and somatostatin analogues can inhibit TSH secretion from the tumor, as well as decrease tumor size. Given her history of atrial fibrillation, control of hyperthyroidism is the first step. Thus, octreotide

long-acting release (Answer C), a somatostatin analogue, is the correct treatment to administer now. Octreotide is generally successful at normalizing thyroid hormone levels and can reduce tumor size (which is important since it is invading the cavernous sinus). Surgery to debulk the pituitary tumor may be considered on an elective basis when she is clinically stable.

Cabergoline (Answer A) has not been shown to be effective for TSH-secreting tumors.

Methimazole (Answer B) could decrease thyroid hormone levels and help manage hyperthyroidism, but it will have either no effect on the size of the TSH-secreting tumor or it could potentially facilitate tumor growth.

Radiation therapy (Answer D) may take up to 10 years for effect and is associated with hypopituitarism in approximately 30% to 40% of cases.

Although radioactive iodine (Answer E) could treat her hyperthyroidism, it would take months to work and would not treat her TSH-secreting pituitary tumor.

EDUCATIONAL OBJECTIVE
Treat TSH-secreting tumors on the basis of the physiology and regulation of TSH secretion.

REFERENCE(S)

Teramoto A, Sanno N, Tahara S, Osamura YR. Pathological study of thyrotropin-secreting pituitary adenoma: plurihormonality and medical treatment. *Acta Neuropathol.* 2004;108(2):147-153. PMID: 15185102

Beck-Peccoz P, Persani L, Mannavola D, Campi I. TSH-secreting adenomas. *Best Pract Res Clin Endocrinol Metab.* 2009;23(5);597-606. PMID: 19945025

Beck-Peccoz P, Giavoli C, Lania A. A 2019 update on TSH-secreting pituitary adenomas. *J Endocrinol Invest.* 2019;42(12):1401-1406. PMID: 31175617

21 ANSWER: A) Increase in polyuria and polydipsia

Cortisol and thyroid hormone deficiencies increase the sensitivity of vasopressin receptors to vasopressin. Thus, when these hormones are replaced, the small amount of vasopressin still being secreted in a patient with partial diabetes insipidus may no longer be sufficient to effect water reabsorption, and subclinical diabetes insipidus may manifest with polyuria and polydipsia (Answer A). This is particularly the case with administration of glucocorticoids. The converse of excessive vasopressin secretion with hyponatremia (Answer D) is certainly not going to occur.

Although pharmacologic dosages of glucocorticoids can impair libido (Answer B) and erectile function, typical replacement dosages do not.

Institution of steroids should not cause orthostatic hypotension (Answer C). Administration of levothyroxine alone without glucocorticoids could cause hypotension if it unmasks adrenal insufficiency.

EDUCATIONAL OBJECTIVE
Explain the effects of thyroid hormone and cortisol on vasopressin action.

REFERENCE(S)

Iida M, Takamoto S, Masuo M, Makita K, Saito T. Transient lymphocytic panhypophysitis associated with SIADH leading to diabetes insipidus after glucocorticoid replacement. *Intern Med.* 2003;42(10):991-995. PMID: 14606714

Huang CH, Chou KJ, Lee PT, Chen CL, Chung HM, Fang HC. A case of lymphocytic hypophysitis with masked diabetes insipidus unveiled by glucocorticoid replacement. *Am J Kidney Dis.* 2005;45(1):197-200. PMID: 15696461

Sala E, Moore JM, Amorin A, et al. Natural history of Rathke's cleft cysts: a retrospective analysis of a two centres experience. *Clin Endocrinol (Oxf).* 2018;89(2):178-186. PMID: 29781512

Lin M, Wedemeyer MA, Bradley D, et al. Long-term surgical outcomes following transsphenoidal surgery in patients with Rathke's cleft cysts. *J Neurosurg.* 2018;130(3):831-837. PMID: 29775155

22 **ANSWER: A) Obtain a semen analysis**
The first thing to establish in this patient is whether he is truly infertile. Although one might expect that he would be, given his panhypopituitarism and being on testosterone replacement, he may have adequate sperm counts and morphology for fertility. Drincic et al found adequate spermatogenesis for fertility in about 50% of such men. Therefore, the first management step is to obtain a semen analysis (Answer A).

If he has azoospermia or oligospermia, he might respond to hCG injections and may also need FSH injections. Trying these therapies (Answers C and D) before assessing his fertility status would be inappropriate. Clomiphene (Answer B), an estrogen receptor antagonist, would not be expected to be useful in stimulating gonadotropin production in a patient with hypopituitarism.

The chances for fertility in a patient such as this are well over 50% and suggesting adoption at this point (Answer E) would be premature.

EDUCATIONAL OBJECTIVE
Evaluate for infertility in men with hypopituitarism.

REFERENCE(S)

Drincic A, Arseven OK, Sosa E, Mercado M, Kopp P, Molitch ME. Men with acquired hypogonadotropic hypogonadism treated with testosterone may be fertile. *Pituitary.* 2003;6(1):5-10. PMID: 14674718

Farhat R, Al-zidjali F, Alzahrani AS. Outcome of gonadotropin therapy for male infertility due to hypogonadotrophic hypogonadism. *Pituitary.* 2010;13(2):105-110. PMID: 19838805

Thyroid Board Review
Jacqueline Jonklaas, MD, PhD, MPH

1 **ANSWER: B) Measure TPO antibodies**

This pregnant woman has mildly elevated TSH and normal free T_4 and thus has subclinical hypothyroidism. The best approach is to determine whether she has TPO antibodies (Answer B) because this would direct her therapy. Current American Thyroid Association guidelines recommend that pregnant patients with a TSH value above the reference range who also have positive TPO antibodies should be treated with levothyroxine. The Endocrine Society guidelines also recommend treatment with levothyroxine in such a scenario, although the American College of Obstetricians and Gynecologists does not. If she were not currently pregnant, a TPO antibody titer could still be obtained, and it could be discussed with the patient whether to monitor her thyroid status or to consider treatment.

Measuring TSH again at the same laboratory (Answer D) is unlikely to provide further helpful information. When managing thyroid disorders during pregnancy, the American Thyroid Association recommends using a pregnancy trimester-specific TSH reference range. The upper limit of such reference ranges is usually lower than that of the nonpregnant reference range. When such a reference range is not available, the American Thyroid Association recommends using a TSH value of approximately 4.0 mIU/L as the upper limit of the reference range. This usually represents a reduction in the upper limit of the nonpregnancy reference range of about 0.5 mIU/L.

Measuring TSH at a laboratory that provides a pregnancy-specific reference range (Answer C) is also unlikely to be helpful, as the value for the upper limit would probably be lower than the patient's current TSH concentration of 5.1 mIU/L.

Her total T_4 value (Answer A) would most likely be elevated due to the effect of estrogen on hepatic synthesis of thyroxine-binding globulin and therefore is unlikely to assist with decision-making.

Initiation of levothyroxine (Answer E) may ultimately be the best approach for this patient, but this is premature until TPO-antibody status has been assessed. Current American Thyroid Association guidelines recommend considering treatment for pregnant patients with TSH values between 4.0 and 10.0 mIU/L and negative TPO antibodies (weak recommendation based on low-quality evidence).

EDUCATIONAL OBJECTIVE
Recommend the best approach to managing subclinical hypothyroidism during pregnancy.

REFERENCE(S)
Alexander EK, Pearce EN, Brent GA, et al. 2017 Guidelines of the American Thyroid Association for the diagnosis and management of thyroid disease during pregnancy and the postpartum. *Thyroid.* 2017;27(3):315-389. PMID: 28056690

De Groot L, Abalovich M, Alexander EK, et al. Management of thyroid dysfunction during pregnancy and postpartum: an Endocrine Society clinical practice guideline. *J Clin Endocrinol Metab.* 2012;97(8):2543-2565. PMID: 22869843

Thyroid Disease in Pregnancy: ACOG Practice Bulletin, Number 223. *Obstet Gynecol.* 2020;135(6):e261-e274. PMID: 32443080

2 **ANSWER: A) Bone marrow suppression**

Mild bone marrow suppression (Answer A) can be seen following radioactive iodine treatment in patients of all age groups and it is usually minor and resolves spontaneously. Empiric selection of radioactive iodine doses is more likely to exceed maximum tolerated activities in older patients than in younger patients. Thus, dosimetric calculation of the appropriate dose may be safer in older age groups. Adverse effects of radioactive iodine include salivary, lacrimal, and nasal symptoms, bone marrow suppression, reproductive impact, and secondary malignancies. In a study of patients older than 70 years who received a mean activity of 136 mCi, a significant decrease in platelets, white blood cells, and hemoglobin was seen within 3 months of the radioactive iodine administration, all of which remained decreased but within the reference range 12 months after treatment. Platelet suppression was only seen with activities greater than 100 mCi. In a study that specifically studied dosimetrically guided therapy, a nadir in white blood cell and platelet counts was observed 1 month after therapy, which then gradually returned to baseline over a 5-year period.

This patient apparently experienced a much greater degree of bone marrow suppression than has typically been reported, particularly after initial therapy. Laboratory test results are shown in the Table.

The patient's epistaxis appears to be a consequence of thrombocytopenia, thus bone marrow suppression is correct.

Elevated creatinine (Answer B) can be seen associated with protocols involving radioactive iodine administration using endogenous hypothyroidism, but it would not be expected with an rhTSH protocol. Furthermore, elevated creatinine would not be expected to cause epistaxis.

Case reports of intranasal and maxillary sinus metastases from papillary thyroid cancer (Answers C and D) have been reported to be associated with epistaxis but would not be suspected here based on absence of radioactive iodine accumulation in these areas on the posttherapy whole-body scan.

Distant metastases (such as skeletal metastases [Answer E]) do not appear to be associated with more bone marrow suppression and thrombocytopenia in the cited studies, although age and radioactive iodine activity may be influencing factors.

EDUCATIONAL OBJECTIVE
Appreciate that bone marrow suppression may occur follow administration of radioactive iodine therapy, especially in older individuals.

REFERENCE(S)
Duskin-Bitan H, Leibner A, Amitai O, et al. Bone-marrow suppression in elderly patients following empiric radioiodine therapy: real-life data. *Thyroid.* 2019;29(5):683-691. PMID: 31084551

Bikas A, Schneider M, Desale S, et al. Effects of dosimetrically guided I-131 therapy on hematopoiesis in patients with differentiated thyroid cancer. *J Clin Endocrinol Metab.* 2016;101(4):1762-1769. PMID: 26900639

3 ANSWER: B) Long-term methimazole therapy
Practice patterns with respect to the choice of therapy for Graves disease have differed over time and according to geographic area. Radioactive iodine therapy was historically favored in the United States and thionamide therapy was favored in Europe. The difference in practice patterns has decreased over time, and overall methimazole has become a more commonly used therapy. The other trend has involved the length of initial methimazole therapy. Current American Thyroid Association guidelines from 2016 suggest an initial period of methimazole therapy of approximately 12 to 18 months with consideration for discontinuing therapy if TSH and TRAb concentrations are normal at that time.

Time	White blood cell count	Platelet count	Hemoglobin	Hematocrit
Before radioactive iodine	6700/μL (SI: 6.7 × 10⁹/L)	215 × 10³/μL (SI: 215 × 10⁹/μL)	13 g/dL (SI: 130 g/L)	39% (0.39)
3 weeks after radioactive iodine	4300/μL (SI: 4.3 × 10⁹/L)	78 × 10³/μL (SI: 78 × 10⁹/μL)	11 g/dL (SI: 111 g/L)	35% (0.35)
12 months after radioactive iodine	4500/μL (SI: 4.5 × 10⁹/L)	120 × 10³/μL (SI: 120 × 10⁹/μL)	...	...

Individuals who have been treated with methimazole to render them euthyroid can often be maintained in the euthyroid state with much lower methimazole dosages than were initially required. Recent studies have shown that long-term low-dosage methimazole treatment is safe and patients may require maintenance dosages as low as 2.5 to 3.5 mg. Such long-term therapy for 5 to 10 years or more may lead to even greater remission rates. In addition, quality of life appears to be better in those receiving long-term methimazole than in those treated with radioactive iodine therapy. Long-term methimazole treatment (Answer B) would be a reasonable approach for this patient.

For this patient, neither of the surgical options offered is ideal. Thyroid lobectomy (Answer E) is likely to be associated with continued or recurrent hyperthyroidism and total thyroidectomy (Answer D) carries a small risk (3%-6%) of damage to the recurrent or superior laryngeal nerves with potential voice impairment, which could affect this patient's job performance.

Some recent studies suggest that quality of life may be worse in patients treated with radioactive iodine than in those treated with surgery or antithyroidal drugs. As this patient specifically mentions a concern about quality of life, radioactive iodine therapy (Answer C) may not be the best choice and could potentially exacerbate Graves orbitopathy.

A 1-year retrial of methimazole (Answer A) may also not be the most suitable option for this patient, as his TRAb level is elevated, so he may have a risk of recurrent hyperthyroidism, which he wishes to avoid.

EDUCATIONAL OBJECTIVE

Appreciate the data demonstrating the efficacy and favorable adverse effect profile of long-term methimazole therapy for Graves disease.

REFERENCE(S)

Ross DS, Burch HB, Cooper DS, et al. 2016 American Thyroid Association guidelines for diagnosis and management of hyperthyroidism and other causes of thyrotoxicosis. *Thyroid.* 2016;26(10):1343-1421. PMID: 27521067

Azizi F, Abdi H, Amouzegar A. Control of Graves' hyperthyroidism with very long-term methimazole treatment: a clinical trial. *BMC Endocr Disord.* 2021;21(1):16. PMID: 33446181

Azizi F, Amouzegar A, Tohidi M, et al. Increased remission rates after long-term methimazole therapy in patients with Graves' disease: results of a randomized clinical trial. *Thyroid.* 2019;29(9):1192-1200. PMID: 31310160

Törring O, Watt T, Sjölin G, et al. Impaired quality of life after radioiodine therapy compared to antithyroid drugs or surgical treatment for Graves' hyperthyroidism: a long-term follow-up with the thyroid-related patient-reported outcome questionnaire and 36-item short form health status survey. *Thyroid.* 2019;29(3):322-331. PMID: 30667296

4 ANSWER: E) Teprotumumab

A 7-item clinical assessment score can be used for initial assessment of a patient with thyroid eye disease. One of the potential shortcomings of this score system is that the responses are binary and the severity of each item cannot be conveyed (eg, mild vs moderate vs significant redness of the eyelids). Changes in severity of thyroid eye disease over time can be reflected in a 10-item activity score (*see table on the next page*). This patient has recent-onset, moderately severe thyroid eye disease. His initial clinical activity score was 4.

Based on his presentation, teprotumumab (Answer E) would be a reasonable therapy for this patient. Teprotumumab is a fully human IGF-1 receptor inhibitory monoclonal antibody. This agent has undergone 2 randomized controlled clinical trials that demonstrated its efficacy for active moderate thyroid eye disease. Its beneficial effect appears to be particularly convincing for patients with significant proptosis. Mean proptosis improved by 2.5 mm and 3.3 mm from baseline in the study eye in the teprotumumab group in these 2 clinical trials reported in 2017 and 2020, respectively. The main drawback to the use of teprotumumab is its extremely high cost. Other questions are about the proportion of patients in whom the improvements will be durable and the role of teprotumumab in patients with inactive eye disease. Concerns with this drug include deterioration of glucose control in those with diabetes and hearing impairment.

Table. Clinical Activity Score for Thyroid Eye Disease

7-Item Clinical Activity Score (for clinical evaluation)	Patient score
Spontaneous retrobulbar pain	
Pain on attempted up or lateral gaze	
Redness of the eyelids	1
Redness of the conjunctiva	1
Swelling of the eyelids	1
Inflammation of the caruncle and/or plica	
Conjunctival edema (chemosis)	1
Total (maximum score 7)	4
10-Item Clinical Activity Score (assesses for changes over time)	
Increase of at least 2 mm in proptosis	1
Decrease of at least 8 degrees in any direction	
Decrease in visual acuity by 2 lines	
Total (maximum score 10)	5

Adapted from Dolman PJ. Ophthal Plast Reconstr Surg, 2018;34(4S Suppl 1). © The American Society of Ophthalmic Plastic and Reconstructive Surgery, Inc.

Surgical intervention for thyroid eye disease, including orbital decompression surgery (Answer C), is usually initiated in inactive thyroid eye disease to reduce intraorbital pressure and proptosis by removing the enlarged orbital tissues. It is generally not recommended when thyroid eye disease has not yet stabilized.

Selenium (Answer D) may have some role in mild active eye disease. However, it has been less studied in areas such as the United States that are selenium-sufficient and should not be the main therapy for a patient whose proptosis is worsening.

High-dosage intravenous glucocorticoids (Answer B) are considered the preferred therapy for patients who have active moderate to severe eye disease with prominent components of soft-tissue inflammation and diplopia. These features are not prominent in this particular patient; he has mild soft-tissue inflammation and no diplopia.

Azathioprine (Answer A) does not have proven efficacy for thyroid eye disease and also has notable adverse effects.

EDUCATIONAL OBJECTIVE
Review the treatment options available for moderately severe thyroid eye disease.

REFERENCE(S)
Dolman PJ. Grading severity and activity in thyroid eye disease. *Ophthalmic Plast Reconstr Surg.* 2018;34(4S Suppl 1):S34-S40. PMID: 29952931

Douglas RS, Kahaly GJ, Patel A, et al. Teprotumumab for the treatment of active thyroid eye disease. *N Engl J Med.* 2020;382(4):341-352. PMID: 31971679

Smith TJ, Kahaly GJ, Ezra DG, et al. Teprotumumab for thyroid-associated ophthalmopathy. *N Engl J Med.* 2017;376(18):1748-1761. PMID: 28467880

5 **ANSWER: B) Follow-up thyroid ultrasonography in approximately 1 year**
The results of FNA biopsy cytology may yield benign (Bethesda II) or malignant (Bethesda VI) results. Such results are directly useful for determining a patient's management. However, approximately 25% of thyroid nodule aspirates may be classified as indeterminate for malignancy, as occurred in this patient's case. Additional testing may be helpful for cases of indeterminate cytology; genetic testing, RNA-based classifier, and microRNA classifier approaches are all available.

Genetic testing may include testing for strong driver variants (*BRAF* V600E pathogenic variant, *RET* fusions, and *TERT* promoter variants), the more common weak driver variants (*RAS*), as well as other pathogenic variants and fusions with low frequencies and uncertain predictive value for malignancy. The strong driver variants are highly predictive of malignancy, with robust positive predictive values. RNA-based risk classifiers have been particularly useful for ruling out the need for surgery due to their high negative predictive value. MicroRNA testing has shown promise for improving diagnostic accuracy in preliminary testing when it is combined with mutation testing.

This patient wishes to avoid surgery if her cancer risk is low, and testing did not reveal any pathogenic variants. Commercial testing panels for pathogenic variants include Thyroseq v3, Thyroseq v2, and ThyGeNEXT. The negative predictive values of Thyroseq v3 and Thyroseq v2 are reported as 0.96 (95% CI, 0.83-0.88) and 0.95 (95% CI, 0.85-1.00), respectively, in a recent meta-analysis. Results from ThyGeNEXT suggest a negative predictive value of 0.84 (95% CI, 0.77-0.91) with adjustment for disease prevalence in Bethesda II, IV, and V nodules. Regardless of which mutation testing was used for this patient, these negative predictive values are sufficiently high for her to avoid a total thyroidectomy (Answer D). Furthermore, right lobectomy (Answer C) can also be avoided; the number of false-negative results with ThyroSeq v3 and v2 is extremely low. However, because a small number of false-negative results are reported, no further follow-up (Answer A) is not wise, particularly in a young patient, and follow-up ultrasonography (Answer B) to assess for changes in the size or appearance of the patient's nodule is indicated.

The remaining answer option, ultrasonography to assess for cervical adenopathy (Answer E), is not necessary in the setting of low likelihood of malignancy.

Preliminary data suggest that combining both ThyGeNEXT testing and microRNA testing in a multiplatform test, as was done for this patient, improves both positive and negative predictive value. Refinements in RNA-based classifiers have also improved the performance of this diagnostic test.

EDUCATIONAL OBJECTIVE
Explain the role of mutation analysis and microRNA testing in informing decisions about management of thyroid nodules.

REFERENCE(S)
Silaghi CA, Lozovanu V, Georgescu CE, et al. Thyroseq v3, Afirma GSC, and microRNA panels versus previous molecular tests in the preoperative diagnosis of indeterminate thyroid nodules: a systematic review and meta-analysis. *Front Endocrinol (Lausanne).* 2021;12:649522. PMID: 34054725

Jug R, Foo W-C, Jones C, Ahmadi S, Jiang XS. High-risk and intermediate-high-risk results from the ThyroSeq v2 and v3 thyroid genomic classifier are associated with neoplasia: independent performance assessment at an academic institution. *Cancer Cytopathol.* 2020;128(8):563-569. PMID: 32339438

Lupo MA, Walts AE, Sistrunk JW, et al. Multiplatform molecular test performance in indeterminate thyroid nodules. *Diagn Cytopathol.* 2020;48(12):1254-1264. PMID: 32767735

Vuong HG, Nguyen TPX, Hassell LA, Jung CK. Diagnostic performances of the Afirma Gene Sequencing Classifier in comparison with the Gene Expression Classifier: a meta-analysis. *Cancer Cytopathol.* 2021;129(3):182-189. PMID: 32726885

6 **ANSWER: D) Proceed with surgery**

There are cross-sectional studies demonstrating that TSH values are positively associated with obesity and BMI values, such that in one study an increase in TSH values was observed for every 1 quartile increase in BMI. In another study, approximately 10% of patients with elevated BMIs also had TSH values above the upper limit of the reference range, compared with 5.8% of those with a normal weight. BMI-specific TSH reference ranges have been proposed.

It has also been shown that bariatric surgery, with associated weight loss, leads to normalization of TSH values. Free T_4 values, however, do not appear to be associated with BMI and are not affected by weight loss following bariatric surgery. Total T_3 levels may decrease after bariatric surgery. Decreased leptin stimulation of the thyroid axis with a decrease in serum TSH has been proposed to occur after weight loss.

In the patient presented here, it would appear that her mildly elevated TSH is most likely a consequence of her obesity, especially because her TPO antibodies are not elevated. There is no rationale for delaying bariatric surgery based on her thyroid function tests and her surgery can proceed as planned (Answer D).

Significant weight loss is not associated with treatment of mild hypothyroidism. Therefore, levothyroxine (Answer A) would not reduce this patient's degree of obesity.

Further laboratory evaluation with measurement of either leptin (Answer B) or reverse T_3 (Answer C) is not actionable. Leptin levels may decrease after bariatric surgery and reverse T_3 levels may also increase, but assessment of these levels before bariatric surgery does not provide additional useful information.

The patient's TSH concentration is not useful for determining the most appropriate bariatric surgery to choose (Answer E).

EDUCATIONAL OBJECTIVE

Explain how obesity *per se* can alter TSH and that this is likely to be a consequence rather than a cause of obesity.

REFERENCE(S)

Cho WK, Nam HK, Kim JH, et al. Thyroid function in Korean adolescents with obesity: results from the Korea National Health and Nutrition Examination Survey VI (2013-2015). *Int J Endocrinol.* 2018;2018:6874395. PMID: 30250485

Kitahara CM, Platz EA, Ladenson PW, Mondul AM, Menke A, Berrington de González A. Body fatness and markers of thyroid function among U.S. men and women. *PLoS One.* 2012;7(4):e34979. PMID: 22511976

Guan B, Chen Y, Yang J, Yang W, Wang C. Effect of bariatric surgery on thyroid function in obese patients: a systematic review and meta-analysis. *Obes Surg.* 2017;27(12):3292-3305. PMID: 29039052

Juiz-Valiña P, Outeiriño-Blanco E, Pértega S, Varela-Rodriguez BM, García-Brao MJ, Mena E, et al. Effect of weight loss after bariatric surgery on thyroid-stimulating hormone levels in euthyroid patients with morbid obesity. *Nutrients.* 2019;11(5):1121. PMID: 31137484

Chikunguwo S, Brethauer S, Nirujogi V, et al. Influence of obesity and surgical weight loss on thyroid hormone levels. *Surg Obes Relat Dis.* 2007;3(6):631-635; discussion 5-6. PMID: 18023816

7 ANSWER: A) Measure free T$_4$

When this patient's missing medical records were located, it became apparent that he had undergone transsphenoidal surgery for a nonfunctional pituitary adenoma. Following surgery, he initially took levothyroxine, hydrocortisone, and testosterone replacement. However, to simplify the regimen for his family, his glucocorticoid replacement was changed from twice-daily hydrocortisone to once-daily prednisone. He self-discontinued his testosterone some time ago.

While testosterone measurement (Answer B) and pituitary MRI (Answer E) could both be indicated, neither is an initial step and would not shed light on his thyroid status.

Similarly, he is not at risk of glucocorticoid deficiency while taking prednisone, so a cosyntropin-stimulation test (Answer D) is not indicated now. If testing his adrenal axis to assess for return of corticotroph function were contemplated, prednisone would need to be held.

Even without his medical records, testosterone deficiency is suggested by his reduced hematocrit, and hypothyroidism is suggested by his symptoms and possibly by his nonpalpable thyroid gland. The hand tremor is most likely a nonspecific finding. Given that he has inadequately treated central hypothyroidism, the patient probably has both a low free T_4 concentration (Answer A) and low total T_3 concentration (Answer C). However, total T_3 is neither sensitive nor specific for diagnosing hypothyroidism.

This patient's central hypothyroidism was confirmed by a low free T_4 concentration of 0.4 ng/dL (5.1 pmol/L). When treating central hypothyroidism, TSH does not need to be monitored. Free T_4 can be kept in the upper one-third to upper half of the reference range for a younger individual without significant medical problems. A free T_4 value in the middle of this normal range might be safer for this older patient.

EDUCATIONAL OBJECTIVE

Explain why serum TSH values cannot be used to adjust therapy for central hypothyroidism and that checking this parameter could potentially be misleading.

REFERENCE(S)

Slawik M, Klawitter B, Meiser E, et al. Thyroid hormone replacement for central hypothyroidism: a randomized controlled trial comparing two doses of thyroxine (T4) with a combination of T4 and triiodothyronine. *J Clin Endocrinol Metab.* 2007;92(11):4115-4122. PMID: 17711927

Ferretti E, Persani L, Jaffrain-Rea ML, Giambona S, Tamburrano G, Beck-Peccoz P. Evaluation of the adequacy of levothyroxine replacement therapy in patients with central hypothyroidism. *J Clin Endocrinol Metab.* 1999;84(3):924-929. PMID: 10084572

Klose M, Marina D, Hartoft-Nielsen ML, et al. Central hypothyroidism and its replacement have a significant influence on cardiovascular risk factors in adult hypopituitary patients. *J Clin Endocrinol Metab.* 2013;98(9):3802-3810. PMID: 23796569

8 ANSWER: E) Thyroidectomy

This patient's experience is not uncommon; there is a tendency for patients to gain weight after undergoing thyroidectomy. Two meta-analyses have examined this issue. One study documented weight gain of 4.7 lb (2.13 kg) approximately 2 years after patients underwent thyroidectomy for various reasons.

Study	N	Mean	SE	95% CI	Weight Change	Weight (fixed)	Weight (random)
Glick (2018)	79	0.06	0.78	[-1.46, 1.58]		0.1%	5.7%
Lombardi (2017)	155	0.16	0.03	[0.09, 0.23]		68.0%	6.3%
Singh Ospina (2018)	157	0.32	0.57	[-0.80, 1.44]		0.2%	6.0%
Kormas (1998)	8	0.50	0.81	[-1.09, 2.09]		0.1%	5.7%
Sohn (2015)	700	0.50	0.12	[0.27, 0.73]		5.9%	6.3%
Lang (2015)	581	1.16	0.14	[0.89, 1.43]		4.3%	6.3%
Weinreb (2011)	102	1.51	0.77	[0.00, 3.02]		0.1%	5.7%
Rotondi (2014)	267	1.60	0.25	[1.11, 2.09]		1.3%	6.3%
Zihni (2017)	30	1.60	0.69	[0.24, 2.96]		0.2%	5.8%
Bel Lassen (2016)	225	1.65	0.31	[1.04, 2.26]		0.8%	6.2%
Ozdemir (2010)	22	2.00	0.53	[0.96, 3.04]		0.3%	6.0%
Kedia (2016)	291	2.35	0.50	[1.37, 3.33]		0.3%	6.1%
Polotsky (2011)	153	2.70	0.37	[1.97, 3.43]		0.6%	6.2%
Jonklaas (2011)	120	3.10	0.30	[2.51, 3.69]		0.9%	6.2%
Schneider (2014)	204	4.70	0.07	[4.56, 4.84]		16.6%	6.3%
Tigas (2000)	57	6.10	0.72	[4.69, 7.51]		0.2%	5.8%
Dale (2001)	13	10.27	2.56	[5.25, 15.29]		0.0%	2.9%
Fixed effect model	3164	1.07		[1.02, 1.13]		100.0%	
Random effects model		2.13		[0.95, 3.30]			100.0%

Heterogeneity: $\chi^2_{16} = 3554.67$ ($p = 0$)

Meta-analysis of weight changes following total thyroidectomy across the studies (3164 patients, 17 studies).

Huynh CN et al. *J Clin Endocrinol Metab,* 2021;106(1) © Endocrine Society.

Another study found weight gain of 2.1 to 2.4 lb (0.94 to 1.07 kg) at 1 to 2 years of follow-up. Weight gain was less in patients undergoing surgery for thyroid cancer and greater in those undergoing surgery for hyperthyroidism, perhaps due to potential TSH-suppressive therapy and the preceding hyperthyroidism, respectively. One of the individual studies documented a mean 1-year weight gain of 6.8 lb (3.1 kg [standard deviation 3.3 kg]) in those undergoing thyroidectomy for benign thyroid disease, compared with a mean weight gain of 4.9 lb (2.2 kg) over 1 year in those with nonsurgical hypothyroidism. The weight gain within the surgical group was greater in menopausal women than in premenopausal women or men.

For this patient, factors that could not be contributing to her weight gain include menopausal status (Answer B) (as the patient is still experiencing regular menses) and suboptimally treated hypothyroidism after thyroidectomy (Answer C) (as the patient was promptly started on levothyroxine). Her TSH value (Answer D) is also not the culprit because it lies within the lower part of the reference range and is very similar to her prethyroidectomy value. Synthetic combination therapy with both levothyroxine and liothyronine (Answer A) does not usually achieve weight loss if serum TSH is maintained within the reference range. Thus, the best answer choice is thyroidectomy (Answer E), although studies examining whether this is mediated by inability of synthetic thyroid hormone to restore normal physiology, advancing patient age, or other factors are still needed.

EDUCATIONAL OBJECTIVE

Describe the weight changes that may ensue as patients are treated for postsurgical hypothyroidism.

REFERENCE(S)

Jonklaas J, Nsouli-Maktabi H. Weight changes in euthyroid patients undergoing thyroidectomy. *Thyroid.* 2011;21(12):1343-1351. PMID: 22066482

Singh Ospina N, Castaneda-Guarderas A, Hamidi O, et al. Weight changes after thyroid surgery for patients with benign thyroid nodules and thyroid cancer: population-based study and systematic review and meta-analysis. *Thyroid.* 2018;28(5): 639-649. PMID: 29631475

Huynh CN, Pearce JV, Kang L, Celi FS. Weight gain after thyroidectomy: a systematic review and meta-analysis. *J Clin Endocrinol Metab.* 2021;106(1): 282-291. PMID: 33106852

9 ANSWER: E) Recurrent papillary thyroid cancer

Positive thyroglobulin antibodies occur in approximately 15% to 20% of patients with differentiated thyroid cancer and are most common in those with underlying autoimmune thyroid disease. If present, these thyroglobulin antibodies compromise the ability to follow thyroglobulin as a tumor marker. Immunochemiluminometric assays may underestimate thyroglobulin levels, and radioimmunoassays may overestimate thyroglobulin levels. However, regardless of the direction of the error, measurement of thyroglobulin levels is problematic in patients with thyroglobulin antibodies. Although not shown in all studies, thyroglobulin antibody trends appear to have a prognostic significance, thus serving as a surrogate tumor marker. A decline in thyroglobulin antibodies is generally reassuring and indicative of no residual disease. A stable level of thyroglobulin antibodies is also reassuring, although it may indicate persistent disease. An increasing level of thyroglobulin antibodies usually indicates progression of residual disease or disease recurrence.

In this patient, her increasing thyroglobulin antibodies most likely signify recurrent or residual papillary thyroid cancer (Answer E). It is possible that she has distance metastases. However, persistent or recurrent disease in cervical lymph nodes is the most likely scenario. The location of this patient's suspected recurrent or residual disease could be identified by cervical ultrasonography, iodine scanning, or fluorodeoxyglucose PET scanning if necessary.

There is no particular reason to suspect that this patient has developed radioactive iodine–refractory disease (Answer C), as her nodal disease was initially iodine-avid.

The patient received a ^{131}I dose of 150 mCi and had no subsequent evidence of remnant on either iodine scanning or neck ultrasonography, making autoimmune processes in the thyroid remnant (Answer A) unlikely.

If the patient had developed a second autoimmune disease (Answer B), autoantibodies to that tissue, rather than thyroid tissue would be anticipated.

Thyroglobulin itself can be measured using a mass spectrometry assay. This has been suggested as one possible approach when a patient has thyroglobulin antibodies. However, not using this assay (Answer D) would not account for rising thyroglobulin antibody titers.

EDUCATIONAL OBJECTIVE
Explain the prognostic significance of decreasing, stable, and increasing concentrations of thyroglobulin antibodies.

REFERENCE(S)
Spencer CA, Takeuchi M, Kazarosyan M, et al. Serum thyroglobulin autoantibodies: prevalence, influence on serum thyroglobulin measurement, and prognostic significance in patients with differentiated thyroid carcinoma. *J Clin Endocrinol Metab.* 1998;83(4):1121-1127. PMID: 9543128

de Meer SGA, Vorselaars WMCM, Kist JW, et al. Follow-up of patients with thyroglobulin-antibodies: Rising Tg-Ab trend is a risk factor for recurrence of differentiated thyroid cancer. *Endocr Res.* 2017;42(4):302-310. PMID: 28509618

Reverter JL, Rosas-Allende I, Puig-Jove C, et al. Prognostic significance of thyroglobulin antibodies in differentiated thyroid cancer. *J Thyroid Res.* 2020;2020:8312628. PMID: 32351680

Hsieh C-J, Wang P-W. Sequential changes of serum antithyroglobulin antibody levels are a good predictor of disease activity in thyroglobulin-negative patients with papillary thyroid carcinoma. *Thyroid.* 2014;24(3):488-493. PMID: 23971786

10

ANSWER: A) Defer assessment of the patient's thyroid nodule until initial treatment for lung cancer has been completed

The American College of Radiology TI-RADS (Thyroid Imaging, Reporting, and Data System) is used to assess the risk for malignancy of thyroid nodules and to determine whether to proceed to a thyroid nodule biopsy. The TI-RADS system assesses nodules based on their composition, echogenicity, shape, margins, and echogenic foci as visualized on ultrasonography. The incidentally identified thyroid nodule in this vignette is TI-RADS level 5. This highly suspicious category usually leads to a biopsy for thyroid nodules that are 1 cm or larger.

Such incidentally found fluorodeoxyglucose PET–positive thyroid nodules may be identified in about 2% of fluorodeoxyglucose PET scans performed for nonthyroid malignancies such as breast cancer, lung cancer, melanoma, and colon cancer. While this thyroid nodule appears likely to be thyroid cancer and would be biopsied now (Answer D) in the absence of other diagnoses with a significant adverse impact on the patient's prognosis, this may not be the wisest approach given the gravity of his lung cancer diagnosis and the nodule's small size. This patient has a high mortality risk from his lung cancer and a thyroid nodule biopsy could be deferred until his response to his lung cancer therapy has been assessed (Answer A). One study of patients from a cancer referral center documented a 5-year survival rate for patients with lung cancer. Not only would proceeding with further treatment for thyroid cancer have a relatively minor effect on this patient's overall survival compared with the impact from his lung cancer, it would also burden him with the stress of having a second malignancy. Thus, this patient's thyroid nodule biopsy can be deferred until initial treatment for his lung cancer has been completed. He could also be a candidate for active surveillance if papillary thyroid cancer is confirmed.

Measuring free T_4 (Answer B) is not necessary because he has a normal TSH concentration.

Serum thyroglobulin measurement (Answer C) would not be indicated before thyroidectomy even if thyroid cancer were confirmed, as it would not provide useful information about thyroid cancer burden with the thyroid gland still in place.

The tissue from the patient's lung biopsy does not need to be stained for thyroglobulin (Answer E) because thyroglobulin-positivity is specific for thyroid cancer.

In a recent study of patients who had a fluorodeoxyglucose PET–positive incidental thyroid nodule, thyroid ultrasonography was performed in 42%, biopsy was performed in 32%, and thyroid surgery was performed in 6%. One patient died of medullary thyroid cancer.

EDUCATIONAL OBJECTIVE
Consider patient comorbidities and prognosis in decision-making concerning FNA biopsy of small suspicious thyroid nodules.

REFERENCE(S)
Tessler FN, Middleton WD, Grant EG, et al. ACR Thyroid Imaging, Reporting and Data System (TI-RADS): white paper of the ACR TI-RADS Committee. *J Am Coll Radiol.* 2017;14(5):587-595. PMID: 28372962

Piek MW, de Boer JP, Vriens MR, et al. Retrospective analyses of 18FDG-PET/CT thyroid incidentaloma in adults: incidence, treatment, and outcome in a tertiary cancer referral center. *Thyroid.* 2021;31(11):1715-1722. PMID: 34340567

11

ANSWER: D) Raloxifene

Concomitant use of raloxifene (Answer D) has been reported to decrease levothyroxine absorption, although the mechanism is unknown. However, based on limited data, raloxifene does not appear to increase thyroxine-binding globulin levels, but rather it seems to be associated with reduced levothyroxine absorption in some patients. In one study, a 6-hour levothyroxine absorption test showed reduced levothyroxine absorption with simultaneous coadministration of levothyroxine and raloxifene. Separating the levothyroxine and raloxifene doses by 12 hours will alleviate the problem.

Medication nonadherence (Answer C) is a very common cause of TSH elevations in levothyroxine-treated patients and may be associated with conditions such as depression. However, given this patient's history of long-term levothyroxine dosage stability, together with new raloxifene use, nonadherence is a less likely explanation in this setting.

Taking supplemental calcium (Answer A) concomitantly with levothyroxine can decrease levothyroxine absorption by up to 60%, but taking it 4 hours apart from the levothyroxine would not be expected to affect levothyroxine requirements, and the bedtime timing of calcium intake adopted by this patient should avoid any impaired absorption.

Celiac sprue (Answer B) can cause levothyroxine malabsorption, and, because this often co-occurs in patients with autoimmune thyroid disease, sprue is an important etiology to exclude in hypothyroid patients who require higher-than-expected levothyroxine dosages. However, new-onset celiac sprue is less likely than raloxifene use to be the culprit in this patient, especially given that she is asymptomatic.

Vitamin D supplementation (Answer E) is not known to interfere with levothyroxine absorption.

EDUCATIONAL OBJECTIVE
Identify raloxifene as an agent that may alter levothyroxine requirements.

REFERENCE(S)
Garwood CL, Van Schepen KA, McDonough RP, Sullivan AL. Increased thyroid-stimulating hormone levels associated with concomitant administration of levothyroxine and raloxifene. *Pharmacotherapy.* 2006;26(6):881-885. PMID: 16716142

Liwanpo L, Hershman JM. Conditions and drugs interfering with thyroxine absorption. *Best Pract Res Clin Endocrinol Metab.* 2009;23(6):781-792. PMID: 19942153

Skelin M, Lucijanić T, Amidžić Klarić D, et al. Factors affecting gastrointestinal absorption of levothyroxine: a review. *Clin Ther.* 2017;39(2):378-403. PMID: 28153426

Siraj ES, Gupta MK, Reddy SSK. Raloxifene causing malabsorption of levothyroxine. *Arch Intern Med.* 2003;163(11):1367-1370. PMID: 12796075

12 ANSWER: E) Thyroglobulin measurement in the FNA rinse

Multiple studies have described the utility of thyroglobulin washout values from FNA biopsy samples in patients such as the one described in this vignette. This test has the best performance in patients who have undergone thyroidectomy and is thought to be less subject to interference from circulating thyroglobulin antibodies. The higher the aspirate thyroglobulin level, the more accurate the result. Various cutoffs have been proposed for the most accurate thyroglobulin concentration in washout fluid for diagnosing nodal metastases. Washout thyroglobulin concentrations greater than 10 ng/mL (>10 µg/L) and greater than 1.0 ng/mL have been validated. A meta-analysis found a sensitivity of 96.9% and a specificity of 94.1% from pooled studies using cutoffs between 1 and 50 ng/mL (thus, Answer E is correct).

Ultrasonographic findings suggestive of metastatic lymph nodes include long axis greater than 1 cm, round rather than oval shape, cystic appearance, the presence of hyperechoic punctuations, and peripheral rather than central vascularity. However, ultrasonography (Answer B) is less sensitive and specific than FNA biopsy thyroglobulin washout for distinguishing between benign and malignant lymph nodes. FNA biopsy cytology alone, without thyroglobulin washout (Answer A), may miss metastatic cancer in up to 20% of cases.

Stimulated serum thyroglobulin (Answer D) would most likely be elevated in the setting of recurrent disease at any site, but it would not be specific to metastatic disease in the enlarged lymph node.

PET-CT scanning (Answer C) is typically used in the setting of serum thyroglobulin elevation and negative whole-body scan, but it is less sensitive than ultrasonography for the detection of nodal metastases.

EDUCATIONAL OBJECTIVE
Describe the utility of thyroglobulin washout in evaluating cervical lymph nodes in patients with thyroid cancer.

REFERENCE(S)

Kim MJ, Kim EK, Kim BM, et al. Thyroglobulin measurement in fine-needle aspirate washouts: the criteria for neck node dissection for patients with thyroid cancer. *Clin Endocrinol (Oxf)*. 2009;70(1):145-151. PMID: 18466347

Leboulleux S, Girard E, Rose M, et al. Ultrasound criteria of malignancy for cervical lymph nodes in patients followed up for differentiated thyroid cancer. *J Clin Endocrinol Metab*. 2007;92(9):3590-3594. PMID: 17609301

Morita S, Mizoguchi K, Suzuki M, Lizuka K. The accuracy of (18)[F]-fluoro-2-deoxy-D-glucose-positron emission tomography/computed tomography, ultrasonography, and enhanced computed tomography alone in the preoperative diagnosis of cervical lymph node metastasis in patients with papillary thyroid carcinoma. *World J Surg*. 2010;34(11):2564-2569. PMID: 20645089

Moon JH, Kim YI, Lim JA, et al. Thyroglobulin in washout fluid from lymph node fine-needle aspiration biopsy in papillary thyroid cancer: large-scale validation of the cutoff value to determine malignancy and evaluation of discrepant results. *J Clin Endocrinol Metab*. 2013;98(3):1061-1068. PMID: 23393171

Grani G, Fumarola A. Thyroglobulin in lymph node fine-needle aspiration washout: a systematic review and meta-analysis of diagnostic accuracy. *J Clin Endocrinol Metab*. 2014;99(6):1970-1982. PMID: 24617715

13 ANSWER: E) TSH resistance

This patient's thyroid function test results might suggest subclinical hypothyroidism, but he has no goiter, findings on thyroid ultrasonography are normal, and TPO antibodies are negative. This case is typical of inactivating pathogenic variants in the gene encoding the TSH receptor, which cause TSH resistance (Answer E). This situation may be more common than once realized. One study found that 4 of 10 patients with findings similar to those of this patient had inactivating variants in the TSH receptor gene. There is an autosomal dominant pattern of inheritance, but with variable clinical expression. In one study, 64% of offspring were found to be affected. TSH resistance can occur

through additional genetic abnormalities. Defects in *PAX8* gene expression have also been linked to TSH resistance.

Resistance to TSH can either be compensated with normal thyroid hormone levels or uncompensated with low thyroid hormone levels. Whereas uncompensated patients require treatment with levothyroxine, treatment is not thought to be required in compensated patients, such as the one in this vignette.

Although the most common cause of subclinical hypothyroidism is Hashimoto thyroiditis (Answer C), this patient has negative TPO antibodies, no goiter, and homogeneous echotexture on ultrasonography, which, taken together, virtually exclude this disorder.

Adrenal insufficiency (Answer A) can be associated with an isolated mild TSH elevation due to an absence of the tonic suppressive effect of corticosteroids, but generally not to this degree. Furthermore, this patient has no clinical evidence to support a diagnosis of adrenal insufficiency.

Patients with resistance to thyroid hormone (Answer D) have elevated, rather than normal, levels of thyroid hormones.

Selenium excess (Answer B) does not cause thyroid dysfunction.

EDUCATIONAL OBJECTIVE
Distinguish TSH resistance from subclinical hypothyroidism.

REFERENCE(S)

Alberti L, Proverbio MC, Costagliola S, et al. Germline mutations of TSH receptor gene as cause of nonautoimmune subclinical hypothyroidism. *J Clin Endocrinol Metab*. 2002;87(6):2549-2555. PMID: 12050212

Grasberger H, Mimouni-Bloch A, Vantyghem MC, et al. Autosomal dominant resistance to thyrotropin as a distinct entity in five multigenerational kindreds: clinical characterization and exclusion of candidate loci. *J Clin Endocrinol Metab*. 2005;90(7): 4025-4034. PMID: 15870119

Grasberger H, Refetoff S. Resistance to thyrotropin. *Best Pract Res Clin Endocrinol Metab*. 2017;31(2):183-194. PMID: 28648507

14 ANSWER: E) Zoledronic acid

Bisphosphonate therapy (Answer E) has been shown to reduce pain intensity and analgesic requirements in patients with differentiated thyroid cancer with metastases to bone. Bisphosphonates also reduce the frequency of skeletal complications and delay the time to development of those complications in such patients. Although no randomized controlled trial data are available, the data to date in patients with thyroid cancer who have bone involvement, as well as those pertaining to patients with nonthyroidal cancer and metastatic disease to bone, are sufficient to warrant this therapy. The dosing used by Orita et al in their prospective single arm study was zoledronic acid, 4 mg intravenously monthly, for 3 to 31 months (on average 14 doses). Multimodality treatments, including stereotactic radiation therapy and radiofrequency ablation, may also improve survival in these patients.

Total-body irradiation (Answer D), used in some hematologic malignancies, would not be indicated for focal metastatic disease.

Teriparatide (Answer C) is not recommended for use in patients with skeletal malignancies.

Systemic chemotherapy (Answer B) is ineffective in the treatment of thyroid cancer.

Dosimetry-based radioiodine (Answer A) is incorrect because the patient has already been shown to have non–radioiodine-avid disease.

Recent data have shown that the RANKL inhibitor denosumab is superior to zoledronic acid for reducing skeletal-related adverse effects in patients with metastases from solid tumors such as breast and prostate cancers. Denosumab may also be superior for managing skeletal metastases from thyroid cancer.

EDUCATIONAL OBJECTIVE

Discuss the benefits of bisphosphonate therapy in patients with bone metastases from thyroid cancer.

REFERENCE(S)

Wu D, Gomes Lima CJ, Moreau SL, Kulkarni K, Zeymo A, Burman KD, et al. Improved Survival After Multimodal Approach with. *Thyroid.* 2019;29(7):971-978. PMID: 31017051

Nervo A, Ragni A, Retta F, et al. Bone metastases from differentiated thyroid carcinoma: current knowledge and open issues. *J Endocrinol Invest.* 2021;44(3):403-419. PMID: 32743746

Chen C, Li R, Yang T, et al. Denosumab versus zoledronic acid in the prevention of skeletal-related events in vulnerable cancer patients: a meta-analysis of randomized, controlled trials. *Clin Ther.* 2020;42(8):1494-1507.e1. PMID: 32718784

Orita Y, Sugitani I, Takao S, Toda K, Manabe J, Miyata S. Prospective evaluation of zoledronic acid in the treatment of bone metastases from differentiated thyroid carcinoma. *Ann Surg Oncol.* 2015;22(12):4008-4013. PMID: 25762482

15 ANSWER: D) Repeated surveillance testing in 1 year

This patient has microscopic local invasion of tumor and positive central compartment lymph node disease. According to the AJCC-8 staging system (American Joint Committee on Cancer, 8th edition), her tumor is classified as T3, N1, M0, stage I. After surgery and radioiodine therapy, the patient has persistent elevation of serum thyroglobulin, but this is down-trending over time. According to current recommendations for restratification of risk on the basis of response to initial therapy, she has had an acceptable response to therapy, with an unstimulated thyroglobulin value less than 1.0 ng/mL (<1.0 μg/L) and stimulated thyroglobulin value less than 10 ng/mL (<10 μg/L). Numerous studies have demonstrated progressive spontaneous decreases in thyroglobulin over years after initial therapy. The best option in this patient is to continue to monitor without intervention or additional unnecessary testing (Answer D).

PET-CT (Answer C) can be considered in patients with cancer who are at high risk and have elevated serum thyroglobulin (>10 ng/mL [>10 μg/L]) and a negative whole-body scan. However, such imaging is not indicated in this patient who has low and declining serum thyroglobulin values.

Noncontrast chest CT (Answer A) is the most sensitive test for small lung metastases and may be performed in patients with cancer who are at high risk and have elevated or rising serum thyroglobulin values.

Neck MRI (Answer B) is occasionally useful for visualization of metastatic disease that is not well visualized by ultrasonography or contrast neck CT, but this is not the case here.

There is no evidence for spurious thyroglobulin measurements. Assessing serum thyroglobulin over time with the same assay (rather than switching to a different assay [Answer E]) is preferred because of interassay variability.

EDUCATIONAL OBJECTIVE
Recommend an appropriate surveillance strategy for differentiated thyroid cancer.

REFERENCE(S)
Tuttle RM, Alzahrani AS. Risk Stratification in Differentiated Thyroid Cancer: From Detection to Final Follow-up. *J Clin Endocrinol Metab.* 2019;104(9):4087-4100. PMID: 30874735

Haugen BR, Alexander EK, Bible KC, et al. 2015 American Thyroid Association management guidelines for adult patients with thyroid nodules and differentiated thyroid cancer: the American Thyroid Association Guidelines Task Force on Thyroid Nodules and Differentiated Thyroid Cancer. *Thyroid.* 2016;26(1):1-133. PMID: 26462967

16 ANSWER: C) TSH, 0.2 mIU/L; total T$_4$, 2.5 µg/dL (SI: 32.2 nmol/L); total T$_3$, 25 ng/dL (SI: 0.4 nmol/L); free T$_4$, 0.5 ng/dL (SI: 6.4 pmol/L)

This patient has been admitted to the intensive care unit for sepsis and multiorgan failure and his condition is deteriorating. He would be expected to have the classic changes in thyroid hormone levels and TSH that occur as a result of an acute nonthyroidal illness of this severity. The most prevalent and pronounced change of thyroid function during nonthyroidal illness is a low T$_3$ level, present in 70% or more of hospitalized patients, and it may be considered the most characteristic feature of euthyroid sick syndrome. Total T$_4$ is frequently low in patients with severe nonthyroidal illness, and a very low T$_4$ value portends a poor prognosis. Free T$_4$ generally remains in the normal range, but it may be frankly low in gravely ill patients, such as the patient in this case. TSH is frequently normal early in illness, but it may also be decreased in critical illness and then elevated during the recovery stages (generally <20 mIU/L). Using the process of elimination, only Answers B and C have a low T$_3$ value. Answer B has a slightly elevated serum TSH level, which can be seen in the recovery stage after a nonthyroidal illness, but this patient is unfortunately not recovering. Answer C, with more severe alterations in T$_3$, as well as depressions in both total and free T$_4$, is a better fit for this particular moribund patient. Low T$_3$ concentrations are a predictor of poor outcomes, including mortality, in patients hospitalized in the intensive care unit.

EDUCATIONAL OBJECTIVE
Identify expected thyroid function test patterns seen during severe nonthyroidal illness.

REFERENCE(S)
Farwell AP. Nonthyroidal illness syndrome. *Curr Opin Endocrinol Diabetes Obes.* 2013;20(5):478-484. PMID: 23974778

Van den Berghe G. Non-thyroidal illness in the ICU: a syndrome with different faces. *Thyroid.* 2014;24(10):1456-1465. PMID: 24845024

Shigihara S, Shirakabe A, Kobayashi N, et al. Clinical significance of low-triiodothyronine syndrome in patients requiring non-surgical intensive care - tri-iodothyronine is a comprehensive prognostic marker for critical patients with cardiovascular disease. *Circ Rep.* 2021;3(10):578-588. PMID: 34703935

17 ANSWER: E) Thyroid lobectomy

All of the options provided could achieve euthyroidism in this patient with a toxic adenoma. However, if she opts for therapy with antithyroid medication (Answer B) she will be committed to lifelong treatment because toxic nodules do not remit.

Thyroid lobectomy for toxic adenoma (Answer E) results in a high cure rate (treatment failure of <1%) with only a 2% to 3% risk for postoperative hypothyroidism.

Radioactive iodine treatment for toxic adenoma (Answer C) results in a higher risk for hypothyroidism than does thyroid lobectomy, with progressively increasing rates of hypothyroidism that approach 60% at 20 years. The risk for posttreatment hypothyroidism is higher in patients with underlying thyroid autoimmunity, such as a patient who is TPO-antibody positive.

Ethanol injection (Answer A) is not routinely recommended as a treatment for toxic adenoma because of high rates of thyroid pain and other complications.

Finally, radiofrequency ablation (Answer D) is potentially appealing for this patient because of low reported complication rates and a very low risk for permanent hypothyroidism. However, radiofrequency ablation may have a lower success rate with resolving hyperthyroidism due to toxic nodules with success rates of 24% to 74%. It may be more suitable for patients with nodules smaller than 3 cm in size.

EDUCATIONAL OBJECTIVE
Summarize factors in decision-making regarding available treatment modalities for toxic nodules.

REFERENCE(S)
Orloff LA, Noel JE, Stack BC Jr, et al. Radiofrequency ablation and related ultrasound-guided ablation technologies for treatment of benign and malignant thyroid disease: an international multidisciplinary consensus statement of the American Head and Neck Society Endocrine Surgery Section with the Asia Pacific Society of Thyroid Surgery, Associazione Medici Endocrinologi, British Association of Endocrine and Thyroid Surgeons, European Thyroid Association, Italian Society of Endocrine Surgery Units, Korean Society of Thyroid Radiology, Latin American Thyroid Society, and Thyroid Nodules Therapies Association. *Head Neck*. 2022;44(3):633-660. PMID: 34939714

Ross DS, Burch HB, Cooper DS, et al. 2016 American Thyroid Association guidelines for diagnosis and management of hyperthyroidism and other causes of thyrotoxicosis. *Thyroid*. 2016;26(10):1343-1421. PMID: 27521067

18 ANSWER: D) Increase the levothyroxine dosage to 500 mcg daily

Absorption of levothyroxine occurs in the distal small intestine. Patients with short bowels due to surgery or extensive small-bowel disease may experience malabsorption of levothyroxine. One study of 5 patients with surgically shortened small bowels (undergone removal of portions of jejunum and ileum) documented diminished levothyroxine absorption in each patient, despite the presence of an intact duodenum. Another study demonstrated an increased levothyroxine dosage requirement (as high as 600 mcg daily) in a patient after a jejunoileal bypass procedure, with a diminished requirement following surgical reversal. Therefore, the distal small bowel is probably the most important site for absorption of levothyroxine. Variable effects on levothyroxine dosing have been reported following Roux-en-Y gastric bypass surgery, with most patients actually requiring lower dosages postoperatively than preoperatively, most likely due to reduced body weight. A subset of patients requires very high levothyroxine dosages postoperatively, however, due to malabsorption. The patient in this vignette needs a higher levothyroxine dosage (Answer D).

Changing to once-weekly levothyroxine (Answer B), changing to liothyronine (Answer A), or switching brands of levothyroxine (Answer E) ignores the basic problem of malabsorption. Giving parenteral levothyroxine (Answer C) is unnecessarily aggressive.

EDUCATIONAL OBJECTIVE
Evaluate the need for high levothyroxine requirements following small-bowel resection.

REFERENCE(S)
Azizi F, Belur R, Albano J. Malabsorption of thyroid hormones after jejunoileal bypass for obesity. *Ann Intern Med*. 1979;90(6):941-942. PMID: 443690

Stone E, Leiter LA, Lambert JR, Silverberg JD, Jeejeebhoy KN, Burrow GN. L-thyroxine absorption in patients with short bowel. *J Clin Endocrinol Metab*. 1984;59(1):139-141. PMID: 6725518

Gadiraju S, Lee CJ, Cooper DS. Levothyroxine dosing following bariatric surgery. *Obes Surg.* 2016;26(10):2538-2542. PMID: 27475799

19 ANSWER: A) Iatrogenic subclinical hyperthyroidism

In large studies, subclinical hypothyroidism has been associated with increased cardiovascular risk and subtly increased symptom scores. Adverse effects of subclinical hypothyroidism have been most clearly demonstrated when the serum TSH concentration is 10.0 mIU/L or greater. However, very large-scale trials would likely be required to demonstrate benefits, and no intervention trial to date has demonstrated a consistent improvement in sense of well-being or energy level (Answer D), weight reduction (Answer E), or improvement in cognitive function (Answer B) with treatment of subclinical hypothyroidism when the baseline TSH is less than 10.0 mIU/L. While some, but not all, studies have shown decreases in LDL cholesterol following initiation of levothyroxine treatment for subclinical hypothyroidism, HDL cholesterol (Answer C) is typically not altered in patients with subclinical hypothyroidism. Current recommendations in the absence of unequivocal evidence for treatment benefit are to treat subclinical hypothyroidism when the TSH concentration is consistently greater than 10.0 mIU/L and to individualize treatment decisions when the TSH concentration is between 5.0 and 10.0 mIU/L. Analysis of the NHANES-III population survey (Third National Health and Nutrition Examination Survey) has shown that normal elderly patients without goiter or serologic evidence of Hashimoto thyroiditis have a rightward shift in the upper normal limit for TSH, with the upper 95% CI ranging to approximately 7.5 mIU/L in octogenarians. However, the TSH value of 8.9 mIU/L in this patient is most likely truly abnormal. Patients with positive TPO antibodies, such as this one, are at higher risk for overt hypothyroidism and may be particularly good candidates for levothyroxine therapy to prevent this progression. It is important to monitor treatment appropriately because iatrogenic subclinical hyperthyroidism (Answer A) is clearly

detrimental, and studies have shown that 14% to 21% of individuals taking levothyroxine are overtreated.

EDUCATIONAL OBJECTIVE
Describe the limited evidence for benefit of levothyroxine initiation when the TSH concentration is less than 10.0 mIU/L.

REFERENCE(S)

Hennessey JV, Espaillat R. Diagnosis and management of subclinical hypothyroidism in elderly adults: a review of the literature. *J Am Geriatr Soc.* 2015;63(8):1663-1673. PMID: 26200184

Javed Z, Sathyapalan T. Levothyroxine treatment of mild subclinical hypothyroidism: a review of potential risks and benefits. *Ther Adv Endocrinol Metab.* 2016;7(1):12-23. PMID: 26885359

Baumgartner C, Blum MR, Rodondi N. Subclinical hypothyroidism: summary of evidence in 2014. *Swiss Med Wkly.* 2014;144:w14058. PMID: 25536449

Stott DJ, Rodondi N, Kearney PM, et al; TRUST Study Group. Thyroid hormone therapy for older adults with subclinical hypothyroidism. *N Engl J Med.* 2017;376(26):2534-2544. PMID: 28402245

Surks MI, Boucai L. Age- and race-based serum thyrotropin reference limits. *J Clin Endocrinol Metab.* 2010;95(2):496-502. PMID: 19965925

Pearce EN. Update in lipid alterations in subclinical hypothyroidism. *J Clin Endocrinol Metab.* 2012;97(2):326-333. PMID: 22205712

20 ANSWER: A) Repeat thyroid function tests in 3 to 6 months

Subclinical hyperthyroidism, in which serum TSH values are low but thyroid hormone levels remain normal, is relatively common, affecting approximately 1.5% of the US adult population. About 5% of patients progress to overt hyperthyroidism, an outcome that is more likely when TSH is fully suppressed. Up to one-third of patients with subclinical hyperthyroidism spontaneously become euthyroid again; this is most common when the underlying cause of their hyperthyroidism is Graves disease and when the baseline TSH concentration is between 0.1 and

0.4 mIU/L. Subclinical hyperthyroidism has been associated with increased risk for all-cause and cardiovascular mortality, atrial fibrillation, osteoporosis, and fracture. However, there is currently limited evidence for treatment benefit, particularly in younger individuals, and treatment confers some risks. Current guidelines recommend observation with monitoring of thyroid function (Answer A) rather than treatment (Answers B and E) for asymptomatic patients younger than 65 years who do not have cardiac disease or osteoporosis in whom the TSH is persistently lower than normal but 0.1 mIU/L or greater.

β-adrenergic blockade (Answer D) might be useful in the setting of hyperthyroid symptoms or tachycardia, but this patient has neither.

Thyroid ultrasonography (Answer C) is not necessary at this point, given the relatively unremarkable thyroid examination. If performed, ultrasonography might show increased vascularity of the thyroid gland suggestive of Graves disease. However, Graves disease is already evident based on the elevated thyroid-stimulating immunoglobulin value.

EDUCATIONAL OBJECTIVE

List indications for treatment of subclinical hyperthyroidism.

REFERENCE(S)

Ross DS, Burch HB, Cooper DS, et al. 2016 American Thyroid Association guidelines for diagnosis and management of hyperthyroidism and other causes of thyrotoxicosis. *Thyroid.* 2016;26(10):1343-1421. PMID: 27521067

Carle A, Andersen SL, Boelaert K, Laurberg P. Management of endocrine disease: subclinical thyrotoxicosis: prevalence, causes and choice of therapy. *Eur J Endocrinol.* 2017;176(6):R325-R337. PMID: 28274949

Vadiveloo T, Donnan PT, Cochrane L, Leese GP. The Thyroid Epidemiology, Audit, and Research Study (TEARS): the natural history of endogenous subclinical hyperthyroidism. *J Clin Endocrinol Metab.* 2011;96(1):E1-E8. PMID: 20926532

21 ANSWER: D) Thyroid ultrasonography with color Doppler

This patient developed thyrotoxicosis shortly after discontinuing amiodarone. This drug is very rich in iodine, with a 100-mg tablet containing an amount of iodine that is approximately 250 times the recommended daily iodine requirement. Amiodarone can persist for months in tissues such as liver and lung, and amiodarone-induced thyrotoxicosis may actually occur after drug discontinuation. Amiodarone-induced thyrotoxicosis has been categorized as type 1 or iodine-induced hyperthyroidism (occurs in individuals with underlying thyroid disease) or as type 2 which is an inflammatory, destructive thyroiditis. Among the answers provided, thyroid ultrasonography with color Doppler (Answer D) is most likely to establish whether this is type 1 amiodarone-induced thyrotoxicosis (iodine-induced hyperthyroidism) vs type 2 (destructive thyroiditis). Thyroidal vascularity is typically diffusely increased in type 1 amiodarone-induced thyrotoxicosis, but absent in type 2. Recent reports suggest that ^{99m}Tc-sestamibi, although not among the provided choices, would also be a reasonable option for distinguishing between the 2 entities.

Radioactive iodine uptake (Answer A) is typically low in both type 1 and type 2 amiodarone-induced thyrotoxicosis due to the high levels of nonradioactive iodine present in amiodarone.

An initial study in the 1990s suggested that IL-6 (Answer B), a marker for inflammation, was elevated in type 2 amiodarone-induced thyrotoxicosis and low in type 1, but this test has subsequently been shown to be of very poor utility in distinguishing between the 2 types.

TPO antibodies (Answer C) do not discriminate between the 2 entities.

Measurement of urinary iodine (Answer E) would also not distinguish between the types of amiodarone-induced thyrotoxicosis, as this patient would still be expected to have an elevated iodine load from amiodarone regardless of the etiology of his thyrotoxicosis.

EDUCATIONAL OBJECTIVE

Explain testing modalities for distinguishing between the 2 types of amiodarone-induced thyrotoxicosis.

REFERENCE(S)

Danzi S, Klein I. Amiodarone-induced thyroid dysfunction. *J Intensive Care Med.* 2015;30(4):179-185. PMID: 24067547

Bogazzi F, Bartalena L, Martino E. Approach to the patient with amiodarone-induced thyrotoxicosis. *J Clin Endocrinol Metab.* 2010;95(6):2529-2535. PMID: 20525904

Tomisti L, Urbani C, Rossi G, et al. The presence of anti-thyroglobulin (TgAb) and/or anti-thyroperoxidase antibodies (TPOAb) does not exclude the diagnosis of type 2 amiodarone-induced thyrotoxicosis. *J Endocrinol Invest.* 2016;39(5):585-591. PMID: 26759156

Wang J, Zhang R. Evaluation of 99mTc-MIBI in thyroid gland imaging for the diagnosis of amiodarone-induced thyrotoxicosis. *Br J Radiol.* 2017;90(1071):20160836. PMID: 28106465

22   ANSWER: C) Radioiodine therapy with rhTSH

CT shows a substernal goiter with mass effect on the trachea. The patient is symptomatic, with positional dyspnea, most likely due to the compression of his trachea by the symmetrically enlarged thyroid when he lies on his side. The best option is radioiodine therapy with rhTSH (Answer C). Various doses of rhTSH can be used, and this treatment can decrease goiter size by approximately 27% to 46% at 6 months and 32% to 62% at 12 months. rhTSH-assisted treatment with radioiodine in a patient with an intact thyroid needs to be closely monitored because of acute release of thyroid hormone from the gland under the influence of rhTSH and temporary swelling of thyroid tissue. Although radioiodine therapy can be administered without the assistance of rhTSH (Answer D), there is less goiter shrinkage, so this is not the best choice in this patient with compressive symptoms. The magnitude of the shrinkage without rhTSH is 3% to 36% at 6 months and 19% to 46% at 12 months. However, the risk of eventual hypothyroidism is greater when rhTSH is used.

This euthyroid patient's thyroid mass is unlikely to respond significantly to levothyroxine suppressive therapy (Answer A), and suppressing serum TSH would be inadvisable in an older individual.

Thermal ablation (Answer E) would not reduce the size of this very large substernal goiter, and no intervention (Answer B) is inappropriate given his symptomatic disease.

EDUCATIONAL OBJECTIVE

Recommend a management approach to address a symptomatic goiter when surgery is contraindicated.

REFERENCE(S)

Bahn RS, Castro MR. Approach to the patient with nontoxic multinodular goiter. *J Clin Endocrinol Metab.* 2011;96(5):1202-1212. PMID: 21543434

Fast S, Nielsen VE, Bonnema SJ, Hegedüs L. Dose-dependent acute effects of recombinant human TSH (rhTSH) on thyroid size and function: comparison of 0.1, 0.3 and 0.9 mg of rhTSH. *Clin Endocrinol (Oxf).* 2010;72(3):411-416. PMID: 19508679

Bonnema SJ, Hegedüs L. Radioiodine therapy in benign thyroid diseases: effects, side effects, and factors affecting therapeutic outcome. *Endocr Rev.* 2012;33(6):920-980. PMID: 22961916

Nielsen VE, Bonnema SJ, Boel-Jørgensen H, Grupe P, Hegedüs L. Stimulation with 0.3-mg recombinant human thyrotropin prior to iodine 131 therapy to improve the size reduction of benign nontoxic nodular goiter: a prospective randomized double-blind trial. *Arch Intern Med.* 2006;166(14):1476-1482. PMID: 16864757

Xu C, Wang P, Miao H, et al. Recombinant human thyrotropin-stimulated radioiodine therapy in patients with multinodular goiters: a meta-analysis of randomized controlled trials. *Horm Metab Res.* 2020;52(12):841-849. PMID: 32961564

Lee YY, Tam KW, Lin YM, et al. Recombinant human thyrotropin before (131)I therapy in patients with nodular goitre: a meta-analysis of randomized controlled trials. *Clin Endocrinol (Oxf).* 2015;83(5):702-710. PMID: 25370124

23 ANSWER: D) Parathyroid cyst

The classic description of parathyroid cyst fluid is clear, colorless, liquid that contains extremely high PTH levels. When such fluid is obtained during biopsy of what appears to be a thyroid nodule, the fluid should be sent for PTH analysis. Parathyroid cysts (Answer D) can be functioning or nonfunctioning. Serum calcium and PTH levels may also be elevated if the patient has hyperparathyroidism due to a functioning parathyroid cyst. Surgery is generally recommended for functioning parathyroid cysts, whereas conservative therapy, aspiration, sclerotherapy, or surgery can be pursued for nonfunctioning cysts.

Branchial cleft cysts (Answer B) are located laterally in the neck, and thyroglossal duct cysts (Answer E) are generally located at the midline adjacent to the hyoid bone.

Follicular thyroid cancer (Answer C) is not generally prone to cystic change, but conversely this is a common finding in patients with papillary thyroid cancer.

Aberrant salivary gland tissue with cystic degeneration (Answer A) is a very rare disorder and cases do not occur within or juxtaposed to the thyroid.

EDUCATIONAL OBJECTIVE
Recognize the typical presentation of a parathyroid cyst.

REFERENCE(S)
Wani S, Hao Z. Atypical cystic adenoma of the parathyroid gland: case report and review of the literature. *Endocr Pract.* 2005;11(6):389-393. PMID: 16638726

Xu P, Xia X, Li M, Guo M, Yang Z. Parathyroid cysts: experience of a rare phenomenon at a single institution. *BMC Surg.* 2018;18(1):9. PMID: 29409478

Chaabouni MA, Achour I, Thabet W, et al. Parathyroid cyst: a rare entity. *SAGE Open Med Case Rep.* 2021;9:2050313X211066648. PMID: 34987819

24 ANSWER: A) Atypia of undetermined significance

The Bethesda System for Reporting Thyroid Cytopathology, which was introduced in 2007 and updated in 2017, distributes thyroid FNA biopsy results into 1 of 6 categories: I = nondiagnostic or unsatisfactory (Answer D); II = benign (Answer B); III = atypia of undetermined significance (AUS) or follicular lesion of undetermined significance (FLUS) (Answer A); IV = follicular neoplasm or suspicious for a follicular neoplasm; V = suspicious for malignancy (Answer E); and VI = malignant (Answer C). The atypia category includes several different subtype descriptions, one of which applies in this patient's case, consisting of focal features suggestive of papillary thyroid carcinoma, including nuclear grooves, prominent nucleoli, elongated nuclei or cytoplasm, and/or intranuclear cytoplasmic inclusions in an otherwise predominantly benign-appearing sample (thus, Answer A is correct). The malignancy rate for such lesions is expected to be 6% to 18%, assuming that noninvasive follicular thyroid neoplasm with papillary-like nuclear features (NIFTP) is not classified as a malignancy. If NIFTP is instead considered to be a cancer, then the risk for malignancy in this group is 10% to 30%.

Nodules suspicious for malignancy (Answer E) are characterized by the presence of some suspicious features, but not enough to lead to a definitive diagnosis. The risk of malignancy in these nodules is 45% to 60% if NIFTP is not considered to be malignant. If NIFTP is considered to be a malignancy, then the risk of malignancy is 50% to 75%.

Nodules interpreted as malignant (Answer C) have classic papillary cancer features such as true papillae, psammoma bodies, and intranuclear cytoplasmic inclusions and, in contrast to nodules with atypia of undetermined significance, cells throughout the specimen, not just focally, exhibit nuclear grooves, prominent nucleoli, and elongated nuclei. The risk for malignancy in these lesions is 94% to 96%.

EDUCATIONAL OBJECTIVE
Classify results from thyroid FNA biopsy according to the Bethesda System for Reporting Thyroid Cytopathology.

REFERENCE(S)

Cibas ES, Ali SZ. The 2017 Bethesda System for Reporting Thyroid Cytopathology. *Thyroid.* 2017;27(11):1341-1346. PMID: 29091573

Strickland KC, Howitt BE, Marqusee E, et al. The impact of noninvasive follicular variant of papillary thyroid carcinoma on rates of malignancy for fine-needle aspiration diagnostic categories. *Thyroid.* 2015;25(9):987-992. PMID: 26114752

Bongiovanni M, Spitale A, Faquin WC, Mazzucchelli L, Baloch ZW. The Bethesda System for Reporting Thyroid Cytopathology: a meta-analysis. *Acta Cytol.* 2012;56(4):333-339. PMID: 22846422

25 ANSWER: E) Stop liothyronine and increase the levothyroxine dosage to 150 mcg daily

This patient's recent prepregnancy TSH value was normal. However, most women require an increase of 25% to 30% in thyroid hormone dosages with pregnancy, due largely to increased thyroxine-binding globulin levels. The goal of therapy in the first trimester is a TSH concentration less than 2.5 mIU/L. Whether levothyroxine/liothyronine combination therapy improves quality of life in selected patients remains controversial. However, levothyroxine/liothyronine combination therapy is not recommended for pregnant women because it is primarily maternal T_4, not T_3, that crosses the placenta. This concern would apply to either synthetic combination therapy or "natural" combination therapy that uses desiccated thyroid extract. Therefore, normalizing maternal TSH on combination therapy could potentially result in fetal hypothyroxinemia (thus, Answers A, B, C, and D are incorrect). In converting from combination therapy with levothyroxine/liothyronine to levothyroxine monotherapy (Answer E), it is important to remember that liothyronine is approximately 3 times more potent metabolically than levothyroxine, and therapeutic equivalence for 10 mcg of liothyronine is achieved with 30 mcg levothyroxine.

EDUCATIONAL OBJECTIVE

Recommend appropriate thyroid hormone replacement in early pregnancy.

REFERENCE(S)

Jonklaas J, Bianco AC, Bauer AJ, et al. Guidelines for the treatment of hypothyroidism: prepared by the American Thyroid Association task force on thyroid hormone replacement. *Thyroid.* 2014;24(12):1670-1751. PMID: 25266247

Yassa L, Marqusee E, Fawcett R, Alexander EK. Thyroid hormone early adjustment in pregnancy (the THERAPY) trial. *J Clin Endocrinol Metab.* 2010;95(7):3234-3241. PMID: 20463094

Calvo RM, Jauniaux E, Gulbis B, et al. Fetal tissues are exposed to biologically relevant free thyroxine concentrations during early phases of development. *J Clin Endocrinol Metab.* 2002;87(4):1768-1777. PMID: 11932315

Celi FS, Zemskova M, Linderman JD, et al. The pharmacodynamic equivalence of levothyroxine and liothyronine: a randomized, double blind, cross-over study in thyroidectomized patients. *Clin Endocrinol (Oxf).* 2010;72(5):709-715. PMID: 20447070

26 ANSWER: C) Perform a whole-body radioactive iodine scan

The differential diagnosis for thyrotoxicosis with low radioactive iodine uptake includes subacute thyroiditis painless postpartum or sporadic thyroiditis (unlikely given the duration of thyrotoxicosis); factitious thyroiditis; drug-induced thyroiditis; iodine-induced hyperthyroidism (excluded by the normal urinary iodine concentration); and very rarely struma ovarii or widely metastatic follicular thyroid carcinoma.

In struma ovarii, radioactive iodine uptake will be low in the neck, but uptake will be increased in the pelvis (thus, Answer C is correct). Struma may be suspected in patients with low radioactive iodine thyrotoxicosis who have a pelvic mass or in women with suspected inflammatory thyroiditis when the thyrotoxicosis is persistent and the expected hypothyroid phase does not occur.

Measuring the erythrocyte sedimentation rate (Answer B) would be used to diagnose subacute thyroiditis, but this is unlikely given the duration of thyrotoxicosis and lack of thyroid tenderness. It is also less likely in the setting of primarily T_3

toxicosis, as thyroiditis usually presents as a T_4-predominant thyrotoxicosis.

Inquiring about exogenous thyroid hormone sources (Answer A) is incorrect because exogenous thyroid hormone use is excluded by the elevated serum thyroglobulin.

Starting methimazole (Answer E) would control the patient's hyperthyroidism but would not help determine the correct diagnosis.

Performing thyroidectomy (Answer D) is not indicated, as it would not cure the thyrotoxicosis, which is of extrathyroidal origin.

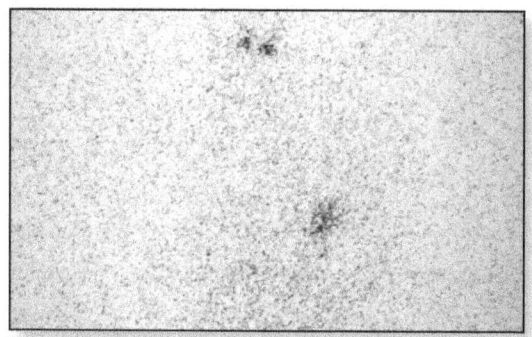

Whole-body ^{123}I scan, showing salivary and pelvic uptake, but no uptake in the thyroid.

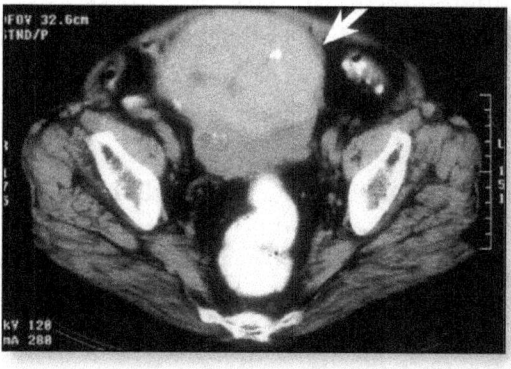

CT showing struma ovarii (arrow).

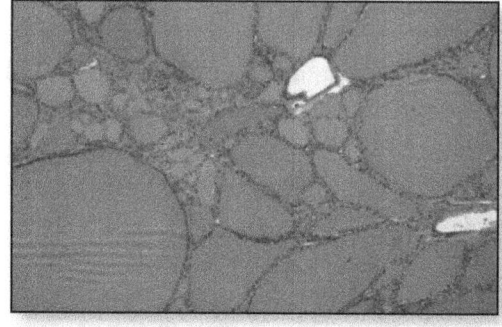

Surgical specimen from the pelvic mass showing typical thyroid follicles (hematoxylin and eosin stain).

EDUCATIONAL OBJECTIVE
Perform the differential diagnosis for thyrotoxicosis with low thyroidal radioactive iodine uptake and recognize the need to test for struma ovarii in an unusual case.

REFERENCE(S)

Shanbhogue AK, Shanbhogue DK, Prasad SR, Surabhi VR, Fasih N, Menias CO. Clinical syndromes associated with ovarian neoplasms: a comprehensive review. *Radiographics.* 2010;30(4):903-919. PMID: 20631359

Ross DS. Syndromes of thyrotoxicosis with low radioactive iodine uptake. *Endocrinol Metab Clin North Am.* 1998;27(1):169-185. PMID: 9534035

27   ANSWER: B) Graves disease

This patient has moderate thyrotoxicosis recognized in the first trimester and persisting into the early second trimester. The primary differential is between Graves disease and gestational thyrotoxicosis. Gestational thyrotoxicosis is the most frequent cause of hyperthyroidism in the first trimester. It is typically seen in women with hyperemesis gravidarum and is caused by markedly elevated serum β-hCG levels. The concentration of β-hCG correlates with the severity of nausea, and gestational thyrotoxicosis is unusual in women without clinically significant nausea and vomiting. Gestational thyrotoxicosis resolves spontaneously as β-hCG levels fall after weeks 10 to 12 of gestation. Reference ranges for hCG concentrations during pregnancy are available from some studies such as the Generation R study. Graves disease is far more likely in this vignette because the thyrotoxicosis is not resolving after 12 weeks' gestation, the T_3 concentration is relatively elevated compared with the T_4 level, and she has no nausea and vomiting (thus, Answer B is correct and Answer A is incorrect).

Serum thyroglobulin levels would be low with surreptitious thyroid hormone ingestion (Answer E).

Subacute thyroiditis (Answer D) is unlikely in the absence of thyroid pain or tenderness.

Molar pregnancy (Answer C), a form of gestational trophoblastic disease, generally presents with abnormal vaginal bleeding, an enlarged uterus, and a positive pregnancy test resulting from β-hCG elevation. Hyperthyroidism occurs in approximately 5% of women with gestational trophoblastic disease due to hCG stimulation of the TSH receptor (1 U of hCG is equivalent to approximately 0.001 U of TSH).

EDUCATIONAL OBJECTIVE
Perform the differential diagnosis for thyrotoxicosis in the first trimester of pregnancy.

REFERENCE(S)
Cooper DS, Laurberg P. Hyperthyroidism in pregnancy. *Lancet Diabetes Endocrinol.* 2013;1(3):238-249. PMID: 24622372

Alexander EK, Pearce EN, Brent GA, et al. 2017 Guidelines of the American Thyroid Association for the diagnosis and management of thyroid disease during pregnancy and the postpartum. *Thyroid.* 2017;27(3):315-389. PMID: 28056690

Korevaar TIM, Steegers EAP, de Rijke YB, et al. Reference ranges and determinants of total hCG levels during pregnancy: the Generation R Study. *Eur J Epidemiol.* 2015;30(9):1057-1066. PMID: 25963653

28 ANSWER: D) Thyroid hormone therapy with a target TSH level between 0.5 and 2.0 mIU/L

In this vignette, a solitary intrathyroidal papillary carcinoma was identified at the time of thyroid lobectomy. The patient has no evidence of metastatic disease or aggressive histology. The risk of tumor persistence or recurrence in unifocal, intrathyroidal papillary carcinoma is extremely low (1% to 2%). The risk for tumor-related mortality is essentially zero. Thyroid lobectomy provides sufficient treatment. The 2015 American Thyroid Association guidelines on the management of thyroid nodules and thyroid cancer explicitly recommend against the use of radioiodine remnant ablation in this setting because it has not been shown to improve either overall or disease-free survival.

Completion thyroidectomy with or without remnant ablation with radioiodine (Answers A and B) is overly aggressive for this clinical circumstance.

The guidelines also specifically recommend against ablation of a remaining lobe without completion thyroidectomy in any patient with thyroid cancer (Answer C) because long-term outcomes of this approach are unknown.

Levothyroxine therapy with a low-normal TSH target (Answer D) is the best option. Suppression of the serum TSH below 0.5 mIU/L (Answer E) is not necessary to improve outcomes.

EDUCATIONAL OBJECTIVE
Manage unifocal intrathyroidal papillary carcinoma.

REFERENCE(S)
Haugen BR, Alexander EK, Bible KC, et al. 2015 American Thyroid Association management guidelines for adult patients with thyroid nodules and differentiated thyroid cancer: the American Thyroid Association guidelines task force on thyroid nodules and differentiated thyroid cancer. *Thyroid.* 2016;26(1):1-133. PMID: 26462967

Tarasova VD, Tuttle RM. Current management of low risk differentiated thyroid cancer and papillary microcarcinoma. *Clin Oncol (R Coll Radiol).* 2017;29(5):290-297. PMID: 28087101

Tuttle RM, Alzahrani AS. Risk stratification in differentiated thyroid cancer: from detection to final follow-up. *J Clin Endocrinol Metab.* 2019;104(9):4087-4100. PMID: 30874735

29 ANSWER: D) Neck ultrasonography

Medullary thyroid cancer accounts for fewer than 5% of thyroid cancer cases in the United States; approximately 80% of these cases represent sporadic, nonfamilial disease. The 2015 American Thyroid Association guidelines for the management of medullary thyroid cancer recommend that *RET* proto-oncogene testing be offered to all patients with a preoperative (or postoperative) diagnosis of medullary thyroid cancer. The guidelines state that "patients presenting with a thyroid nodule and a cytological or histological diagnosis of medullary thyroid cancer should have a physical examination, determination of serum levels of calcitonin and CEA, and genetic testing for a *RET* germline pathogenic variant. The presence of a pheochromocytoma and hyperparathyroidism should be excluded in patients with hereditary medullary thyroid cancer." This patient's plasma metanephrine levels are normal, which effectively rules out pheochromocytoma, and thus she does not need adrenal imaging (Answer A). Hyperparathyroidism has also been ruled out, and therefore a sestamibi scan (Answer E) is not warranted.

Neck ultrasonography (Answer D) to assess for the presence of local metastases is important before thyroidectomy to determine whether neck dissection is warranted. This patient's baseline serum calcitonin concentration less than 500 pg/mL (<146 pmol/L) suggests that distant metastases will not be present. However, if this patient's preoperative ultrasonography demonstrates extensive disease in the neck, or if she had signs or symptoms suggestive of distant metastases, imaging with chest CT to detect lung or mediastinal metastases and imaging with MRI or 3-phase contrast-enhanced multidetector CT to detect liver metastases would then be recommended. MRI of the liver (Answer C) is thus not recommended at this stage of her evaluation.

Fluorodeoxyglucose-PET (Answer B) is poorly sensitive for medullary cancer and is not recommended for the detection of distant disease.

EDUCATIONAL OBJECTIVE
In a patient with medullary thyroid cancer, perform neck ultrasonography before proceeding to thyroid surgery.

REFERENCE(S)
Wells SA Jr, Asa SL, Dralle H, et al; American Thyroid Association Guidelines Task Force on Medullary Thyroid Carcinoma. Revised American Thyroid Association guidelines for the management of medullary thyroid carcinoma. *Thyroid.* 2015;25(6):567-610. PMID: 25810047

Moraitis AG, Martucci VL, Pacak K. Genetics, diagnosis, and management of medullary thyroid carcinoma and pheochromocytoma/paraganglioma. *Endocr Pract.* 2014;20(2):176-187. PMID: 24449662

30 ANSWER: D) Somatic activating variant in the gene encoding the TSH receptor

The thyroid scan shows a large, right-sided autonomous thyroid nodule with suppression of the left lobe, which is only faintly visible in the image. Most such nodules examined have somatic activating variants in the genes encoding the TSH receptor (Answer D) or the G$_s$ alpha subunit, leading to constitutive activation and hyperfunction within the nodule. When an autonomous nodule grows to a large enough mass (classically described as 3 cm or more in maximal diameter), overt hyperthyroidism may occur, as occurred in this patient. Because the TSH becomes suppressed in the face of elevated thyroid hormone values, the activity of the contralateral lobe is suppressed.

In addition to somatic variants affecting only the "hot" thyroid nodule, as described in this case, germline pathogenic variants (Answer B) that would affect the entire thyroid and all other cells of the body can also occur. This leads to an inherited form of thyrotoxicosis due to a germline activating variant in the gene encoding the TSH receptor, which presents with diffuse thyrotoxicosis evident in infancy or later in life as nonautoimmune thyrotoxicosis with a diffuse goiter and increased radioactive iodine uptake throughout the thyroid gland. This is not the case in this vignette.

Activating variants in the gene encoding the sodium-iodide symporter (Answer A) have not been reported as a source of thyroid autonomy.

Inactivating variants in the gene encoding the G$_s$-alpha subunit (Answer C) would not lead to enhanced hormonogenesis.

Hemiagenesis (Answer E) is excluded by the thyroid scan image showing bilateral thyroid tissue.

EDUCATIONAL OBJECTIVE
Identify common patterns on thyroid scans and describe the pathogenesis of a solitary hot nodule.

REFERENCE(S)

Nishihara E, Amino N, Maekawa K, et al. Prevalence of TSH receptor and Gsalpha mutations in 45 autonomously functioning thyroid nodules in Japan. *Endocr J.* 2009;56(6):791-798. PMID: 19550078

Hébrant A, van Staveren WC, Maenhaut C, Dumont JE, Leclère J. Genetic hyperthyroidism: hyperthyroidism due to activating TSHR mutations. *Eur J Endocrinol.* 2011;164:1-9. PMID: 20926595

Ross DS, Burch HB, Cooper DS, et al. 2016 American Thyroid Association guidelines for diagnosis and management of hyperthyroidism and other causes of thyrotoxicosis. *Thyroid.* 2016;26(10):1343-1421. PMID: 27521067

31 ANSWER: B) <3%

The image shows a spongiform nodule with clearly defined margins. A nodule's appearance is defined as spongiform when more than half of nodule volume is composed of microcystic spaces. This ultrasound pattern strongly suggests that the nodule is benign, with less than 3% risk of malignancy (Answer B). Because of the low risk for malignancy in these nodules, current American Thyroid Association guidelines recommend consideration of FNA biopsy for spongiform nodules 2 cm or larger but note that these can also be followed with observation without proceeding with FNA biopsy.

Intermediate suspicion patterns associated with a 10% to 20% risk of malignancy (Answer D) include hypoechoic nodules with smooth margins but without microcalcifications, extrathyroidal extension, or a taller-than-wide shape.

Low suspicion nodules are those that are isoechoic or hyperechoic without microcalcifications, irregular margins, or taller-than-wide shape. Low suspicion nodules have 5% to 10% risk of malignancy (Answer C).

Nodules with a high risk of malignancy of 70% to 90% (Answer E) include those that are hypoechoic with irregular margins, have microcalcifications, have taller-than-wide shape, or have evidence of extrathyroidal extension.

Purely cystic nodules with no solid component are considered benign with less than 1% risk of malignancy (Answer A). The risk of malignancy within these nodules overlaps with the estimate of less than 3% described for spongiform nodules in the 2015 American Thyroid Association Guideline for management of thyroid nodules and thyroid cancer. However, due to the negligible risk of malignancy of less than 1%, no biopsy is recommended unless needed to manage compression or cosmetic issues caused by the cystic nodule.

EDUCATIONAL OBJECTIVE
Interpret the malignancy risk associated with different thyroid ultrasonographic patterns.

REFERENCE(S)

Haugen BR, Alexander EK, Bible KC, et al. 2015 American Thyroid Association Management guidelines for adult patients with thyroid nodules and differentiated thyroid cancer: the American Thyroid Association Guidelines Task Force on Thyroid Nodules and Differentiated Thyroid Cancer. *Thyroid.* 2016;26(1):1-133. PMID: 26462967

Durante C, Grani G, Lamartina L, Filetti S, Mandel SJ, Cooper DS. The diagnosis and management of thyroid nodules: a review. *JAMA.* 2018;319(9):914-924. PMID: 29509871

32 ANSWER: C) Perform thyroid lobectomy

Nondiagnostic FNA biopsy results describe samples that contain only cyst fluid or in which there are insufficient cells for diagnosis; this occurs in 2% to 16% of FNA biopsy attempts. Repeated FNA biopsy is typically recommended when this occurs, and repeated aspiration is diagnostic 60% to 80% of the time when nodules are not predominantly cystic. The risk of malignancy in repeatedly nondiagnostic nodules with suspicious ultrasonographic features such as irregular margins, taller-than-wide shape, hypoechogenicity, or microcalcifications is approximately 25%, whereas the risk of malignancy is only about 4% in nodules lacking those concerning features.

If this nodule did not have a high-suspicion ultrasonographic pattern, either continued close observation (Answer D) or diagnostic lobectomy would be appropriate options. However, in the presence of both high-suspicion ultrasonographic features and significant nodule growth (20% in at least 2 dimensions), thyroid surgery (Answer C) is the more appropriate choice.

^{18}F-fluorodeoxyglucose PET/CT uptake (Answer B) in thyroid nodules confers an increased risk for thyroid cancer (about 33%), but this imaging would not provide a definitive diagnosis.

Molecular markers (Answer E) are unlikely to provide additional diagnostic information in the absence of an adequate cellular biopsy.

Whether serum calcitonin (Answer A) should be routinely measured in the workup of thyroid nodules remains controversial, but this will not provide a definitive diagnosis in the case.

In some studies, core-needle biopsy, an option that was not provided in this vignette, may improve rates of diagnosis in nodules with repeatedly nondiagnostic FNA biopsy.

EDUCATIONAL OBJECTIVE
Manage thyroid nodules that have repeatedly nondiagnostic cytopathology.

REFERENCE(S)

Haugen BR, Alexander EK, Bible KC, et al. 2015 American Thyroid Association management guidelines for adult patients with thyroid nodules and differentiated thyroid cancer: the American Thyroid Association guidelines task force on thyroid nodules and differentiated thyroid cancer. *Thyroid*. 2016;26(1):1-133. PMID: 26462967

Moon HJ, Kwak JY, Choi YS, Kim EK. How to manage thyroid nodules with two consecutive non-diagnostic results on ultrasonography-guided fine-needle aspiration. *World J Surg*. 2012;36(3):586-592. PMID: 22228400

Park CJ, Kim EK, Moon HJ, Yoon JH, Park VY, Kwak JY. Thyroid nodules with nondiagnostic cytologic results: follow-up management using ultrasound patterns based on the 2015 American Thyroid Association Guidelines. *AJR Am J Roentgenol*. 2018;210(2):412-417. PMID: 29091005

33 ANSWER: D) Levothyroxine therapy with a goal TSH between 0.5 and 2.0 mIU/L

This patient's histopathology would formerly have been described as encapsulated follicular variant of papillary thyroid carcinoma, but this has been renamed to noninvasive follicular thyroid neoplasm with papillary-like nuclear features (NIFTP). This redefinition was an expert consensus made on the basis of a retrospective review of 109 patients with NIFTP who did not receive radioactive iodine and who were observed for 10 to 26 years; all of these patients were alive without evidence for tumor recurrence at the end of follow-up. Long-term prospective studies have not been performed. NIFTP is currently best understood as a premalignant lesion. Secondary diagnostic criteria for NIFTP include lack of the *BRAF* V600E variant or other high-risk variants in *TERT* or *TP53*.

Calcitonin production is not a characteristic of thyroid follicular cells and measuring serum calcitonin (Answer E) would have no role in this patient's evaluation. It can only be diagnosed based on surgical pathology, when there has been close examination of the entire lesion and tumor capsule.

NIFTP is believed to be associated with a very low risk for tumor recurrence. Because this is considered low risk, completion thyroidectomy with or without radioactive iodine ablation (Answers A and B) is not warranted.

TSH-suppressive levothyroxine therapy (Answer C) confers some risks of bone and cardiac toxicity and is unlikely to confer any benefit given the absent recurrence risk in these lesions.

Levothyroxine therapy with a low-normal TSH target (Answer D) is the best option. The most appropriate follow-up surveillance strategy is currently unknown, although periodic ultrasonography and serum thyroglobulin assessment can be considered.

EDUCATIONAL OBJECTIVE
Identify noninvasive follicular thyroid neoplasm with papillary-like nuclear features and explain its prognostic implications.

REFERENCE(S)

Nikiforov YE, Seethala RR, Tallini G, et al. Nomenclature revision for encapsulated follicular variant of papillary thyroid carcinoma: a paradigm shift to reduce overtreatment of indolent tumors. *JAMA Oncol.* 2016;2(8):1023-1029. PMID: 27078145

Haugen BR, Sawka AM, Alexander EK, et al. American Thyroid Association guidelines on the management of thyroid nodules and differentiated thyroid cancer task force review and recommendation on the proposed renaming of encapsulated follicular variant papillary thyroid carcinoma without invasion to noninvasive follicular thyroid neoplasm with papillary-like nuclear features. *Thyroid.* 2017;27(4):481-483. PMID: 28114862

Baloch ZW, Harrell RM, Brett EM, Randolph G, Garber JR; AACE Endocrine Surgery Scientific Committee and Thyroid Scientific Committee. American Association of Clinical Endocrinologists and American College of Endocrinology disease state commentary: managing thyroid tumors diagnosed as noninvasive follicular thyroid neoplasm with papillary-like nuclear features. *Endocr Pract.* 2017;23(9):1150-1155. PMID: 28920749

Nikiforov YE, Baloch ZW, Hodak SP, et al. Change in diagnostic criteria for noninvasive follicular thyroid neoplasm with papillarylike nuclear features. *JAMA Oncol.* 2018;4(8):1125-1126. PMID: 29902314

www.ingramcontent.com/pod-product-compliance
Lightning Source LLC
Chambersburg PA
CBHW080410190526
45161CB00003B/196